Children, Media, and Technology

An accessible introduction to children, media, and technology that centers questions of access, diversity, equity, and inclusion to provide a timely and much-needed text for communication and media studies students and scholars.

This book covers several long-standing as well as contemporary issues and controversies pertaining to media and youth, such as violence, cyberbullying, and online harassment; body image disturbances and beauty norms; and responses to increasingly sophisticated marketing strategies. It also fully explores the ways in which media and technology use enriches the lives of children and teens and empowers them, with positive implications for their sense of self; learning and education; sociality, friendships, and respect for others; and knowledge of and action in the world around them. In each of these lines of inquiry, up-to-date theory and research findings relevant to diverse young media users and questions of access, equity, representation, and inclusion make this a distinct approach to enhance students' understanding of children, media, and technology.

This is an essential text for students of Media and Communication Studies taking courses such as Children and Media; Children, Teens, and Media; and Children, Adolescents, and Media, as well as similar classes being taught in related departments.

Erica Scharrer is Professor of Communication at the University of Massachusetts Amherst where she studies the role of media in the lives of adolescents. She is the co-author of *Quantitative Research Methods in Communication: The Power of Numbers for Social Justice* with Srividya Ramasubramanian and *Media and the American Child* with George Comstock. Scharrer is also the editor of the *Media Effects/Media Psychology* volume of the *International Encyclopedia of Media Studies*, among other books and articles.

Shining a unique light on the field of young people and media, this special edited volume focuses on social justice issues and broadens our perspective through contributions from a variety of perspectives and social contexts. A most timely text in an era of cultural and technological turmoil!

– **Dafna Lemish**, *Rutgers University*

Featuring contributions from leading scholars across the globe, this book offers critical insights into how technology intersects with equity and diversity in young lives. It addresses crucial social issues such as identity, body image, and commercialization, making it a vital resource for those seeking to understand the challenges and opportunities media presents for children today.

– **Patti M. Valkenburg**, *University of Amsterdam*

Children, Media, and Technology
Access, Equity, Diversity, and Inclusion

Edited by Erica Scharrer

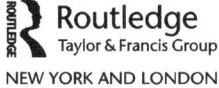
NEW YORK AND LONDON

Designed cover image: Getty Images

First published 2025
by Routledge
605 Third Avenue, New York, NY 10158

and by Routledge
4 Park Square, Milton Park, Abingdon, Oxon, OX14 4RN

Routledge is an imprint of the Taylor & Francis Group, an informa business

© 2025 selection and editorial matter, Erica Scharrer; individual chapters, the contributors

The right of Erica Scharrer to be identified as the author of the editorial material, and of the authors for their individual chapters, has been asserted in accordance with sections 77 and 78 of the Copyright, Designs and Patents Act 1988.

All rights reserved. No part of this book may be reprinted or reproduced or utilised in any form or by any electronic, mechanical, or other means, now known or hereafter invented, including photocopying and recording, or in any information storage or retrieval system, without permission in writing from the publishers.

Trademark notice: Product or corporate names may be trademarks or registered trademarks, and are used only for identification and explanation without intent to infringe.

ISBN: 978-1-032-59133-9 (hbk)
ISBN: 978-1-032-59053-0 (pbk)
ISBN: 978-1-003-45312-3 (ebk)

DOI: 10.4324/9781003453123

Typeset in Sabon
by KnowledgeWorks Global Ltd.

To GGSB with so much love

Contents

List of Contributors ix

PART I
Landscapes/Contexts 1

1 Introduction 3
   ERICA SCHARRER

2 Access/Use 16
   DEVINA SARWATAY AND USHA RAMAN

3 Representation 36
   SINDY R. SUMTER, IRENE I. VAN DRIEL,
   AND CHERRIE JOY F. BILLEDO

4 Parents/Caregivers 65
   WONSUN SHIN

5 Media Literacy Education 84
   SRIVIDYA RAMASUBRAMANIAN, SHANNON BURTH,
   AND PATRICK R. JOHNSON

6 Policies 100
   SUN SUN LIM AND BECKY PHAM

PART II
Interpretations/Implications   117

7 Social Identity   119
   L. MONIQUE WARD, JASMINE BANKS,
   ENRICA BRIDGEWATER, AND MIRANDA REYNAGA

8 Body Image   143
   JENNIFER STEVENS AUBREY, HEATHER GAHLER,
   AND KAUSUMI SAHA

9 Aggression   162
   MARINA KRCMAR, TONI LANE HINES,
   AND OLIVIA BUCKLEY

10 News/Politics   185
   LYNN SCHOFIELD CLARK

11 Learning   209
   FASHINA ALADÉ

12 Advertising/Commercialization   229
   REGINA JIHEA AHN

Index   251

Contributors

Regina Jihea Ahn (PhD) is an Assistant Professor of Strategic Communication at University of Miami School of Communication, USA. Her research spans consumer socialization, media literacy, and social media dynamics. She explores vulnerabilities in diverse demographics, including children, older adults, and patients. She aims to explore these topics from a cross-cultural perspective, advocating for fostering critical thinking skills.

Fashina Aladé (PhD) is an Assistant Professor of Advertising & Public Relations and Human Development & Family Studies at Michigan State University, USA. Her work lies at the intersection of media effects, developmental psychology, and early childhood education, with a focus on the impact of representations of race and culture on young children's learning from educational media.

Jennifer Stevens Aubrey (PhD) is a Professor of Communication at the University of Arizona, USA. Her research focuses on media effects on emotional, mental, and physical health in adolescents and young adults.

Jasmine Banks is a PhD candidate in the Department of Psychology at the University of Michigan, USA. She examines the intricacies of Black digital spaces at the intersection of race, identity, and culture, focusing on the digital manifestations of African-American traditions, meaning-making processes, and their role and impact on everyday life.

Cherrie Joy (Chei) F. Billedo (PhD, VU University, the Netherlands) is an Assistant Professor at the Amsterdam School of Communication Research (ASCoR) at the University of Amsterdam, the Netherlands. She is broadly interested in representation in media science, social media use among minoritized social groups, and media representation effects among young people.

Enrica Bridgewater is a joint Communication and Media and Psychology PhD student at the University of Michigan, USA. Her research interests include representations of minoritized communities in entertainment media; media contributions to identity development and psychological well-being across the lifespan; and the role of algorithms in shaping children's digital content.

Olivia Buckley (BA, Wake Forest University) is currently a Clinical Associate at DBT Works outside of Boston, MA, USA. She graduated from Wake Forest University in 2024 with a double major in Communications and Psychology. She conducted research with Marina Krcmar and with professors in Psychology during her time at Wake Forest University.

Shannon Burth (MA, Syracuse University) is a Mass Communication doctoral student at Syracuse University, USA. Her scholarship addresses media literacy, critical thinking, identity, representation, and inequalities. Her identity-focused research explores intersectional disability studies and representations.

Lynn Schofield Clark (PhD) is Distinguished Professor of Media, Film, and Journalism Studies and Director of the Estlow Center for Journalism and New Media at the University of Denver, USA. She teaches on social media, journalism, AI, and youth media cultures, and is the award-winning author (with Regina Marchi) of *Young People and the Future of News*, as well as *The Parent App, From Angels to Aliens*, and several other books and articles.

Heather Gahler is a PhD candidate in Communication at the University of Arizona, USA. Her research examines media effects on body image among diverse groups.

Toni Lane Hines (MA, Wake Forest University '25) is a graduate student at Wake Forest University, USA and mother of an amazing little boy to whom she accredits her interest in children media effects. After graduating Summa Cum Laude from undergrad, Toni received a full scholarship to continue her education at Wake Forest University and attributes her success to Christ.

Patrick R. Johnson (PhD, University of Iowa) is an Assistant Professor of Journalism in the Diederich College of Communication at Marquette University, USA. His scholarship focuses on the intersection of news literacy, journalism practice, sex and sexuality, LGBTQ rights, and journalism education.

Marina Krcmar (PhD, University of Wisconsin-Madison) is a Professor at Wake Forest University, USA. She has published over 100 chapters and articles that have appeared in *Journal of Communication, Human Communication Research, Media Psychology, Communication Research*, and many other journals. Her books: *Living Without the Screen* and *Communication Theory and Research: An Advanced Introduction* were published by Routledge.

Sun Sun Lim (PhD) is Vice President, Partnerships & Engagement and Lee Kong Chian Professor of Communication and Technology at Singapore Management University, Singapore. She has extensively researched the social impact of technology, authoring over 100 academic publications including *Transcendent Parenting: Raising Children in the Digital Age* (Oxford University Press, 2020).

Becky Pham is a PhD candidate (Communication) at the Annenberg School for Communication and Journalism, University of Southern California, USA. She researches how families, youth, and communities of immigrant background use digital media and consume popular culture, and how their media engagement shapes their communication and lived experience.

Usha Raman (PhD) is a Professor at the Department of Communication, University of Hyderabad, India where she teaches and researches in the areas of digital cultures, science and health communication, feminist media studies, and children and media.

Srividya Ramasubramanian (PhD, Penn State University) is Newhouse Professor & Endowed Chair at Syracuse University, USA. Her scholarship focuses on anti-racism, decolonizing pedagogy, trauma-informed approaches, and critical media effects.

Miranda Reynaga is a PhD candidate in the Personality & Social Contexts Area of Psychology at the University of Michigan, USA. Her research examines how television media influence adolescents' and emerging adults' sexual socialization, with a particular focus on beliefs about gender and sexuality.

Kausumi Saha is a PhD student in Communication at the University of Arizona, USA. Her research examines adolescent identity and fandoms.

Devina Sarwatay (PhD) is Presidential Fellow at Department of Media, Culture and Creative Industries, School of Communication and Creativity at City St George's, University of London, UK. She studies young people and digital cultures. Her latest work is published in *Information Communication and Society*, *Media International Australia*, *Journal of Communication*, and Wiley and Routledge Handbooks.

Wonsun Shin (PhD) is an Associate Professor in Media and Communications at the University of Melbourne, Australia. Areas of research include youth and digital media, parental mediation, and marketing communications. She has numerous publications in international journals and has co-authored *Screen Obsessed: Parenting in the Digital Age* and *Screen Smart: Growing Up in the Digital Age.*

Sindy R. Sumter (PhD, Leiden University, The Netherlands) is an Associate Professor at the Amsterdam School of Communication Research (ASCoR) at the University of Amsterdam, the Netherlands. Her research focuses on the way digital (mobile) technologies and entertainment media can shape social interactions and identity formation of tweens, teens, and young adults.

Irene I. van Driel (PhD, Indiana University Bloomington, USA) is an Assistant Professor at the Amsterdam School of Communication Research (ASCoR) at the University of Amsterdam, the Netherlands. She is interested in the crossroads of media use and youth identity development and her current research focuses on inclusive technology for youth.

L. Monique Ward (PhD) is an Arthur F. Thurnau Professor of Psychology at the University of Michigan, USA. Her research examines media and parental contributions to gender and sexual socialization, with a particular emphasis on sexual objectification. Her work also explores the intersections between gender ideologies, body image, race, and sexuality.

Part I
Landscapes/Contexts

1 Introduction

Erica Scharrer

What would an ideal media and technology landscape for children look like? What would it *not* look like? If you picture a world in which media and technology serve the interests of children, a scenario in which spending time with media and tech is an entirely enriching and supportive experience for kids, what features or conditions would be present or absent? How would your answers to those questions change for adolescents rather than children? How well do you think the current media and technology landscape serves the interests of children and teens? What are some benefits of growing up within our present media and tech cultures and systems? What are some drawbacks? What changes would be needed to maximize the positives and minimize the negatives, and how can those changes be made?

Asking these questions is an excellent way to begin reading this book. In a world that is fair, just, and equitable, everyone should be able to experience conditions that allow them to thrive. Yet, historic and enduring systems of power show that this is often not the case. In this book, we delve into important themes about the ways in which media and technology help to empower and/or disempower young people. We explore the role of media and technology in the lives of children and teens and seek answers to the critical questions of whose interests are served or not served in contemporary media and technology systems and practices.

Today's generation of young people is understood to consist of ardent users of media and technology, and yet *access* to reliable, fast, and up-to-date devices and the content and affordances that they offer remains uneven, with a persistent divide between the "haves" and the "have nots." When media and technology *are* accessed, a fair question is whether young people will have the opportunity to see or connect with media characters, media personalities, or fellow media users that represent the full, complex, varied, and nuanced experiences of *diverse* young people themselves. The question of *inclusion* in media and tech content and practices is a topic of vital importance, as are its implications. The goal of *equity* in representation of social groups (such as groups defined by gender, race, ethnicity, ability, and/or sexual identity) as well as in access to the opportunities that media and technology afford is also key. Questions of access, equity, diversity, and inclusion are critically important in working toward change that allows all people to thrive.

This book covers a number of long-standing as well as current issues and controversies pertaining to media and youth, such as potential links between media and technology use and wellbeing; violence, aggression, and cyberbullying; body image disturbances and beauty norms; and responses to increasingly sophisticated marketing strategies. Yet, this book also fully explores the ways in which media and technology use enriches the lives of children and teens and empowers them, with positive implications for their development, education, sociality, friendships, respect for others, and knowledge of and action in the world around them. Looking not just at interactions between media/tech and young media/tech users but also at the larger systems in which those interactions take shape, this book's contents bridge micro-level and macro-level analyses. In each of these lines of inquiry, up-to-date theory and research findings relevant, in particular, to young media users and questions of access, equity, diversity, and inclusion make this a distinct approach to understanding children, media, and technology.

There is no doubt that media and technology are at the center of young people's lives. Some researchers show this through statistics generated from surveys of older children and adolescents or surveys of the parents or caregivers of those too young to fill out questionnaires. In the United States in 2021, for instance, a Common Sense Media report showed an average of 8 hours and 39 minutes per day among 13- to 18-year-olds and 5 hours and 33 minutes per day among 8- to 12-year-olds spent using entertainment screen media (including watching videos, playing games, using social media, creating content, browsing websites, and engaging in other digital activities; Rideout et al., 2022). The same dataset also estimated that 42% of 10-year-olds, 53% of 11-year-olds, 71% of 12-year-olds, and 90% or more of those aged 16 or older have their own smartphone. In Pew Research Center 2023 data in the United States, 46% of teens said they are online "almost constantly" and another 47% said they are online several times a day (Anderson et al., 2023).

In a Global Kids Online (2019) project, a collaborative initiative between UNICEF and principal investigator Sonia Livingstone at the London School of Economics and Political Science, data were collected from 11 countries: Albania, Argentina, Brazil, Bulgaria, Chile, Ghana, Italy, Montenegro, the Philippines, South Africa, and Uruguay from 2016 to 2018. In total, researchers surveyed nearly 15,000 children aged 9 to 17 who use the internet, together with one parent, and found that the young people spend an average of two hours per day online on a weekday and approximately double that on a weekend. Qi et al. (2023) studied

53 published articles in which the screen time of children aged 6 to 14 was measured in samples of school children from multiple locations in Europe, Asia, the Americas, Australia, and Africa. The average screen time across all of the children studied in the articles was 2 hours and 77 minutes per day. Clearly, around the globe, children are spending substantial amounts of time with various forms of media.

In their prominent book on *Media/Society*, Croteau et al. (2018) identify four key components of media studies: technology, institutions, content, and users. Studying the topic of children and media requires considering each of these factors and the interplay among them. First, it is useful to think about **technologies** and their development, understandings, and uses within particular conditions/contexts. The study of media and tech companies and/or **industries** or **institutions**—including their economic and ownership structures, their platforms and practices, and their regulation—is also vital. For the topic of children and media, therefore, we might study mobile apps used by preschoolers or TikTok, BeReal, or other social media platforms used by adolescents and who or what is behind those media forms.

The **content** that is produced by media and tech companies as well as by their users is an important area of study, as well. The concept of **representation**, for instance, calls for an understanding that media do not merely reflect reality but rather selectively portray or depict (or literally *re*-present) people, events, ideas, etc. (Buckingham, 2015). What becomes media content, then, is not inevitable nor is it an accurate reflection of the "real world," but rather it reflects decisions that have been made about what to include and what to exclude and how to frame, depict, represent, or portray. For children and media, therefore, we might ask questions such as how climate change—a grave concern among many young people—is discussed in the news, or what sorts of comments are posted to "get ready with me" posts on TikTok or Instagram and we might explore the implications of those questions for individuals or for society at large.

Finally, it is crucial to study **media users**, as well, including what motivates them to spend time with particular media selections, what they like and why they like it, and how they interpret or make sense of media texts (like a movie, a commercial, etc.), platforms (such as whether they think they spend too much time on social media), and representations or other aspects of content that they see. Importantly, for instance, we can study how children and teens make meaning from/interpret media as well as whether they might be influenced by media in some way. Interactions with media and technology have the potential to shape young people's identities, values, points of view, and ways of being in the world. **Media effects** is the study of the ways in which the thoughts, feelings, attitudes, values, and behaviors of media users may be affected by media. Studying young media users, therefore, might vary from how they express their fandom of particular musical artists, graphic novels, television programs, or films to whether playing violent video games can contribute to feeling desensitized to aggression.

Studying Young People's Lives: Connections to Media and Technology

There are also multiple perspectives on how to study childhood and adolescence and taking one or more of those perspectives will help shape the kinds of questions that scholars ask about youth and media in their research. ***Developmental psychology***, for instance, is a field that examines changes across the life span, the ways that people change, grow, or develop over time. Researchers using this perspective often study how children's minds develop in association with outside factors including the contexts in which they live and learn, such as the family, school, the media, and society. In other words, they study the interrelationships between the growing self and the social world.

Strasburger et al. (2009) put forth factors that make children unique and are likely to be relevant to their interactions with media. First, by virtue of their age, children have fewer first-hand experiences to use to understand, analyze, evaluate, and critique media practices or media content. If stereotypes are apparent in TV shows or films, for instance, children may not have had the opportunity yet in their lives to meet and interact with a large and diverse number of people that they can call upon to recognize and resist those media stereotypes. Second, and somewhat relatedly, children may have fewer experiences with the media, again because of the limited number of years that they have been able to assemble such experiences. For example, young people may not have the same experiences with what constitutes trustworthy news or information that adults have acquired throughout their lives and so they may be less able to identify disinformation online. Finally, children have been likened to sponges, taking everything in, asking questions, and being eager to learn. They may look to the media for models, cues, and information, then, which can be an enriching and educational experience in some cases and a limited or distorted experience in other cases.

A developmental psychology approach understands adolescence as a stage in life characterized by a great deal of change. Adolescents may be increasingly independent or at least more desiring of their own independence, and that factor is likely to create a scenario in which much of their media use occurs without the direct supervision or knowledge of a parent or caregiver or another adult. Indeed, peers are widely thought of as increasingly central figures in teens' lives, and friends, romantic partners, classmates, and others can become more influential than parents/caregivers at this time, a pattern that makes peer-to-peer communication via social media, for instance, particularly important for adolescents. Adolescence can also be a period in which boundaries are tested, experimentation occurs, and "risky" behaviors might be attempted, and developmental specialists suggest that adolescents, compared to adults, may be particularly likely to think no harm will come to them if they so engage. Media depictions that show minimal consequences for risky behaviors like vaping or alcohol or drug use might have a particular impact among this age group, therefore. Adolescence is also considered a crucial time for the development of identity as well as an interest in social and political issues, all of which can also set the stage for unique interactions with media. Teens might engage in political expression about issues that they care about online, for instance, or they may look for support online for something that they are struggling with and to find people who understand.

One key question among those approaching the study of children and media from a developmental psychology-informed perspective is how and when children develop the ability to distinguish fantasy from reality (Strasburger et al., 2009). Researchers have found, for instance, that children under the age of four may still think that characters on TV are real, and even as they begin a bit later in childhood to know that characters are not real, they may still respond as if they are (such as knowing that the witch in *Wizard of Oz* is not real but still finding her scary). As they mature, children use different ways of judging the realism of television content, including using information about genre or production values (like an animated program not being real) and eventually—with some studies showing this capacity begins at about age eight—comparing whether things that happen on TV are possible in real life. By early adolescence, young people can not only assess whether TV content is possible, they can assess whether it's plausible or probable.

Some have observed that a developmental psychology-based approach to childhood studies considers children as in the stage of becoming an adult rather than in their own stage of being who they are, and some have critiqued this approach for focusing too strongly on what children cannot yet do (Lemish, 2015). For instance, we might observe that, in general, children under the age of eight struggle to understand that a commercial is an attempt to persuade them to like a product, like an ad, or want to buy something. Is that observation too focused on children's supposed deficits? The developmental approach has also been critiqued for making claims that are supposed to apply to most young people although those claims are mostly based on research gathered from mostly White, middle class, Western samples of children and adolescents (Tatlow-Golden & Montgomery, 2021).

The developmental psychology perspective is, therefore, sometimes positioned as different from a ***sociocultural approach*** to the study of childhood. In a sociocultural approach, rather than centering general stages during which most children or teens tend to do this or that, there is greater specificity and relativism. Childhood is thought of as a social construction, not something that is the same for everyone but rather is imagined and experienced differently in different historical, cultural, economic, or political contexts. Emphasis is placed on the capacity of children, and researchers studying children are urged to take a child-centered approach, listening to how children make sense of the world around them, assuming they have the ability to understand and explain their experiences (to researchers and beyond), and taking their experiences seriously.

In this way of approaching the study of childhood and adolescence, there is often pushback against the assumption of risk pertaining to youth and media. Rather than suggesting that children and teens need policies or practices to protect them from harm associated with the use of social media, video games, or other media forms, this way of thinking argues that "we must take into account the way in which children explore and constitute their physical, social and virtual identities and networks, on an unprecedented global scale" (Tsaliki, 2022, p. 479). Harms are not conceived as solved at the individual level (by young people interacting with media making "better" decisions, for instance), but rather at the macro/societal level as they are understood in relation to broad social issues such as misogyny, racism, sexism, classism, or homophobia. The use of media and technology for play (and the right of children to engage in play) is an example of what researchers taking a sociocultural approach might study, as are the ways in which media and technology allow young people to engage in civic participation.

A *children's rights* approach to childhood and adolescence is another important perspective. The children's rights approach argues that children's well-being is centered when they are able to have social, economic, cultural, and civic/political rights. Among its key principles are non-discrimination, putting the best interests of the child first in anything that affects them, giving children the right to survival and development, and respecting the views of the child in matters that affect them. The children's rights framework stems from the 1989 United Nation's Convention on the Rights of the Child in which an international treaty to establish children's rights was adopted. The UNICEF (2024) website explains: "Contained in this treaty is a profound idea: that children are not just objects who belong to their parents and for whom decisions are made, or adults in training. Rather, they are human beings and individuals with their own rights. The Convention says childhood is separate from adulthood, and lasts until 18; it is a special, protected time, in which children must be allowed to grow, learn, play, develop, and flourish with dignity. The Convention went on to become the most widely ratified human rights treaty in history and has helped transform children's lives."

Children's rights perspectives, then, can be thought of as a balance between a children-as-vulnerable and a children-as-agentic perspective.

The perspective acknowledges the ways that children's capacities change and grow over time and argues that corporations and governments have a duty to take children's best interests into account. Protecting children from harm is built into the rights document, as is facilitating their rights to expression, leisure, and well-being. The treaty has been ratified in 196 countries, making it the single most agreed-upon human rights treaty in history (UNICEF, 2024). The United States, however, is the only UN member state that has not signed on, with concerns about sovereignty and legalities often positioned as justification (Chapman et al., 2023).

There are a number of ways that the UN Convention on the Rights of the Child components relate to young people's interactions with media and technology. One right specified in the treaty, for example, is the right of children to play, and in the language of the Rights document, play is expressly defined on the child's own terms rather than through the lens of an adult. Livingstone et al. (2023), for instance, found among a large sample of 6- to 17-year-olds in the UK that design features of digital play that the researchers called "rights respecting"—such as features that protected their privacy, allowed for easy access, and featured "age-appropriate" play—were strongly associated with enjoyment. Another right included in the UN Convention on the Rights of the Child treaty is the right to privacy, which is, of course, an important topic pertaining to young people's use of digital media and will be discussed in multiple chapters of this book.

Different Research Traditions for Studying Young People and Media

Historically, there have been at least two main approaches to studying children and media in the communication field—cultural studies and media effects/media psychology—and in this book, authors are likely to draw from one or both of these main approaches. In the *cultural studies* tradition, most closely connected to a sociocultural approach to childhood as explained above, attention is paid to the central idea that different media users will make sense of and respond to media texts differently. Media users are assumed to be active rather than passive in interactions with media and technology and, in this tradition, researchers often place an emphasis on the agency of young people rather than their vulnerability to media influence. The cultural studies tradition is associated with qualitative methods where in-depth features of media texts and the forces and factors behind how those texts take shape are examined. When young people are studied in cultural studies research their answers to open-ended questions via interviews, focus groups, or through a questionnaire or other writing or drawing exercise as well as detailed analyses of the media they produce are examined to understand their experiences, views, etc.

The cultural studies tradition seeks to understand media practices, institutions, texts, and audiences in the context of historical, cultural, political, and economic conditions. Indeed, in critical cultural studies—drawing from feminist, postcolonial, queer, and critical race theories as well as Marxist thought—media industries, media texts, and media users are examined in relation to power structures in society. This approach to research seeks to identify and challenge systems that maintain unequal distribution of power in society, including those associated with race, class, gender, sexuality, and other social group formations. This connects directly to this book's focus on access, equity, diversity, and inclusion.

In the *media effects/media psychology* tradition, most closely associated with a developmental psychology approach to the study of childhood as explained above, attention is paid to the ways in which media shape how young people think, feel, and act. As in the cultural studies tradition, this tradition can also seek to understand how children and teens make sense of the media, but in this case, doing so is typically considered from a psychological rather than a sociocultural perspective. Interpreting or making sense of media—itself an indication that media users are interacting actively with/through media rather than passively—is mostly considered as processing, with an emphasis on how the human brain takes in and responds to information or other stimuli in the world. A media effects/media psychology perspective can certainly understand young people's interactions with media and technology as being shaped by social and cultural forces and factors (as will be explained below). But the chief difference is that the emphasis is still on the individual and their thoughts, emotions, attitudes, values, and behaviors rather than on broader-scale groups, communities, societies, or systems. Quantitative research is often used in this field, and when media texts are studied, a large sample is examined and broad patterns (like what percentage of main characters on popular streaming television shows are characters of color) are identified. When children and teens are studied, tools such as survey research or experiments are used to look for statistical patterns between media and technology use and particular outcomes (as well as/alongside other factors).

There is a growing interest in *quantitative criticalism*, using quantitative methods in a manner that helps identify and/or seeks to address inequalities and injustices in the world (Scharrer & Ramasubramanian, 2021). Drawing from the same critical theory-based framework described above that has been central to critical cultural studies, in quantitative criticalism, numbers-based research and statistics are used to show the stark realities of social conditions and social problems as well as to mark and measure progress toward positive social change. The nature of statistics as representing a widely shared experience is harnessed toward social justice ends. For example, researchers can use quantitative methods like surveys or experiments to study the ways in which having characters who look like them on television can empower young media users of color. In this way, too, research from this tradition in the study of children, media, and technology has an important role in understanding access, equity, diversity, and inclusion.

Whether we are studying children's interpretations of media (how they make sense of what they encounter) or the effects of media on children, it is vital to remember that there are no one-size-fits-all, universal experiences. Interactions between media/tech and young people are complex. Different young people can have different ways of making sense of and responding to media. This is in large part because, of course, there is tremendous diversity in who young people are, and that diversity matters for how they look at the world, including in the ways in which they interact with media and technology and the implications of those interactions. And, of course, as young people are situated within particular contexts, systems, and conditions of power, their lived experiences can differ widely, as well.

This attention to context and complexity has always been centered in the critical cultural studies tradition. Yet in the media effects tradition, as well, even some of the very first inquiries into the ways that children are influenced by media have been approached with the understanding that not all children will respond the same way to the same media texts. There has also been an understanding that the features of media texts themselves are important to consider since what they show or what they don't show and how they depict people, actions, etc. will also shape effects. In the famous Bobo doll studies in the 1960s that studied whether preschoolers can learn aggression from television, for instance, differences by the gender of the children who participated in the studies and differences in depictions such as whether the actor modeling the aggression looked more like a person or a cartoon character were explored (Bandura et al., 1961; 1963). The concept of *identification* is central to these very early studies, and that concept can be understood as an interaction between media users and media texts. Different media users have the potential to identify with different media characters and whether, how, or for whom media have effects can be contingent on processes such as this.

Across the decades, media effects studies have gotten much more sophisticated. Drawing on the large and growing body of research evidence that has accumulated over time, the **Differential Susceptibility to Media Influence (DSMM)** framework points out, for instance, that whether or not or the degree to which media will affect individuals is based on a host of factors (Valkenburg & Peter, 2013). Some of those factors have to do with individuals themselves, and Valkenburg and Peter organize those into three types: *dispositional* (anything that varies from person to person, such as their identities, attitudes or values, or moods), *developmental* (anything that has to do with media users' growth/development of their thinking, their emotions, or their social interactions), and *social* (anything that has to do with contexts such as friends or peers, families, school, home, or the wider cultural and its norms).

The DSMM framework also suggests that media effects can be *direct* (media shape some outcome among individuals) or *indirect* (media shape some other factor which then shapes some outcome among individuals). The framework shows further that media uses and media effects can be interrelated or mutually reinforcing. For instance, a teen who holds certain ideas about masculinity might select particular YouTubers to watch, and watching the content created by those YouTubers might, in turn, contribute to the teen's ideas about masculinity. Finally, the DSMM accounts for the idea that media effects can be weaker or stronger as *media influence interacts with the influence of other factors*. For example, if a teen is already feeling left out from a friend group and sees social media content of peers having fun, the co-occurrence of those two factors (already feeling left out + seeing the post) would be likely to have a particular effect on their feelings. From the Bobo doll experiments to today, then, there is *not* an assumption that all children will be affected by media the same way or even that all children will be affected at all.

The Contents of This Book

Centering the interrelated questions of access, diversity, equity, and inclusion in this book on children, media, and technology brings a unique perspective, allowing for the exploration of media practices, access, use, content, and influence as understood within wider conditions associated with power in society. To take such an approach, the authors of the chapters of this book will try to avoid the temptation of easy answers. Although some of the chapter authors may draw more heavily from one or more of the theories, foundations, and methods described in this introduction, they will balance questions of **negative** roles of media and technology in young people's lives with **positive** roles. Across all of the chapters of this book, then, the goal is to complicate or move past old assumptions that pit **agency** against **vulnerability** in kids' interactions with media and technology, finding that kids can be *both* capable, creative, and contented media users *and* at risk for media influence and that even understandings of kids as empowered media users must still be considered in the context of larger systems of power. They will recognize the ways in which young people make meaning from media *and* the ways in which media shapes their thoughts, attitudes, and behavior. Across chapters, authors will draw from **quantitative** research that looks for broad patterns in large research samples as well as **qualitative** research that studies more focused phenomena in depth within smaller samples. When studying children, adolescents, media, and technology, thinking in absolutes or using an either/or perspective will only tell a part of the story. In this book, the chapter authors have made a concerted effort to tell as comprehensive of a story as possible within the confines of the length considerations of a single chapter.

This book is organized into two interrelated sections. The first section is about the media and technology **LANDSCAPES/CONTEXTS** as experienced by children and adolescents. This section seeks to answer the questions: How are children and teens using media and technology in their daily lives? Who or what will they encounter when doing so? Who or what will they likely *not* encounter? And how do key people, entities, and contexts like parents/caregivers at home, educators at school, organizations in the community, or governments at the state level help shape those encounters? In *Chapter 2 Access/Use*, Devina Sarwatay and Usha Raman explore factors that shape whether media forms/platforms are within or outside of the reach of particular young people in particular contexts. The chapter shows that despite structural barriers in equitable access to the digitally connected world, young people are creative in finding ways to use media and technology in their daily lives. In *Chapter 3 Representation*, Sindy R. Sumter, Irene I. van Driel, and Cherrie Joy F. Billedo discuss the theories and research findings about media representations of gender, racial/ethnic, and sexual identities—both in terms of inclusion or positive depictions and exclusion or negative depictions—in media forms popular with youth. In *Chapter 4 Parents/Caregivers*, Wonsun Shin focuses on the family as a key context for young people's interactions with media. Parental practices for negotiating media and tech in kids' lives are discussed, including as shaped by social and cultural contexts. In *Chapter 5 Media Literacy Education*, Srividya Ramasubramanian, Shannon Burth, and Patrick R. Johnson discuss the transformative and empowering potential of media literacy efforts taking place inside as well as outside of school. The authors review educational initiatives that invite young people to both critique and create media, including allowing especially those from minoritized social groups to tell their own stories. Finally, in *Chapter 6 Policies*, Sun Sun Lim and Becky Pham introduce the ways in which governmental bodies or other organizations have put policies into place to regulate digital media with the rights, protections, or interests of young media users in mind.

The next section of the book is titled **INTERPRETATIONS/IMPLICATIONS** and explores media use, meaning making/interpretation, and effects within the landscapes and contexts laid out in the first section. Chapters in this section proceed theme by theme in discussing issues and topics of enduring interest in the role of media and technology in young people's lives. In *Chapter 7 Social Identity*, L. Monique Ward, Jasmine Banks, Enrica Bridgewater, and Miranda Reynaga introduce important questions about how children and teens use media to explore and express their identity, with a focus on gender and racial/ethnic identities. The implications of representations in various media forms are discussed, as are the ways in which especially marginalized or minoritized youth can seek and find connection and support through social media and other media forms. In **Chapter 8 Body Image**, Jennifer Stevens Aubrey, Heather Gahler, and Kausumi Saha provide an in-depth look at the role of media in defining—or challenging—social norms or cultural ideals pertaining to appearance and bodies, with an emphasis on gender, race, and disability. In **Chapter 9 Aggression**, Marina Krcmar, Toni Lane Hines, and Olivia Buckley cover the decades-long controversies around violence in the media (especially TV, movies, video games) and associations with outcomes related to aggression as well as the development of moral reasoning among youth with a focus on how violent media represent social groups. Cyberbullying and other online harms are also discussed, with particular attention to the ways in which societal-level power dynamics shape who or what is targeted in online aggression. In **Chapter 10 News/Politics**, Lynn Schofield Clark explores the ways in which young people use media and technology to learn about events, public figures, and new developments in the world and to engage in political expression and participation in social movements amid changing platforms, business models, and the spread of disinformation. In **Chapter 11 Learning**, Fashina Aladé reviews the uses and effects of media designed with the express purpose of educating youth and/or encouraging their prosocial development. Educational apps for mobile devices as well as educational television programs are discussed in the chapter, with a connection to income-related divides and diverse characters in educational/prosocial media and the effects of such inclusion. Finally, in **Chapter 12 Advertising and Commercialization** by Regina Jihea Ahn, the presence of brands, ads, and marketing messages in a wide variety of media types is examined, as are outcomes associated with exposure to commercial content. One of the key questions of diversity, equity, and inclusion addressed in the chapter is the targeting of ads by gender, race, or other aspects of social group identity and ethical questions pertaining to blurring entertainment and commercial content in modern marketing practices is discussed.

References

Anderson, M., Faverio, M., & Gottfried, J. (2023). *Teens, social media and technology 2023*. Pew Research Center. https://www.pewresearch.org/internet/2023/12/11/teens-social-media-and-technology-2023/

Bandura, A., Ross, D., & Ross, S. A. (1961). Transmission of aggression through imitation of aggressive models. *Journal of Abnormal Social Psychology, 63*, 575–582. https://doi.org/10.1037/h0045925

Bandura, A., Ross, D., & Ross, S. A. (1963). Imitation of film-mediated aggressive models. *Journal of Abnormal Social Psychology, 66*, 3–11. https://doi.org/10.1037/h0048687

Buckingham, D. (2015). *Developing media literacy: Concepts, processes, and practices*. https://davidbuckingham.net/wp-content/uploads/2015/04/media-literacy-concepts-processes-practices.pdf

Chapman, A. R., Brunelli, L., Forman, L., & Kaempf, J. (2023). Promoting children's rights to health and well-being in the United States. *The Lancet Regional Health–Americas*, 25, 1–6. https://doi.org/10.1016/j.lana.2023.100577

Croteau, D., Hoynes, W., & Childress, C. (2018). *Media/society: Technologies, industries, content and users* (7th ed.). Sage Publications.

Global Kids Online (2019). *Global Kids Online: Comparative Report*. UNICEF Office of Research – Innocenti. https://www.unicef.org/innocenti/media/7011/file/GKO-Comparative-Report-2019.pdf

Lemish, D. (2015). *Children and media: A global perspective*. Wiley-Blackwell.

Livingstone, S., Ólafsson, K., & Pothong, K. (2023). Digital play on children's terms: A child rights approach to designing digital experiences. *New Media & Society*. https://doi.org/10.1177/14614448231196576

Qi, J., Yan, Y., & Yin, H. (2023). Screen time among school-aged children of aged 6–14: A systematic review. *Global Health Research and Policy*, 8(1), 12. https://doi.org/10.1186/s41256-023-00297-z

Rideout, V., Peebles, A., Mann, S., & Robb, M. B. (2022). *Common Sense census: Media use by tweens and teens, 2021*. Common Sense. https://www.commonsensemedia.org/sites/default/files/research/report/8-18-census-integrated-report-final-web_0.pdf

Scharrer, E., & Ramasubramanian, S. (2021). *Quantitative research methods in communication: The power of numbers for social justice*. Routledge.

Strasburger, V. C., Wilson, B. J., & Jordan, A. B. (2009). *Children, adolescents, and the media* (2nd ed.). Sage.

Tatlow-Golden, M., & Montgomery, H. (2021). Childhood studies and child psychology: Disciplines in dialogue? *Children & Society*, 35(1), 3–17. https://doi.org/10.1111/chso.12384

Tsaliki, L. (2022). Constructing young selves in a digital media ecology: Youth cultures, practices and identity. *Information, Communication & Society*, 25(4), 477–484.

UNICEF. (2024). *Convention on the Rights of the Child*. https://www.unicef.org/child-rights-convention/

Valkenburg, P. M., & Peter, J. (2013). The differential susceptibility to media effects model. *Journal of Communication*, 63(2), 221–243. https://doi.org/10.1111/jcom.12024

2 Access/Use

Devina Sarwatay and Usha Raman

Oftentimes in policy circles there is the tendency to assume that childhood is a homogenous experience for young people everywhere: children are born, they grow up and go to school, and eventually become adults who take their place in the world. However, young people are just as much part of an intricate world and live lives that are as complicated as any adult's. There is no one experience of childhood as research has shown us repeatedly. Variations in age, gender, income, race, and other socioeconomic factors mean that children have varied life experiences, and consequently access and use media and technology around them differently. There is also the added layer of parental and other adult mediation that affects how children and adolescents encounter and experience media and technology in their everyday lives, as will be taken up in Chapter 4. This chapter gives a broad overview of how access to and use of media and technology by children and adolescents has been studied. It also demonstrates how contextual nuances play a part in children's access and use practices through four cases, thus proposing a more nuanced, context- and culture-centered view of young people's access to and use of digital media that begins with an acknowledgment of diversity and the attendant need to imagine inclusion in a more expansive manner.

Defining Key Terms

For the purpose of this chapter and in most of the literature reviewed here, the following key terms are defined as follows:

1 *Children and adolescents/Young people*: All individuals from birth until the age of 18 years when they are legally considered to be adults under most systems of governance
2 *Childhood*: The years spent as a child and/or the state of being a child
3 *Media and technology*: All digital and social media which can be used as tools for communication and a variety of other functions in a connected

world including the internet, devices like smartphones, and platforms like TikTok
4 *Access*: The means and opportunity to use and benefit from media and technology
5 *Use*: To put media and technology to use to serve the needs of consumption, production, social and cultural engagement, and sharing content online
6 *Inclusion*: Policy and/or practice of providing/making available access and means of using resources to those who might be otherwise excluded and marginalized
7 *Parental mediation*: Parents' or caregivers' strategies and actions toward regulating young people's media and technology access and use so that they can control, supervise, and advise on children and adolescents' media and technology habits. Usually, parental mediation is categorized as active, restrictive, and co-viewing/co-using

   a *Active parental mediation*: Parents' or caregivers' conscious use of communication and collaborative decision-making with children about their media and technology habits depending on their developmental needs
   b *Restrictive parental mediation*: Parents' or caregivers' strict restrictions and rules about children's media and technology habits
   c *Co-viewing/co-using*: Parents' or caregivers' presence and joint engagement (ideally without criticism) with children in their media and technology habits for a shared experience

8 *Moral panics/Technopanics*: General anxieties about risks and harms arising from the use or exposure to new technologies. Often the perception of the negative impact of technologies/media leads to restrictive parental mediation and the formulation of protectionist policies
9 *Agency*: The sense of being in or having control over your life and its decisions, that is, you have the capacity to think through and act rationally in your everyday lives

Selected Research Trends

As with most resources in the world, access to and use of media and digital technology are characterized by divides and inequalities stemming from a variety of socioeconomic and cultural factors. Apart from broader structural and material factors, these inequalities could be related to gender (Gillwald & Partridge, 2023), income (Goedhart et al., 2019; Marler, 2023), and skill/knowledge (Wang, 2020), among other factors. Children and adolescents within these categories could also face limitations to access and use of technological and cultural resources, with additional challenges posed by their inability to make independent decisions and relative lack of autonomy. Issues such as multigenerational mediation (Nimrod et al., 2023) and restrictive parental mediation (Sarwatay et al., 2022) further limit their exercise of agency, in addition to disadvantages stemming from class or other forms of marginality (Banaji, 2017; Katz & Hightower, 2023), higher vulnerability to online risks and harms (Marchant et al., 2017; Patchin & Hinduja, 2017), and limited literacy/resources to help protect them on platforms and environments not necessarily built for them (Sarwatay et al., 2021; Simone et al., 2019).

Overcoming Barriers

It is well established that digital inequalities more broadly mirror social and cultural inequalities (Helsper, 2021), but young people everywhere demonstrate agency and resistance by negotiating access to use media and technology (Bhatia et al., 2021; Sarwatay & Raman, 2022). Often, they are able to manage access to digital and social media with cheap smartphones and mobile internet plans that are deployed for digital leisure and play (Arora et al., 2023; Nelson, 2021; Rangaswamy & Arora, 2016; Rangaswamy & Cutrell, 2013) even where there are economic barriers. Other challenges may stem from such factors as social background and gender identity (Bhatia et al., 2021; Duek & Moguillansky, 2020; Ringrose et al., 2013) and restrictive parental mediation arising from moral panics or technopanics, given that most media and technology are not child-centered and rarely take into account the needs or vulnerabilities of younger users (Marwick, 2008; Radesky & Hiniker, 2022).

Of course, where there are restrictions, there are also ways to circumvent regulation, and this is something young people often tend to do. For instance, they find creative ways to negotiate their digital presence and to engage in online activism (Sarwatay & Raman, 2022; Subramanian, 2021). Interestingly, some parents actively encourage even underage children to have social media accounts (boyd et al., 2011; Torkington, 2022), and of course, there is the phenomenon of *sharenting* (Lazard, 2022; Leaver, 2020) where parents post content related to their children online, although arguably the latter has more to do with parental use of social media to showcase their own and their children's lives rather than mediating or moderating their children's use—something beyond the scope of the current chapter.

Affordances, Risks, and Literacies

Research across contexts has shown that young people use media and technology for meaning-making, identity curation and creation, self-expression, socialization, creativity, activism, and other purposes like learning and creating and maintaining their networks online (boyd, 2007;

Green, 2021; Hausmann et al., 2017; Livingstone et al., 2017; Nolas et al., 2016; Sarwatay et al., 2022; Sarwatay & Raman, 2022). Despite the predominance of notions of harms and dangers and the desire and assumed responsibility to regulate young people's media and technology access and use (technopanics) in popular media narratives, such studies have made it clear that young people, particularly those who have grown up in a digitally suffused world, have naturally adapted to ways of being digital that evidence their awareness of and negotiation with potential harms, usually defined as digital and/or media literacy (Wuyckens et al., 2022). This is not, however, to minimize the very real dangers of exploitation that children are vulnerable to, or to diminish the need for both policy and design interventions that can address these while also working toward more inclusive and safe online spaces (Livingstone et al., 2017; Reid Chassiakos et al., 2016; Third et al., 2019). However, projects of digital inclusion have sometimes tended to further legitimize and reinforce divides and inequalities. Structural disempowerment is often not acknowledged and accounted for within a techno-utopian frame (Sarkar, 2016; Tripp, 2011), that is, many initiatives promising inclusion end up further marginalizing participants or have a set agenda of what counts as "productive" and/or "valid" use of a particular media/technology initiative limiting open-ended exploration and self-directed learning. Children and childhood are also imagined variously across cultures, leading to different approaches to policy making related to technology and its implementation across commercial, educational, and other spheres (Raman & Kasturi, 2023).

There is an emphasis on authenticity and being yourself online among young people as they use digital and social media for identity and relationship management even as they grow into an awareness of their role as political and social agents (Raman & Verghese, 2014; Sarwatay & Raman, 2022; Zillich & Riesmeyer, 2021). As children and adolescents become more digitally skilled, they learn to seek out better opportunities and combat online risks (Beilmann et al., 2023; Livingstone et al., 2021). Even so, open communication with parents/caregivers, combined with a balance of active and restrictive parental mediation, has shown to have the most positive impact on the ability of young people to learn online self-regulation (Beyens et al., 2019; Sarwatay et al., 2021; Steinfeld, 2021).

Overloaded by the New

While many assume that young people are always eager to experiment with and adopt new technology, this largely depends on several factors with affordances (implicit or built into the design of technology and tools), access, and use being the most important ones. However, with AI (Artificial

Intelligence) and GenAI (Generative AI) tools becoming available for everyday use, we find some students, particularly those in higher education, have mixed responses to this new technology being embedded in our daily lives for fear of losing creativity, for instance (Smolansky et al., 2023). In addition, some young people are also just not interested in using media and technology at this stage of their lives (Brites & Ponte, 2018; Guzman, 2022). Some recent work, including that of sociologist Jonathan Haidt, draws on conversations with young people to suggest that they feel overwhelmed by the presence of social media in their lives, and would welcome restrictions or delays in its use, particularly if this was applied across their peer groups (Haidt, 2024).

Digital Citizenship

On the other hand, as new media and technology become more embedded in our everyday lives, children and adolescents who are usually enthusiastic users often become their parents' teachers in a role reversal (Wang, 2020). The technology—to the extent they have access to it—has become "everyday" for them, necessitating negotiations on multiple fronts even as they find ways to make it their own. Digital citizenship is also becoming the norm across most geographies, often aggressively promoted by the state, thus making it necessary for young people and adults to be more media literate and digitally skilled (Cortesi et al., 2020; Sarwatay et al., 2021; Stevenson et al., 2022). While children have not been seen as a "public" in most countries (Nolas, 2015), their presence and participation in digital spaces makes it imperative for them to be counted and for their experiences to be foregrounded as new digital governance initiatives are launched and existing ones expand to include new young citizens.

Consequently, what emerges is a complex picture when it comes to young people and digital media use. While on one end we have patchy and limited access and irregular media use due to various forms of inequalities and divides, on the other, we have unlimited access to devices, platforms, and the internet leading to overuse and crossing over to young people becoming *produsers* (the merging of producer and user in our digitally connected world) and even "kidfluencers" who can become global stars and risk being exploited for their creativity and labor (Feller & Burroughs, 2021; Simone et al., 2019). Of course, children and adolescents as users of social media are also impacted by other influencers who may be of their generation or older and this too can affect them physiologically or psychologically (Chakola, 2022; De Veirman et al., 2019; Schmuck, 2021). Nonetheless, it is important to note that access and use of media and technology have not found clear-cut negative impacts on young people's well-being, and several scholars have continued to emphasize the equivocal nature of the evidence (Beyens et al., 2021; Bharucha, 2018; McDool et al., 2020; Valkenburg et al., 2022).

Gendered Aspects of Use and Mediation

The gendered aspect in both use and mediation shows a trend of focusing on girls and women where duties and restrictions are concerned (Beyens et al., 2019; Chandrima et al., 2020; Duek & Moguillansky, 2020; Iqbal et al., 2021; Rodríguez-de-Dios et al., 2018). Girls are often expected to present themselves in a certain way and be mindful of their social interactions online. They are also more restricted by parents/caregivers in terms of access and use of media and technology for fear of risks and harms online. Girls often keep their profiles on social media private and have to deal with trolls, bullies, negative comments, and avoid risky interactions (see also Chapter 9). They have to find creative ways in which they can be present online as well as safeguard their online presence and ensure that their parents'/caregivers' regulations are adhered to. This is as true of emerging economies as it is of people in the Global North (Bhatia et al., 2021; Pea et al., 2012; Ringrose et al., 2013). While children and adolescents are participants in many studies and have the opportunity to share their experiences, this also means that there has been a fair amount of focus on the adults and caregivers around these young people and the manner in which they mediate and regulate their wards' online lives. Most of these parental responsibilities fall on the shoulders of mothers. They have to analyze, regulate, monitor, and safeguard young people online sometimes all by themselves, often becoming the "bad guy" and the strict parent. Mothers are in charge of both boys and girls, but with girls, there is the added pressure of societal norms to be followed as well.

Foregrounding Young Voices

Centering children's voices is increasingly being given due importance as our media and technology landscape has drastically transformed (De Wolf & Vanden Abeele, 2020; Rivas-Lara et al., 2023; Sarwatay, 2022; Stoilova et al., 2021; Third et al., 2019) and it is significant to consider experiences of children and adolescents to understand their needs and safeguard their digital futures. This perspective also comes from the realization that a large proportion of today's teens and adolescents have grown up within a hyper-mediatized and technology-saturated environment. Even in contexts where access is limited, there is a pervasive imagination of the online, as a space of interaction and self-making (Barr, 2019; Livingstone, 2020). We are fast moving from the "networked self"

(Papacharissi, 2012) to the "algorithmised self" (Bhandari & Bimo, 2022) or even—one might speculate—the "synthetic" self. Hence, it becomes important to study children and adolescents in this highly mediated and technologized environment, especially through a culture-centered approach. Foregrounding their voices and recognizing that access and use can be fraught irrespective of contexts will help us include diverse perspectives, perceptions, and experiences (Alper et al., 2016; Banaji, 2016; Ephraim, 2013) so that young people's digital rights can be protected (CRC, 2021; Ito et al., 2023; Lupton & Williamson, 2017; Staksrud & Milosevic, 2017; Third et al., 2019).

Current State of Affairs

Access to media and technology has always been tricky for children and adolescents due to multiple reasons. In many cases, if they fail to get access at home, they may depend on schools, informal learning spaces, and peer networks for digital and social media access. The pandemic severely impacted a huge number of children and adolescents with regard to access to media and technology, and consequently, the opportunity to access education and digital skills. COVID-19-related lockdowns also laid bare the stark digital divides within Global North contexts and further exacerbated them in Global South environments.

Access to the internet at home was a dream for nearly two-thirds of children and youth worldwide with high-income countries having 87% of their children online compared to 6% in low-income countries (UNICEF & ITU, 2020) during the pandemic. The rural-urban divide was very apparent as only about a quarter of young people in rural areas had the internet at home compared to 41% of urban dwellers (UNICEF & ITU, 2020). Figure 2.1 on "Percentage of children and young people with internet access at home, by region" shows the stark differences in access across the globe. The graph comes from UNICEF & ITU authors' calculations based on Multiple Indicator Cluster Surveys, Demographic and Health Surveys, and other national household surveys (2010–2020) in the "Report by UNICEF & ITU on how many children and young people have internet access at home?" (UNICEF & ITU, 2020, p. 5)

In Costa Rica, for example, the closure of a government program has left many children without internet access (Pérez-Sánchez, 2024). On the other hand, most young people in Uruguay now have access both at home and in school (Kids Online Uruguay, 2024) and the access gap is closing in Chile (Livingstone, 2023) and in the United States (Anderson et al., 2023) and most young people in the UK have internet access (Ofcom, 2023). However, a significant number of young people in the United

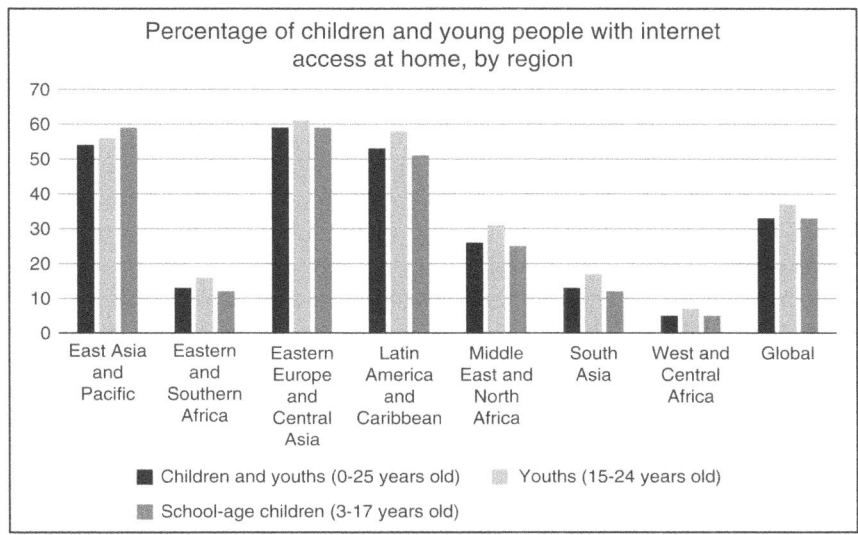

Figure 2.1 Representation of the "Percentage of children and young people with internet access at home."
Source: Data from UNICEF & ITU report, 2020

States are still struggling with access to education technology leading to a digital divide that impacts social inequality (Chandra et al., 2020; Pierce & Cleary, 2024). Education technology or "EdTech" are new media and technology inclusions in teaching-learning environments both in schools/classrooms and at home (used during the pandemic for online classes), for example, interactive projectors and screens, iPads, tablets, Google classrooms, Zoom rooms, Miro boards, MOOCs (massive online open courses), etc. In many countries, smartphones and mobile internet are the gateway to access media and technology and bridge gaps between formal and informal learning and digital access and participation like in Nigeria (Uzuegbunam, 2024), Singapore (Looi et al., 2016), and India (Rangaswamy & Arora, 2016). Overall, it appears that where governments have proactively seen the internet and digital tools as a common good that needs to be offered as a public service, there is a greater degree of access, often facilitated by the state.

Global surveys and statistics show that even younger children (as young as 0–6 years) are spending time on accessing media and technology (Green et al., 2024) with more boys going online than girls in developing economies (Global Kids Online, 2019). Detailed studies focusing on race or caste or class and technology in teens' social media use show that more Black teens use TikTok and Twitter, Hispanic teens prefer WhatsApp, and White teens prefer BeReal in the United States (Anderson et al., 2023), whereas young people from high-income families prefer Instagram and those from middle- and low-income families prefer TikTok and even use it for caste-based activism in India (Sarwatay & Raman, 2022; Subramanian, 2021). The most popular apps for most children are YouTube, TikTok, Instagram, and Snapchat, and nearly all of them are accessed by children on smartphones who have to navigate restrictive parental mediation especially in developing economies because these are considered to be a waste of time or a hindrance to good academic performance (Anderson et al., 2023; Ofcom, 2023; Raman & Kasturi, 2023; Sarwatay & Raman, 2022; Uzuegbunam, 2024). It is important to note here that platforms can come and go according to whatever young people deem to be trending at the moment. So, while BeReal might be the hot, new app when this chapter was initially being written, it might not be so trendy when this book is finally published, much like MySpace was the first big social networking space that now no one has heard about!

Smartphones and mobile media are key technologies that enable young people's access and use. For many young people, mobile use is often linked with age, where younger children usually get their parents'/caregivers' smartphones for a limited time during the day and teenagers begin to get their own devices as a rite of passage of sorts or when they begin to become more independent and have several academic and extra-curricular commitments that they need to fulfil with a certain degree of independence. Naturally, mobile and smartphones and young people's digital cultures are studied with great interest (Goggin, 2013; Ling & Haddon, 2008; Vanden Abeele, 2016) including the use of these devices in learning and leisure as well as parental mediation around mobile and smartphone use of young people (Lim, 2019; Looi et al., 2016; Matthes et al., 2021; Rangaswamy & Arora, 2016). In resource-constrained contexts, young people find ways to maximize smartphone access by co-using the same device with siblings and bartering mobile privileges with completed homework and good academic performance (Sarwatay et al., 2022; Sarwatay & Raman, 2022).

Selected Cases

Our brief review above offers a broad sense of how research in the field has looked at children and adolescents' access to and use of media and technology in their daily lives. Below are four specific research-based cases that we highlight to understand how different media and technology are accessed and used differently by children and adolescents from diverse

Table 2.1 Case study on teens using media for parental socialization.

Case	*Mutual Influence in LGBTQ Teens' Use of Media to Socialize Their Parents (Mares et al., 2022)*
Location/Study type	*USA/Quantitative*
Summary	*Teens encouraged parents to watch LGBTQ-positive media content for socialization and to initiate or model conversations about gender and sexual identities. This served to augment parental receptivity and support of LGBTQ identities that in turn led to improved self-esteem and lower depressive symptoms among the group of American teens studied.*
Remarks	*This study is a great example of combining theory and testing hypotheses to show how teens used media to get their parents to watch and talk about LGBTQ experiences so that they could negotiate their gender and sexual identities and garner parental support for better self-esteem and well-being.*

Source: Authors.

contexts and constraints. Each of these represents a different context, and uses varied theoretical approaches and methods to derive insights.

Case 1: Teens' Use of Media to Socialize Parents

Most research focuses on parental mediation of children's access to and use of technology in their everyday lives, but we would like to highlight one case here where researchers found that teens used media to socialize their parents about gender and sexual identities (see Table 2.1).

Case 2: Adolescents' Use of Smartphones to Cope with Stress

This next case (see Table 2.2) shows how smartphone use can develop into a digital coping mechanism for stress management by adolescents. Researchers not only generated a theory around adolescents' smartphone coping styles using qualitative methods but also created a validated scale (a set of items to include on a survey) to measure how teens strategized their well-being using smartphones.

Case 3: Teens' Digital Expression of Sexuality

The third case (see Table 2.3) relates to research that seeks to understand adolescents' digital expressions of sexuality via sexting, a social practice that has been enabled by access to and use of media and technology at their disposal.

Table 2.2 Case study on teens' smartphone coping styles.

Case	Coping styles among Chinese adolescents: The development and validation of a smartphone coping style scale (Huang et al., 2023)
Location/Study type	China/Mixed methods
Summary	Researchers developed a scale to catalogue Chinese adolescents' smartphone coping styles to understand how smartphone use allowed them to manage stress. They found that teens coped digitally by using smartphones to solve daily problems, seek social support, and distract from negative emotions.
Remarks	This example allows you to see theory generation and testing (smartphone coping style scale) in practice. This study led to the development of a reliable tool to test digital coping of adolescents using smartphones for well-being. Researchers acknowledge the ease of access to media and technology afforded by smartphones to Chinese teens and how it has become a popular means to help them cope with stress. They develop a scale to measure different coping styles, synthesize the distinct elements of these coping strategies, and validate a tool that enables us to capture and understand adolescents' smartphone coping styles for well-being.

Source: Authors.

Table 2.3 Case study on teens' digital sexual practices and perspectives on sex education.

Case	"Send Nudes?": Teens' perspectives of education around sexting, an argument for a balanced approach (Woodley et al., 2024)
Location/Study type	Australia/Qualitative
Summary	Interviews were conducted with teens to understand their perspectives about sexting and relationships and sexuality education to find that prohibition or fear-based strategies are less effective and a sex-positive and balanced approach to sex education works better.
Remarks	This study uses the social constructionism theory to unpack how young people in Australia digitally express and practice their sexuality and to explore what kind of sex education might work better with the kind of socialization they achieve with their level of access to and use of media and technology around them. It analyzes the common practice of "sending nudes" and the associated probable risks and harms that often result in technopanics and moral panics among adults. The response is generally to restrict phone use, whereas this research suggests that mobile-based, positive, communication-oriented practices can enable a more nuanced understanding of a teen digital practice.

Source: Authors.

Table 2.4 Case study on young people's TikTok cultures.

Case	*Exploring children's TikTok cultures in India: Negotiating access, uses, and experiences under restrictive parental mediation (Sarwatay et al., 2022)*
Location/Study type	*India/Qualitative*
Summary	*A qualitative approach and multimodal methods were used to understand young people's TikTok cultures under restrictive parental mediation (i.e., when their parents/caregivers have placed restrictions on their media use). Platform-specific access and use mediated by restrictive parental practices meant that children and adolescents in India found ways to negotiate, demonstrate agency, and resist parental controls to participate in vernacular digital cultures, that is, regional/context-specific everyday digital practices.*
Remarks	*This study uses innovative approaches to understand and analyze children and adolescents' TikTok cultures. Many conceptions of the platform's affordances and related access and use concerns raised by adults and media discourse were contrasted by young people showing how perceptions vary, pointing to the importance of foregrounding young people's voices.*

Source: Authors.

Case 4: Young People's Platformized Digital Cultures

The final case in this chapter (see Table 2.4) helps us understand platform-specific digital cultures of young people and how parental mediation affects children and adolescents' access and use of media and technology due to technopanics and resulting restrictions.

The four cases outlined above point to the multiplicity of ways in which young people make use of digital media to fulfill their own needs, even as it is clear that these are needs not necessarily envisaged by the developers of these tools. While the last case (Sarwatay et al., 2022) points to how children in relatively resource-poor regions find ways to not only access media but actively bend it to their desires, the first one illustrates how another group of young people turn media into a stimulus for conversation with adults. Across all cases, we see instances of innovative routes to access and ingenious and productive use. These cases also take us beyond the numbers on levels of digital media access and types of use among children, giving us a sense of what is actually going on in children's lives.

What Lies Ahead

Globally, there is a preponderance of studies among young people, primarily in the Global North, who have regular and easy access to technology and media. However, in recent years, many more researchers—especially those who acknowledge the presence of diversities and inequalities—are including children and adolescents from the Global South, as well as those from underrepresented communities within the Global North regions. These studies offer compelling evidence of young people's resistance and agency in the face of barriers to further their digital participation and citizenship in an increasingly connected world. These serve as excellent examples of young people's digital cultures, forming in organic and perhaps unexpected ways.

This is not to say that all children and adolescents in resource-advantaged countries have uniform or uninterrupted access and use of media and technology nor that all resource-disadvantaged contexts have equally fraught circumstances, for there are barriers, divides, and inequalities everywhere (Banaji, 2016). Nonetheless, we have a long way to go because many children and adolescents who are differently abled, identify themselves as those belonging to diverse gender and sexual identities, or are living in or escaping from precarity are yet to find expansive representation in research, and, indeed, in the imagination of those who design and deploy technologies.

This is a trend that we also see in media and technology ecosystems that are generally not built with young people at the center of the design or production process, but instead prioritize a certain kind of user, who is:

1 Someone living in a family with disposable income such that media and technology devices are affordable
2 An able-bodied young person who can easily use media and technology without accessibility issues
3 Someone who is skilled and has the capacity to navigate platforms and make use of their affordances

There is a growing call for more research in this area that prioritizes the needs of a diverse range of young people, and this can begin only by understanding the specific contexts in which they encounter media and technology, the specific ways in which they engage with these tools, and the varied ways in which they make them part of their everyday lives.

References

Alper, M., Katz, V. S., & Clark, L. S. (2016). Researching children, intersectionality, and diversity in the digital age. *Journal of Children and Media*, 10(1), 107–114. https://doi.org/10.1080/17482798.2015.1121886

Anderson, M., Faverio, M., & Gottfried, J. (2023). *Teens, social media and technology 2023*. Pew Research Center. https://www.pewresearch.org/internet/2023/12/11/teens-social-media-and-technology-2023/

Arora, P., Alencar, A., Jaramill-Dent, D., Warnes, J., & Pérez-Iglesias, E. (2023). *The digital leisure divide and the forcibly displaced*. UNHCR. https://www.

unhcr.org/innovation/wp-content/uploads/2023/04/The-Digital-Leisure-Divide-Field-Research.pdf

Banaji, S. (2016). *Global research on children's online experiences: Addressing diversities and inequalities* (p. 26). Global Kids Online. http://globalkidsonline.net/wp-content/uploads/2016/05/Guide-10-Diversities-and-inequalities-Banaji.pdf

Banaji, S. (2017). *Children and media in India: Narratives of class, agency and social change*. Routledge. https://www.routledge.com/Children-and-Media-in-India-Narratives-of-Class-Agency-and-Social-Change/Banaji/p/book/9781138344570

Barr, R. (2019). Growing up in the digital age: Early learning and family media ecology. *Current Directions in Psychological Science*, 28(4), 341–346. https://doi.org/10.1177/0963721419838245

Beilmann, M., Opermann, S., Kalmus, V., Vissenberg, J., & Pedaste, M. (2023). The role of school-home communication in supporting the development of children's and adolescents' digital skills, and the changes brought by COVID-19. *Journal of Media Literacy Education*, 15(1), 1–13. https://doi.org/10.23860/JMLE-2023-15-1-1

Beyens, I., Pouwels, J. L., van Driel, I. I., Keijsers, L., & Valkenburg, P. M. (2021). Social media use and adolescents' well-being: Developing a typology of person-specific effect patterns. *Communication Research*, 00936502211038196. https://doi.org/10.1177/00936502211038196

Beyens, I., Valkenburg, P. M., & Piotrowski, J. T. (2019). Developmental trajectories of parental mediation across early and middle childhood. *Human Communication Research*, 45(2), 226–250. https://doi.org/10.1093/hcr/hqy016

Bhandari, A., & Bimo, S. (2022). Why's everyone on TikTok now? The algorithmized self and the future of self-making on social media. *Social Media + Society*, 8(1), 20563051221086241. https://doi.org/10.1177/20563051221086241

Bharucha, J. (2018). Social network use and youth well-being: A study in India. *Safer Communities*, 17(2), 119–131. https://doi.org/10.1108/SC-07-2017-0029

Bhatia, K. V., Arora, P., & Pathak-Shelat, M. (2021). Good girls don't go online: Unpacking the quotidian playful resilience influencing girls' social and digital engagements. *International Journal of Communication*, 15(0), Article 0. https://ijoc.org/index.php/ijoc/article/view/17552

boyd, danah. (2007). Why youth heart social network sites: The role of networked publics in teenage social life. In D. Buckingham (Ed.), *Youth, identity, and digital media* (pp. 119–142). MIT Press. https://doi.org/10.31219/osf.io/22hq2

boyd, danah, Hargittai, E., Schultz, J., & Palfrey, J. (2011). Why parents help their children lie to Facebook about age: Unintended consequences of the 'Children's online privacy protection Act'. *First Monday*, 16(11). https://doi.org/10.5210/fm.v16i11.3850

Brites, M. J., & Ponte, C. (2018). Reasons and circumstances that lead to the non-use of media by young people and their families. *Comunicação e Sociedade*, 34, 411–429. https://doi.org/10.17231/comsoc.34(2018).2956

Chakola, A. (2022). *The impact of social media influencer on the buying behaviour of Gen Z in India* [Masters, National College of Ireland]. https://ncrma.ncirl.ie/6436/

Chandra, S., Chang, A., Day, L., Fazlullah, A., Liu, J., McBride, L., Mudalige, T., Weiss, D., (2020). *Closing the K–12 digital divide in the age of distance learning*. Common Sense Media and Boston Consulting Group. https://www.commonsensemedia.org/sites/default/files/featured-content/files/common_sense_media_report_final_7_1_3pm_web.pdf

Chandrima, R. M., Kircaburun, K., Kabir, H., Riaz, B. K., Kuss, D. J., Griffiths, M. D., & Mamun, M. A. (2020). Adolescent problematic internet use and parental mediation: A Bangladeshi structured interview study. *Addictive Behaviors Reports*, *12*, 100288. https://doi.org/10.1016/j.abrep.2020.100288

Cortesi, S. C., Hasse, A., Lombana, A., Kim, S., & Gasser, U. (2020). Youth and digital citizenship+ (plus): Understanding skills for a digital world. *SSRN Electronic Journal*. https://doi.org/10.2139/ssrn.3557518

CRC. (2021). *OHCHR | General comment No. 25 (2021) on children's rights in relation to the digital environment*. OHCHR. https://www.ohchr.org/en/documents/general-comments-and-recommendations/general-comment-no-25-2021-childrens-rights-relation

De Veirman, M., Hudders, L., & Nelson, M. R. (2019). What is influencer marketing and how does it target children? A review and direction for future research. *Frontiers in Psychology*, *10*, 2685. https://doi.org/10.3389/fpsyg.2019.02685

De Wolf, R., & Vanden Abeele, M. M. P. (2020). Editorial: Children's voices on privacy management and data responsibilization. *Media and Communication*, *8*(4), 158–162. https://doi.org/10.17645/mac.v8i4.3722

Duek, C., & Moguillansky, M. (2020). Children, digital screens and family: Parental mediation practices and gender. *Comunicação e Sociedade*, *37*, Article 37. https://journals.openedition.org/cs/2362

Ephraim, P. E. (2013). African Youths and the dangers of social networking: A culture-centered approach to using social media. *Ethics and Information Technology*, *15*(4), 275–284. https://doi.org/10.1007/s10676-013-9333-2

Feller, G., & Burroughs, B. (2021). Branding kidfluencers: Regulating content and advertising on YouTube. *Television & New Media*, 152747642110528. https://doi.org/10.1177/15274764211052882

Gillwald, A., & Partridge, A. (2023). *Gendered nature of digital inequality: Evidence for policy considerations*. RIA: Research ICT Africa. https://policycommons.net/artifacts/3495819/gendered-nature-of-digital-inequality/4296397/

Global Kids Online. (2019). *Growing up in a connected world: Understanding children's risks and opportunities in a digital age*. UNICEF Office of Research. https://www.unicef-irc.org/growing-up-connected#sectionDownload

Goedhart, N. S., Broerse, J. E., Kattouw, R., & Dedding, C. (2019). 'Just having a computer doesn't make sense': The digital divide from the perspective of mothers with a low socio-economic position. *New Media & Society*, *21*(11–12), 2347–2365. https://doi.org/10.1177/1461444819846059

Goggin, G. (2013). Youth culture and mobiles. *Mobile Media & Communication*, *1*(1), 83–88. https://doi.org/10.1177/2050157912464489

Green, L. (Ed.). (2021). *The Routledge companion to digital media and children*. Routledge.

Green, L., Haddon, L., Livingstone, S., O'Neill, B., Stevenson, K., & Holloway, D. (2024). *Digital media use in early childhood: Birth to six*. Bloomsbury Publishing.

Guzman, A. (2022). Moving human-machine communication forward through the study of non-use and failure. *Communication 1*, *9*(1). https://doi.org/10.7275/1crf-aj68

Haidt, J. (2024). *The anxious generation*. Allen Lane. https://www.penguin.co.uk/books/456971/the-anxious-generation-by-haidt-jonathan/9780241647660

Hausmann, J. S., Touloumtzis, C., White, M. T., Colbert, J. A., & Gooding, H. C. (2017). Adolescent and young adult use of social media for health and its implications. *Journal of Adolescent Health*, *60*(6), 714–719. https://doi.org/10.1016/j.jadohealth.2016.12.025

Helsper, E. (2021). *The digital disconnect: The social causes and consequences of digital inequalities.* SAGE Publications Ltd. https://in.sagepub.com/en-in/sas/the-digital-disconnect/book262151

Huang, S., Lai, X., Ke, L., Qin, X., Yan, J. J., Xie, Y., Dai, X., & Wang, Y. (2023). Coping styles among Chinese adolescents: The development and validation of a smartphone coping style scale. *Journal of Children and Media, 17*(4), 488–505. https://doi.org/10.1080/17482798.2023.2239951

Iqbal, S., Zakar, R., & Fischer, F. (2021). Predictors of parental mediation in teenagers' internet use: A cross-sectional study of female caregivers in Lahore, Pakistan. *BMC Public Health, 21*(1), 317. https://doi.org/10.1186/s12889-021-10349-z

Ito, M., Cross, R., Dinakar, K., & Odgers, C. (Eds.). (2023). *Algorithmic rights and protections for children.* The MIT Press. https://doi.org/10.7551/mitpress/13654.001.0001

Katz, V., & Hightower, B. (2023). How class matters: Examining working-class children's home technology environments from a developmental perspective. *International Journal of Communication, 17*(0), Article 0. https://ijoc.org/index.php/ijoc/article/view/19734

Kids Online Uruguay. (2024). *Children connected – new findings from Uruguay* [Global Kids Online]. http://globalkidsonline.net/uruguay/

Lazard, L. (2022). Digital mothering: Sharenting, family selfies and online affective-discursive practices. *Feminism & Psychology, 32*(4), 540–558. https://doi.org/10.1177/09593535221083840

Leaver, T. (2020). Balancing privacy: Sharenting, intimate surveillance, and the right to be forgotten. In L. Green, D. Holloway, K. Stevenson, T. Leaver, & L. Haddon (Eds.), *The Routledge companion to digital media and children*. Routledge.

Lim, S. S. (2019). *Transcendent parenting: Raising children in the digital age.* Oxford University Press.

Ling, R., & Haddon, L. (2008). Children, youth and the mobile phone. In K. Drotner & S. Livingstone (Eds.), *The international handbook of children, media and culture* (pp. 137–151). SAGE. https://doi.org/10.4135/9781848608436

Livingstone, S. (2020, May 13). Digital by default: The new normal of family life under COVID-19. *Parenting for a digital future.* https://blogs.lse.ac.uk/parenting4digitalfuture/2020/05/13/digital-by-default/

Livingstone, S. (2023). *New findings from Kids Online Chile* [Global Kids Online]. http://globalkidsonline.net/chile2023/

Livingstone, S., Mascheroni, G., & Stoilova, M. (2021). The outcomes of gaining digital skills for young people's lives and wellbeing: A systematic evidence review. *New Media & Society,* 146144482110431. https://doi.org/10.1177/14614448211043189

Livingstone, S., Ólafsson, K., Helsper, E. J., Lupiáñez-Villanueva, F., Veltri, G. A., & Folkvord, F. (2017). Maximizing opportunities and minimizing risks for children online: The role of digital skills in emerging strategies of parental mediation. *Journal of Communication, 67*(1), 82–105. https://doi.org/10.1111/jcom.12277

Looi, C.-K., Lim, K. F., Pang, J., Koh, A. L. H., Seow, P., Sun, D., Boticki, I., Norris, C., & Soloway, E. (2016). Bridging formal and informal learning with the use of mobile technology. In C. S. Chai, C. P. Lim, & C. M. Tan (Eds.), *Future learning in primary schools: A Singapore perspective* (pp. 79–96). Springer. https://doi.org/10.1007/978-981-287-579-2_6

Lupton, D., & Williamson, B. (2017). The datafied child: The dataveillance of children and implications for their rights. *New Media & Society, 19*(5), 780–794. https://doi.org/10.1177/1461444816686328

Marchant, A., Hawton, K., Stewart, A., Montgomery, P., Singaravelu, V., Lloyd, K., Purdy, N., Daine, K., & John, A. (2017). A systematic review of the relationship between internet use, self-harm and suicidal behaviour in young people: The good, the bad and the unknown. *PLOS ONE, 12*(8), e0181722. https://doi.org/10.1371/journal.pone.0181722

Mares, M.-L., Chen, Y. A., & Bond, B. J. (2022). Mutual influence in LGBTQ teens' use of media to socialize their parents. *Media Psychology, 25*(3), 441–468. https://doi.org/10.1080/15213269.2021.1969950

Marler, W. (2023). 'You can't talk at the library': The leisure divide and public internet access for people experiencing homelessness. *Information, Communication & Society, 26*(7), 1303–1321. https://doi.org/10.1080/1369118X.2021.2006742

Marwick, A. E. (2008). To catch a predator? The MySpace moral panic. *First Monday, 13*(6). https://doi.org/10.5210/fm.v13i6.2152

Matthes, J., Thomas, M. F., Stevic, A., & Schmuck, D. (2021). Fighting over smartphones? Parents' excessive smartphone use, lack of control over children's use, and conflict. *Computers in Human Behavior, 116*, 106618. https://doi.org/10.1016/j.chb.2020.106618

McDool, E., Powell, P., Roberts, J., & Taylor, K. (2020). The internet and children's psychological wellbeing. *Journal of Health Economics, 69*, 102274. https://doi.org/10.1016/j.jhealeco.2019.102274

Nelson, E. L. (2021). *Understanding childhood and play in the post-digital age.* University of Glasgow.

Nimrod, G., Elias, N., & Lemish, D. (2023). Like grandmother, like mother? Multigenerational mediation of young children's media use. *International Journal of Communication, 17*(0), Article 0. https://ijoc.org/index.php/ijoc/article/view/20517

Nolas, S.-M. (2015). Children's participation, childhood publics and social change: A review. *Children & Society, 29*(2), 157–167. https://doi.org/10.1111/chso.12108

Nolas, S.-M., Varvantakis, C., & Aruldoss, V. (2016). (Im)possible conversations? Activism, childhood and everyday life. *Journal of Social and Political Psychology, 4*(1), Article 1. https://doi.org/10.5964/jspp.v4i1.536

Ofcom. (2023). *Children and parents: Media use and attitudes report 2023.* Ofcom. https://www.ofcom.org.uk/research-and-data/media-literacy-research/childrens/children-and-parents-media-use-and-attitudes-report-2023

Papacharissi, Z. (2012). A networked self: Identity performance and sociability on social network sites. In F. L. F. Lee, L. Leung, J. L. Qiu, & D. S. C. Chu (Eds.), *Frontiers in new media research* (1st ed., pp. 207–221). Routledge. https://doi.org/10.4324/9780203113417

Patchin, J. W., & Hinduja, S. (2017). Digital self-harm among adolescents. *Journal of Adolescent Health, 61*(6), 761–766. https://doi.org/10.1016/j.jadohealth.2017.06.012

Pea, R., Nass, C., Meheula, L., Rance, M., Kumar, A., Bamford, H., Nass, M., Simha, A., Stillerman, B., Yang, S., & Zhou, M. (2012). Media use, face-to-face communication, media multitasking, and social well-being among 8- to 12-year-old girls. *Developmental Psychology, 48*, 327–336. https://doi.org/10.1037/a0027030

Pérez-Sánchez, R. (2024, February 12). Unveiling digital disparities in Costa Rica. *Global Kids Online.* http://globalkidsonline.net/costa-rica/

Pierce, G. L., & Cleary, P. F. (2024). The persistent educational digital divide and its impact on societal inequality. *PLOS ONE, 19*(4), e0286795. https://doi.org/10.1371/journal.pone.0286795

Radesky, J., & Hiniker, A. (2022). From moral panic to systemic change: Making child-centered design the default. *International Journal of Child-Computer Interaction, 31*(March 2022), 100351. https://doi.org/10.1016/j.ijcci.2021.100351

Raman, U., & Kasturi, S. (Eds.). (2023). *Childscape, mediascape: Children and media in India*. Orient BlackSwan. https://orientblackswan.com/details?id=9789354427305

Raman, U., & Verghese, R. (2014). Indian Youth and social media: Modes of engagement? In *Social media, culture and politics in Asia* (pp. 212–240). Peter Lang Publishing.

Rangaswamy, N., & Arora, P. (2016). The mobile internet in the wild and every day: Digital leisure in the slums of urban India. *International Journal of Cultural Studies*, *19*(6), 611–626. https://doi.org/10.1177/1367877915576538

Rangaswamy, N., & Cutrell, E. (2013). Anthropology, development, and ICTs: Slums, youth, and the mobile internet in urban India. *Information Technologies & International Development*, *9*(2), 51–63.

Reid Chassiakos, Y., Radesky, J., Christakis, D., Moreno, M. A., Cross, C., Hill, D., Ameenuddin, N., Hutchinson, J., Levine, A., Boyd, R., Mendelson, R., & Swanson, W. S.COUNCIL ON COMMUNICATIONS AND MEDIA. (2016). Children and adolescents and digital media. *Pediatrics*, *138*(5), e20162593. https://doi.org/10.1542/peds.2016-2593

Ringrose, J., Harvey, L., Gill, R., & Livingstone, S. (2013). Teen girls, sexual double standards and 'sexting': Gendered value in digital image exchange. *Feminist Theory*, *14*(3), 305–323. https://doi.org/10.1177/1464700113499853

Rivas-Lara, S., Pham, B., & Ulhs, Y. (2023, March 15). Mobilizing teen-centered research findings for teen-oriented storytelling. *Connected Learning Alliance*. https://clalliance.org/blog/mobilizing-teen-centered-research-findings-for-teen-oriented-storytelling/

Rodríguez-de-Dios, I., van Oosten, J. M. F., & Igartua, J.-J. (2018). A study of the relationship between parental mediation and adolescents' digital skills, online risks and online opportunities. *Computers in Human Behavior*, *82*, 186–198. https://doi.org/10.1016/j.chb.2018.01.012

Sarkar, S. (2016). Beyond the "digital divide": The "computer girls" of Seelampur. *Feminist Media Studies*, *16*(6), 968–983. https://doi.org/10.1080/14680777.2016.1169207

Sarwatay, D. (2022). In their voices: Foregrounding young people's social media practices and experiences. In S. Kotilainen (Ed.), *Methods in practice: Studying children and youth online* (pp. 41–44). Leibniz-Institut für Medienforschung | Hans-Bredow-Institut (HBI). https://doi.org/10.21241/ssoar.83031

Sarwatay, D., Lee, J., & Kaye, D. B. V. (2022). Exploring children's TikTok cultures in India: Negotiating access, uses, and experiences under restrictive parental mediation. *Media International Australia*, *186*(1), 48–65. https://doi.org/10.1177/1329878X221127037

Sarwatay, D., & Raman, U. (2022). Everyday negotiations in managing presence: Young people and social media in India. *Information, Communication & Society*, *25*(4), 536–551. https://doi.org/10.1080/1369118X.2021.1988129

Sarwatay, D., Raman, U., & Ramasubramanian, S. (2021). Media literacy, social connectedness, and digital citizenship in India: Mapping stakeholders on how parents and young people navigate a social world. *Frontiers in Human Dynamics*, *3*, 601239. https://doi.org/10.3389/fhumd.2021.601239

Schmuck, D. (2021). Following social media influencers in early adolescence: Fear of missing out, social well-being and supportive communication with parents. *Journal of Computer-Mediated Communication*, *26*(5), 245–264. https://doi.org/10.1093/jcmc/zmab008

Simone, van der H., Verdoodt, V., & Leiser, D. M. (2019). Child labour and online protection in a world of influencers. *SSRN Electronic Journal*. https://doi.org/10.2139/ssrn.3458379

Smolansky, A., Cram, A., Raduescu, C., Zeivots, S., Huber, E., & Kizilcec, R. F. (2023). Educator and student perspectives on the impact of generative AI on assessments in higher education. *Proceedings of the Tenth ACM Conference on Learning @ Scale*, 378–382. https://doi.org/10.1145/3573051.3596191

Staksrud, E., & Milosevic, T. (2017). Adolescents and children in global media landscape: From risks to rights. *Annals of the International Communication Association*, 41(3–4), 235–241. https://doi.org/10.1080/23808985.2017.1387503

Steinfeld, N. (2021). Parental mediation of adolescent internet use: Combining strategies to promote awareness, autonomy and self-regulation in preparing youth for life on the web. *Education and Information Technologies*, 26(2), 1897–1920. https://doi.org/10.1007/s10639-020-10342-w

Stevenson, K., Jayakumar, E., See, H. W., Ryu, Y., & Das, S. (2022). *Children's perspectives of digital citizenship in India, Korea and Australia: Report of findings from children's digital citizenship and safety roundtables* [Application/pdf]. Edith Cowan University/ARC Centre of Excellence for the Digital Child. https://doi.org/10.25958/0J0C-XP24

Stoilova, M., Nandagiri, R., & Livingstone, S. (2021). Children's understanding of personal data and privacy online – A systematic evidence mapping. *Information, Communication & Society*, 24(4), 557–575. https://doi.org/10.1080/1369118X.2019.1657164

Subramanian, S. (2021). Bahujan girls' anti-caste activism on TikTok. *Feminist Media Studies*, 21(1), 154–156. https://doi.org/10.1080/14680777.2021.1864875

Third, A., Collin, P., Walsh, L., & Black, R. (2019). Digital inclusion. In A. Third, P. Collin, L. Walsh, & R. Black (Eds.), *Young people in digital society: Control shift* (pp. 129–174). Palgrave Macmillan UK. https://doi.org/10.1057/978-1-137-57369-8_4

Third, A., Livingstone, S., & Lansdown, G. (2019). Recognizing children's rights in relation to digital technologies: Challenges of voice and evidence, principle and practice. In *Research handbook on human rights and digital technology* (pp. 376–410). Elgar Online. https://www.elgaronline.com/view/edcoll/9781785367717/9781785367717.00029.xml

Torkington, S. (2022). A third of children have adult social media accounts, UK regulator finds: How can we improve child safety online? *World Economic Forum*. https://www.weforum.org/agenda/2022/10/children-digital-safety-social-media/

Tripp, L. M. (2011). 'The computer is not for you to be looking around, it is for schoolwork': Challenges for digital inclusion as Latino immigrant families negotiate children's access to the internet. *New Media & Society*, 13(4), 552–567. https://doi.org/10.1177/1461444810375293

UNICEF & ITU. (2020). *How many children and young people have internet access at home?* UNICEF. https://data.unicef.org/resources/children-and-young-people-internet-access-at-home-during-covid19/

Uzuegbunam, C. E. (2024). Children's access and connection to digital technology. In C. E. Uzuegbunam (Ed.), *Children and young people's digital lifeworlds: Domestication, mediation, and agency* (pp. 77–87). Springer International Publishing. https://doi.org/10.1007/978-3-031-51303-9_5

Valkenburg, P. M., Beyens, I., Pouwels, J. L., van Driel, I. I., & Keijsers, L. (2022). Social media browsing and adolescent well-being: Challenging the "passive social media use hypothesis." *Journal of Computer-Mediated Communication*, 27(1), zmab015. https://doi.org/10.1093/jcmc/zmab015

Vanden Abeele, M. M. P. (2016). Mobile youth culture: A conceptual development. *Mobile Media & Communication*, 4(1), 85–101. https://doi.org/10.1177/2050157915601455

Wang, Y. (2020). Parent–child role reversal in ICT domestication: Media brokering activities and emotional labours of Chinese "study mothers" in Singapore. *Journal of Children and Media*, *14*(3), 267–284. https://doi.org/10.1080/17482798.2020.1725900

Woodley, G. N., Green, L., & Jacques, C. (2024). 'Send nudes?': Teens' perspectives of education around sexting, an argument for a balanced approach. *Sexualities*, 13634607241237675. https://doi.org/10.1177/13634607241237675

Wuyckens, G., Landry, N., & Fastrez, P. (2022). Untangling media literacy, information literacy, and digital literacy: A systematic meta-review of core concepts in media education. *Journal of Media Literacy Education*, *14*(1), 168–182. https://doi.org/10.23860/JMLE-2022-14-1-12

Zillich, A. F., & Riesmeyer, C. (2021). Be yourself: The relative importance of personal and social norms for adolescents' self-presentation on Instagram. *Social Media + Society*, *7*(3), 205630512110338. https://doi.org/10.1177/20563051211033810

3 Representation

Sindy R. Sumter, Irene I. van Driel, and Cherrie Joy F. Billedo

A classic moment in the public discourse about the importance of representation in media occurred in the United States during the fall of 1999. All TV shows announced for the upcoming season featured a White leading character. Media representation advocate groups called for TV boycotts and hosted talk show discussions and soon responses by academics followed (Gray, 2001; Gross, 2001). At that time, networks promised to add roles for people of color, but trending hashtags such as #OscarsSoWhite in 2015 and #OscarsSoMale in 2018 demonstrate that change in the media landscape has been notoriously slow (Molina-Guzmán, 2018).

Youth and media scholars view media as a key socializer, a super peer, or a role model (Elmore et al., 2017). In an ideal world, media offer youth both mirrors and windows (Bishop, 1990). Mirrors serve to reflect youth and their familiar environments, and windows allow them to see people and worlds differing from their own. These mediated mirrors and windows positively impact youth development *if* that media content authentically represents all identities. However, in entertainment media content certain identities are hardly reflected, or *underrepresented*. Moreover, some identities are presented in a narrow, negative, or stereotypical manner, or in other words, *misrepresented*. The underrepresented or misrepresented identities in entertainment media are often identities that have been historically marginalized. As a result, the exclusionary practice of entertainment media contributes to existing inequalities, including gender-, race/ethnicity-, and sexual orientation-based inequality. Under- and misrepresentation of minoritized identity groups is in part attributed to the lack of diversity in media entertainment board and writing rooms, including the video game industry (Kohlburn et al., 2023).

This chapter provides an overview of the current state of mirrors and windows available to youth by discussing relevant media representation and effect theories as well as content analytical research. The chapter focuses on entertainment media popular among youth, i.e., television shows, movies, and games. The prominence of US media content limits insights in media

DOI: 10.4324/9781003453123-4

representation globally; however, young people from countries that are small or have limited resources are known to consume content that is created in the United States (Lustyik, 2013). Finally, the chapter focuses on three identity markers most frequently studied and especially important from a developmental perspective, namely gender, sexual orientation, and race/ethnicity.

Media Representation: Theoretical Approaches

Contemporary theories in the field of youth and media stress the importance of closely examining media *content* to understand media preferences of and media effects on young viewers (Valkenburg & Peter, 2013). In the context of media representation, it is important to realize that young viewers can belong to either majority or minoritized groups, and the same goes for the characters that feature in the media content they consume. This means that the effects of media content depend on the interplay between the identity characteristics of the viewer and those of the media character(s). Media representations of minoritized groups have the potential to shape the expectations those groups set for themselves and affect perceptions majority groups hold of minoritized groups, and vice versa. For example, consider a show like the family sitcom *Black-ish* which is created by Kenya Barris and features a predominantly Black cast. The show revolves around an upper-middle-class family with both parents in well-paid positions as advertising executive and doctor, and the episodes center discussions of Black heritage, culture, and traditions such as Juneteenth—a holiday to celebrate the end of slavery in the United States, and challenges related to growing up in a predominantly White setting. By including these topics in their storylines, this show gives young Black viewers narratives that can inform both their sense of self and perhaps the goals they set, and viewers with different racial/ethnic backgrounds broaden their perceptions of Black people.

To understand the impact media representation may have on youth, it is important to be familiar with some theoretical frameworks. Specifically, *media selection* theories provide information on which types of media and their representations young people gravitate to, while *media effect* theories explain how different types of media representation might affect young people (see also Chapter 7 of this book). We will briefly discuss these two types of theories.

Media Selection Theories

Media selection theories help predict why young people are drawn to particular types of representation in media content, e.g., *social identity theory* by Tajfel and Turner (1979), and *social identity gratifications* by Harwood (1999). These identity-based selection theories argue that people prefer and feel a greater attachment to content that is identity congruent (Scharrer et al., 2022). This means that young people seek out media that feature characters that are like them. This need for identity-congruent media is stronger for minoritized group members than for majority group members. For example, Kukshinov and Shaw (2022) showed that young gamers of color who identified as a gender minority were more likely than White male gamers to select a playable character that resembled them. Researchers theorized that the White male gamers were so accustomed to looking similar to the default characters that they do not experience a need for identity gratification through game characters. Notably, minoritized youth do not only seek out content specific to that identity, as this is only one aspect of who they are, they also experience individual and developmental needs similar to those of majority youth (e.g., Martins et al., 2022).

Media Effect Theories

To explain potential representation effects, researchers frequently refer to three media effect theories, **cultivation theory** (Gerbner, 1969), **social cognitive theory** (Bandura, 1986), and **mediated contact theory** (e.g., Park, 2012).

Cultivation theory argues that the more frequently you see certain media portrayals, the more likely you are to believe that these portrayals reflect reality. For example, as most media depict scientists as men (e.g., Steinke, 2017), this is expected to cultivate the belief that in the real world, most scientists are men. Cultivation theory also states that *all* media, on average, mirror the dominant views in society. Thus, from children's books and games to adult horror movies, similar messages are repeated, resulting in further *mainstreaming* of these views. Mainstreaming implies that since the same broad messages are likely to be present in any sort of media content, those who consume a lot of media—no matter who they are—are likely to converge in their views of the world. In the case of our example, narrow media portrayals are expected to contribute to society's expectations that only boys can become scientists (Steinke, 2017) and that view may be held relatively equally among people of all genders. Consequently, media may reinforce existing inequalities in society.

Similarly, **social cognitive theory** predicts that youth learn from media by observing role models and their behaviors, especially similar role models (Bandura, 1986). When certain groups are underrepresented in media, young people that belong to these groups have access to fewer role models they can identify with. For example, only after the *Hunger Games* movie was released did more girls take up archery; a sport for which until that moment few female role models existed (Crookston, 2018).

Finally, **mediated contact theories** explain how exposure to media content that features positive portrayals of marginalized groups can contribute to prejudice reduction (e.g., Park, 2012). This theory argues that, just like real-life socializing with people who are different from you can promote inclusive attitudes, exposure to such mediated portrayals has similar effects. For example, watching series that feature sexual minority characters is known to reduce homophobic attitudes (e.g., Yan, 2019).

Media Representation: Quantity and Quality Typologies

How media present characters with minoritized and majority backgrounds is important to understand next. Already in the late 1960s, Clark (1969) theorized that representation of minoritized groups, Black US citizens in his research, will change over time in a manner that mirrors the gradual acceptance of a minoritized group by the majority group. It starts with *non-recognition*, or no representation at all, moves to misrepresentation and is expected to culminate in *respect*, a final stage in which the minoritized group is presented similar to the majority group. Despite this theory, reality seems more complex; representation of minoritized characters may regress before it improves and may differ per genre.

Methodologically, content analyses help show how social groups are portrayed in media in terms of *quantity*, and the type of roles, or *quality*. Research assessing the quantity of media representation of identity groups looks at the frequency of roles in entertainment media that feature either minoritized or majority characters. Character prominence is also considered when assessing representation frequency across different roles, such as distinguishing between leading and supporting roles, or between playable and non-playable characters in video games, or by measuring screen time and speaking time. Overall, representation quantity communicates to young viewers how society values a group, with low visibility communicating low value.

Content analyses show roughly four dimensions of representation *quality*: First, the extent to which the minoritized identity plays a *central role in the storyline*, or if they are just like any other main character. Second, how characters *look and behave*, such as personality, interests, appearance, and mannerisms. Third, the *treatment* of characters by others. Are they popular, bullied, or ignored, for instance? *Fourth*, the *social (economic) status* of characters, such as what job they have and how much money they make. These character qualities together reveal how society views the group the character belongs to.

In short, when studying how minoritized groups are portrayed, researchers agree that the state of minority representation varies in quantity and quality of roles over time and across media types and genres. In the section below you will find the quantity and quality of representation in children and adolescent media reviewed for gender, sexual orientation, and race/ethnicity. Adolescent media includes adult media popular among adolescents.

State of Media Representation of Gender, Sexual Orientation, and Race/Ethnicity

Developing your gender identity, experiencing who you are sexually or romantically attracted to, and exploring your racial/ethnic identity are among the most important developmental goals for young people (e.g., Frable, 1997). To some extent, developmental processes are experienced differently by youth that belong to minoritized groups compared to majority groups. For example, youth with minoritized identities are likely to experience discrimination early on and may have less access to identity-empowering environments, including media products that include positive and well-rounded portrayals of people just like them. Below, content analytical research is used to see whether media provide especially minoritized young people with an identity-empowering environment or if it falls short.

Gender Identity Representation in Youth Media[1]

Historically, gender has been understood as synonymous with the sex assigned at birth, i.e., as either male or female based on a binary concept of biological sex. Nevertheless, gender surpasses the confines of assigned sex. As children grow older, they develop their own gender identity, or their deeply felt, inherent sense of being girl/woman/female, boy/man/male, both, or neither (APA, 2022). Although gender identity is invisible, individuals express their gender externally (e.g., name, pronouns, hairstyle, clothing, behaviors). The expression of gender identity is influenced by societal norms, including media (for review see Ward & Grower, 2020).

For many individuals, their gender identity corresponds to the sex assigned at birth, e.g., assigned male at birth and identifies as a man (APA, 2022). These individuals are described as cisgender (or cis). However, there are people who do not identify as cisgender, thus falling into the gender minority category (GLAAD, n.d.). Gender minority individuals are people whose gender identity differs from the sex assigned at birth (transgender), who do not identify strictly as either boy/man or girl/woman (nonbinary), who do not align with any specific gender (agender), or whose gender identity is more fluid than what is typically associated with the traditional gender binary (e.g., genderqueer).

We will review the quantity and quality of cisgender and gender minority representation in children's and adolescents' programming and in video games. Although cisgender women do not hold a statistical minority position in society, in the context of media representation—and more broadly—they share similar *minoritization* experiences (Wingrove-Haugland & McLeod, 2021). Notably, many studies do not assess gender minority representation, thus limiting our insights for these specific groups (Walsh & Leaper, 2020).

Quantity of Minoritized Gender Representation

Children's programming. Historically, there has been a greater representation of boys/men compared to girls/women in children's programming (Lemish & Elias, 2019; Santoniccolo et al., 2023; Ward & Grower, 2020). Although there is a move toward gender equality in children's programming, this progression is not linear and male characters still regularly outnumber female characters in recent TV seasons. For example, while in 2022 female characters comprised 51.1% of leading roles in US children's shows, a year later this decreased to 44.3% (Meyer & Conroy, 2023a). There is little representation of gender minority identities in current children's programming (Hale & Melzer, 2022). In a sample of 99 new US children's programs in 2022, only 0.3% featured nonbinary characters (Meyer & Conroy, 2023a). In 2023, Disney featured its first nonbinary supporting character, Lake Ripple in the animated film "Elemental," voiced by nonbinary actor Ava Kai Hauser.

Adolescent programming. Like children's programming, adolescent programming is historically characterized by male-dominated character portrayals (Ward & Grower, 2020), but currently progressing toward binary gender equality in quantity of leading characters and screen time allocation (e.g., Giaccardi et al., 2019; Screen Australia, 2016). Analyzing three decades of popular films using gender detection algorithms, Mazières and colleagues (2021) showed a clear trend toward more equal representation of women and men over the years. Representations of gender minorities, such as trans and genderqueer/nonbinary individuals, remain sparse. GLAAD showed that while the number of nonbinary characters in TV shows increased between 2021 and 2022, the number of transgender characters decreased during the same time period (Deerwater et al., 2024).

Video games. While children and adolescent programming moves toward binary gender equality, this is not the case for video games. Historically, gender representation in video games has been a male domain (Lucas & Sherry, 2004) and this seems to persist. Recent content analyses still show that female characters are less likely to be leading or playable characters (e.g., Waddell et al., 2022). Gender minority characters are scarce and not typically playable characters. However, there is a gradual increase in gender minority representation (Utsch et al., 2017).

Paper Mario: The Thousand-Year Door, released in 2024, can be considered a positive exemplar of improved representation of gender minorities. Mario is joined by friends, including the purple ghost Vivian, to save Princess Peach. Vivian is a transgender woman, and playable character, whose gender identity was implied in earlier releases but made explicit in the 2024 remake (Vivian, 2024).

Quality of Minoritized Gender Representation

Children's programming. Gender-stereotypical portrayals remain abundant in television and movies created for children (Walsh & Leaper, 2020). Feminine and masculine physical traits are highly differentiated in media targeting infants and toddlers as well as programming for older children (e.g., Aubrey & Roberts, 2020). Generally, female characters have stereotypical appearance features which emphasize femininity such as hair ribbons, make-up, or pink outfits (Lemish & Elias, 2019; Steyer, 2014); whereas physical strength is emphasized for male characters (Hale & Melzer, 2022). For non-physical traits, female characters tend to be portrayed in a more positive light compared to male characters, although still consistent with traditional gender norms including being polite, obedient, and likeable. Male characters, on the other hand, are likely portrayed as aggressive, dominant, adventurous, and funny (Ward & Grower, 2020).

When it comes to professional careers, male characters are more likely to be featured as having paid work compared to female characters. When female characters do work, they hold stereotypical female or secondary occupations, such as assistant to a male character (Ward & Grower, 2020). Moreover, the roles of female characters often revolve around themes of motherhood or caregiving; whereas counterpart themes, such as fatherhood, are less emphasized in male characters. If portrayed in domestic contexts, male characters are often shown to be unskilled and less family oriented (Steyer, 2014; Ward & Grower, 2020).

Although gender stereotypes are still common in Disney films (Coyne et al., 2016; England et al., 2011), over the years the depictions of female leading characters have come to include more counter-stereotypical appearances and personalities. Disney princesses are not solely featured as skinny damsels in distress, but are shown as strong, independent, adventurous heroines (Davis, 2014). For example, Moana, the leading character of a 2016 Disney animation film, has several counter-stereotypical features. Physically, Moana is relatively muscular and in terms of personality, she is seemingly fearless, confident, and adventurous. As the most streamed movie across different platforms in 2023 (Nielsen, 2024), it shows that young audiences appreciate non-stereotypical representation of a Disney princess, or any character for that matter.

Adolescent programming. Stereotypical portrayals of male and female characters are similarly prevalent in films and television designed for or popular among adolescents. This includes an overemphasis on female characters' physical attractiveness and female characters shown as highly invested in their physical appearance (McDade-Montez et al., 2017). They are sexualized and likely recipients of attractiveness-related comments, particularly from male characters (e.g., Gerding & Signorielli, 2014). In the context of heterosexual romantic relationships, male characters are often shown as valuing girls only for their physical attractiveness, whereas their female counterparts engage in self-objectification and ego-stroking of boys (Kirsch & Murnen, 2015). Consequently, media provide young people who are exploring their romantic relationships with narrow scripts, prescribing highly gendered dating strategies and sexual goals.

Considering the quality of representation of gender minority characters, specifically transgender characters, there is a trend from narrow and negative portrayals to more positive portrayals. Stereotypical, negative, and fetishized portrayals were quite common in earlier representations of transgender characters in media (Hale & Melzer, 2022). In recent years, transgender characters have been portrayed in more meaningful narratives (Masanet et al., 2022) and presented in both positive and groundbreaking ways (McLaren et al., 2021). One such character is Elle Argent in *Heartstopper*, a Netflix series. Elle's storyline does not only focus on her trans identity nor is she cast in a one-dimensional supporting role. Instead, *Heartstopper* shows Elle having her own romantic subplot, and experiencing nuanced emotions just like other leading characters. Remarkably, Elle is played by Yasmin Finney, a transwoman of color (Gendergp, 2023).

Video games. Video games remain a fertile ground for the perpetuation of gender stereotypes, especially the sexualization of women (e.g., Lynch et al., 2024; Waddell et al., 2022). The male characters are depicted as hypermasculine, highlighting physical strength and aggression, while female characters are depicted as demure and serve as love interests that need rescuing (Scharrer, 2013). They are physically thin and curvaceous, and frequently scantily clad (Beasley & Collins Standley, 2002; Downs & Smith, 2010). On a few occasions, female characters are presented as powerful and clever. However, power is still sexualized, with female characters being shown as sexually manipulative and dangerous (Tompkins et al., 2020). Binary gender representations have improved somewhat in recent games. For instance, male characters are no longer merely depicted as powerful and strong compared to earlier versions (Gilbert et al., 2023) and female characters are less sexualized (Lynch et al., 2016). Gender minority characters remain scarce, but there are some improvements in terms of gaming options. For example, some games removed gender restrictions on avatars, and the game *Sims 4* includes the customization options of binders and top-surgery scars for transgender characters (Whitehouse et al., 2023).

Sexual Identity Representation in Youth Media

A second major developmental goal for young people is to explore the concept of sexual orientation and to establish their sexual identity (Morgan, 2019). Similar to gender identity, media is a socializing agent with regard to the establishment of one's own sexual identity and one's general understanding of sexual orientation. Media offer young people a view on what romantic relationships look like, who is attracted to whom, and which types of relationships are present and accepted in society (e.g., Ward et al., 2014). To understand the dominant socializing messages, this section reviews the prevalence of sexual minority groups in entertainment media and how these groups are portrayed. Sexual minority groups include all groups, including gay, lesbian, bisexual, and queer, outside of the majority who identify as heterosexual and merely experience opposite-sex attraction (Morgan, 2019). Most studies on sexual minority representation in entertainment media report how many characters can be identified as LGBTQIA+.[2] By grouping characters this way, i.e., collapsing gender and sexual minority representation, it is sometimes difficult to accurately assess sexual minority representation. In this section, the terminology from the cited studies will be used and thus may vary.

Quantity of Sexual Minority Representation

Children's programming. Several studies specifically focus on representation in children's (ages 0–12) entertainment media produced in the United States (e.g., Deerwater et al., 2024; Dennis, 2009; Meyer & Conroy, 2023a) as well as several European countries (i.e., Belgium: Van Wichelen & Dhoest, 2023, Denmark: Thorfinnsdottir & Jensen, 2017; Ireland: Vanlee & Kerrigan, 2021). In children's programming, explicit references to characters' sexual orientation are limited. When reviewing the prevalence of LGBTQIA+ characters in US children's programming from 2018 to 2022, there is a peak in 2019 with 4.9% LGBTQIA+ characters (Meyer & Conroy, 2023a). Prevalence was somewhat lower in 2022 when programming included a little over 2% LGBTQIA+ characters (Meyer & Conroy, 2023a). Similar rates are found in other countries. For example, in Denmark around 2% of sexuality-related references in children's programming involved sexual minority characters (Thorfinnsdottir & Jensen, 2017). The same study showed that none of the 340 families in these programs included non-heterosexual parent(s)/caregiver(s). This is important to reflect upon because more children are growing up in households with same-sex parents, but they have limited opportunities to watch shows that represent their household (e.g., Snyder et al., 2023). Notably, at least one new US children's show included a character in a two-dad household, namely Stacey from *Marvel's Moon Girl and Devil Dinosaur*.

Underrepresentation of sexual minority characters is also seen in children's movies. None of the Disney animation movies released before 2005 included sexual minority characters (e.g., Martin & Kazyak, 2009; Towbin et al., 2004). Disney movies continued to lack explicit and prominent representation of sexual minority characters until the release of *Strange World* in 2023. While the movie *Zootopia* (2016) included a very short scene featuring a gay couple whose sexual orientation could be inferred from the credits only, in *Strange World*, (2023) the leading character is a gay teenage boy, and his sexual orientation is evident from the start.

Adolescent programming. The frequency of sexual minority characters in entertainment media popular among adolescent audiences is somewhat higher compared to children's media. Following the introduction of the first gay teen character in the show *My So-Called Life* in 1994, adolescent programming has come to include more sexual minority characters both in lead as well as supporting roles. GLAAD's monitor of sexual orientation representation showed that the number of recurring LGBTQ characters in scripted series on US's major broadcasting channels increased from 1.1% in season 2007/2008 to 11.9% in season 2021/2022 (Townsend & Deerwater, 2022). While these shows were not specially targeted at adolescent audiences, the GLAAD monitor included many shows that are very popular among adolescents, including *Heartstopper*, *Gossip Girl*, and *One of Us*.

Reports from other countries reveal a consistent underrepresentation of sexual minority groups, especially among lead characters. For example, while over a quarter of Australian TV shows (27%) included at least one sexual minority character, only 5% of the leading characters could be identified as belonging to a sexual minority (Screen Australia, 2016).[3] Moreover, for most shows representation was limited to one character. In German-language programming, less than 2% of recurring characters could be identified as belonging to a sexual minority while 11% of the German population is said to be non-heterosexual (Prommer et al., 2021).

In the context of adolescent media use and sexual identity formation, it is important to realize that sexual minority adolescents will not only watch mainstream media but will also seek out so-called gay and lesbian-oriented (GLO) media for content that matches their identity. GLO content is defined as media content "specifically designed, produced, and marketed for gay and lesbian audiences" (Bond, 2015, p. 39). US GLO television shows, movies, and songs popular among LGB adolescents include more LGB sexual content than heterosexual sexual content (Bond, 2014). However, Bond's content analysis also showed that these interactions most often included adult characters (91%) and only in a few cases, adolescent characters (8%). Hence, sexual minority adolescents are nearly invisible compared to adults in GLO media.

Video games. While gender representation receives ample attention in video game research (e.g., Lynch et al., 2024), insights on sexual minority representation are limited by a lack of research attention. This becomes apparent from the meta-analysis by Waddell et al. (2022); only two of the 30 studies on the demographic composition of game characters published between 1998 and 2021 assessed the prevalence of sexual minority characters. These studies showed an increase in LGBTQ characters over time (i.e., Belmonte, 2017; Shaw et al., 2019), in particular White gay male non-playable characters. This increase did not hold for other sexual minorities and did not generalize to playable characters. While there are some games with at least some sexual minority representation, prevalence percentages reveal persistent underrepresentation. A content analysis of independent games (published in 2013–2022) on the gaming platform *itch.io* revealed that less than 1% of games, namely 2500 of the 530,000 games listed were accompanied by the tag LGBTQ (Ho et al., 2022). About half of the games with this tag featured same-sex relationships between men and a third between women. Similarly, in 2024, less than 2% of games published by large game publishers, such as Nintendo, included sexual minority content (https://glaad.org/glaad-gaming/2024/lgbtq-video-game-content-is-lacking/).

For a long time, game developers avoided sexual minority representation as it was expected to negatively impact sales. As recently as 2014, a game developer said it was highly unlikely that a Triple-A game, produced by a large company with an equally large budget, would ever include an openly queer leading character (LeJacq, 2014). To avoid backlash, sexual minority characters may not be explicitly labeled as such, but their sexual orientation could be derived, e.g., by backstories or afforded by same-sex gaming options (e.g., Shaw et al., 2019). Therefore, standard content analyses might underestimate representation quantity. Shaw and colleagues aim to more carefully monitor the actual frequency of (playable) sexual minority characters with their queer gaming database (https://lgbtqgamearchive.com/). Either way, in comparison to the frequency of sexual minority characters in television and movies, openly queer representation in video games is still lagging.

Quality of Sexual Minority Portrayals

Children and adolescent programming. Entertainment media include a variety of narrow, negative as well as positive portrayals of sexual minority characters and their experiences (e.g., Birchmore & Kettrey, 2022; Colliver, 2020; Dias et al., 2023; Raley & Lucas, 2006). Some portrayals are applicable to all identities (e.g., negative responses to any deviation from heteronormativity, explicitly or implicitly through ridicule), whereas stereotypical portrayals are specific to a particular identity (e.g., gay men primarily being presented as effeminate).

The *narrow* portrayals of sexual minority characters become evident in how specific characters are shown to behave. For example, male gay characters are shown acting feminine and having interests which are traditionally seen as "for women," and a similar recurring narrow portrayal is lesbian women presenting as masculine or butch. It is important to realize that while some gay men or lesbian women might self-present that way, it is problematic when these characteristics are attributed to most gay and lesbian characters. Authentic representation would be more varied. Moreover, gay characters are also presented in a (hyper)sexualized manner (e.g., Pinsof & Haselton, 2017). Although less common, there are examples of counter-stereotypical portrayals of sexual minority characters. For example, in 2021, Marvel introduced a Black gay male superhero and his family, i.e., husband and son, in their universe; the character has a prominent role, is strong, and is a technology and weapons expert.

The *negative* portrayal of LGB characters was explicit in early entertainment programming, in which it was not uncommon for LGB characters to be presented as villains or evil natured (Raley & Lucas, 2006). A second type of negative portrayal of LGB characters reflects more subtle forms of rejection, namely through ridicule. One of the earliest systematic mappings of sexual minority portrayals on TV looked at prime-time television shows aired in 2001, including *Dawson's Creek* and *Buffy the Vampire Slayer* (Raley & Lucas, 2006). At the time, portrayals of sexual minority characters as evil had become nearly absent but shows still included scenes in which LGB characters were made fun of. A similar pattern characterizes children's programming. For example, Thorfinnsdottir and Jensen (2017) concluded that children's programming included few instances of explicit homophobic behavior, but when characters engaged in same-sex intimate behavior, e.g., dancing, this was used for comedic effect.

In addition to the villainous and ridicule tropes, narratives around LGB characters are also characterized by the so-called "bury your gays" trope (Cover & Milne, 2023). This refers to narratives in which belonging to a sexual minority is consistently linked to tragic life experiences, e.g., characters facing rejection by close others, struggling when coming-out, being victimized, and often romantic storylines are short-lived as at least one of the characters die (early) in a season (Marshall, 2010; McInroy & Craig, 2017). Notably, the responses of the media industry to fan outcries about this trope—specifically when sexual minority fan favorites are killed off by writers—have changed over the years. While in the early 2000s producers would be very defensive, emphasizing their creative freedom, in a more recent case producers were more open to public criticisms, acknowledging the impact storylines have on the viewers, especially viewers that belong to minoritized groups (Cover & Milne, 2023).

When looking at how sexual minority characters are portrayed it is not only important that programming moves away from narrow and negative portrayals toward more inclusive and positive portrayals, but that representation progress might also mean that storylines should focus less on characters' sexual orientation. Australian creators, e.g., expressed "*a desire to make LGBTQ+ subjects visible in ways that located their identities as 'backdrop' in which being non-cisgender or non-heterosexual would be depicted as an ordinary part of everydayness.*" (Cover, 2024, p. 127). Some researchers refer to this as queer normality, which means a sexual minority character is just another character in the show similar to their heterosexual counterparts. For example, Vanlee and Kerrigan (2021) found that in domestic Belgian children's programs that featured LGB characters, their storylines did not primarily revolve around coming out or struggles related to their sexual orientation.

Video games. Several case studies show similar misrepresentations in video games. Some games include explicit homophobic content and a clear rejection of non-heteronormative behavior (e.g., Colliver, 2020; Shaw & Friesem, 2016). Examples of ridicule can also be found in games, such as playable characters engaging in cross-dressing serving as comic relief (Shaw & Friesem, 2016). The unique characteristic of many video games is that the player can create queer gameplay and character interactions, even if the creators did not explicitly include queer storylines or characters. The players themselves can create opportunities for sexual orientation-related representation, e.g., through customization of their avatar with LGBTQIA+ symbols. For example, an *Animal Crossing New Horizons* player shared that the game "*[...] helps to normalize queer identities within the video gaming world. By creating custom-made hats/shirts (e.g., featuring rainbows) and visiting strangers' islands, we LGBTIQA+ users help promote awareness of queer identity.*" (Blanco-Fernández & Moreno, 2023, p. 12).

Table 3.1 Does Your Favorite Childhood Movie Pass the Test?

To advocate for change in media entertainment, a key step is to identify and monitor good and problematic practices regarding the quantity and quality of representation. It is not enough to say there is a problem, you also need to show that there is a problem. For this reason, several advocacy initiatives developed representation tests and ratings for specific identity groups.

Examples of representation tests and ratings:

1 Gender: Bechdel-Wallace test for gender representation; Maisy test for sexism in children's media
2 Sexual minority: GLAAD's Vito Russo test for LGBTQ representation
3 Race/ethnicity: DuVernay test for representation of people of color; Chavez Perez test of racial stereotypes; Riz test for Muslim representation
4 Global representation ratings: The Inclusion List by the Annenberg Inclusion Initiative, Authentically Inclusive Representation by the Center for Scholars & Storytellers

These tests can help provide insight into the quantity and quality of media representation of certain groups over time and demonstrate that media products that pass these tests can entice a large enough audience to be profitable. The latter is especially important for media producers who are expected to make more inclusive media products if they are convinced these movies and or TV shows will generate sufficient revenue. Or in the words of actor Billy Porter[4] "I think the bottom line with Hollywood in everything is commerce, […] if it's gonna make money, it's gonna be fine."

The tests can also be used as selection tools. For example, if public broadcasters want to ensure their programming supports gender equality, a gender representation test could be informative. Starting in 2013, Sweden was the first country to experiment with a representation label for movies released in the cinema. The government-supported "A" campaign introduced the A-label for movies that passed the Bechdel-Wallace test. Thus far no other official representation label has been implemented, therefore we may have to be our own judge until that time. Let's try it out. Think back to your favorite childhood movie –

Would your favorite childhood movie pass the Vito Russo test, or maybe the Duvernay test?

The Vito Russo Test for LGBTQ Representation

1. The film contains a character that is identifiably lesbian, gay, bisexual, transgender, and/or queer
2. That character must not be solely or predominantly defined by their sexual orientation or gender identity (i.e., they are comprised of the same sort of unique character traits commonly used to differentiate straight/cisgender characters from one another)
3. The LGBTQ character must be tied to the plot in such a way that the character's removal would have a significant effect, meaning the character is not there to simply provide colorful commentary, paint urban authenticity, or set up a punchline. The character must matter

Original source: https://glaad.org/sri/2021/vito-russo-test/

The Duvernay Test for Representation of People of Color

1. Complex characters: Stories that pass the test must feature at least two characters of color, and they must not be in a romantic relationship together. These characters must have complex lives rather than existing only in relation to White characters
2. Names: The people of color in a story must have names
3. Speaking parts: Characters of color must have dialogue, and their conversations must not be about supporting a White character

Original source: https://www.nytimes.com/2016/01/30/movies/sundance-fights-tide-with-films-like-the-birth-of-a-nation.html

 When you scrutinize the tests and the included questions, you might notice that most of them are mono-identity tests and measure representation quite roughly. This is why some researchers have criticized the tests, arguing that programming that includes misrepresentations can still pass the test (Nguyen, 2023).

Reference

Nguyen, J. K. (2023). The economic case for equality in screenplays: The Bechdel test, female dialogue and box office revenue. *Journal of Screenwriting*, 14(2), 173–190. http://dx.doi.org/10.1386/josc_00124_1

Source | Authors

Racial/Ethnic Identity Representation in Youth Media

Categorizations of people based on race/ethnicity are socially constructed and have changed over time. In academic research, interpretations of the social constructs of *race* and *ethnicity* vary greatly, often overlap, or are even used interchangeably (Martinez et al., 2023). These concepts are further explained in Chapter 7. In this chapter, we use variations of the term race/ethnicity in relation to the third major developmental goal, i.e., racial/ethnic identity development.

Children differentiate between their own racial/ethnic characteristics and that of others as early as infancy (Rogers et al., 2021). With age, the understanding of race/ethnicity becomes more complex and evolves from recognition of physical characteristics, such as skin color and facial features, to awareness of the societal issues, such as inequality and racism, associated with race/ethnicity (Rogers et al., 2021). Successful racial/ethnic identity development is characterized by a clear sense of one's racial/ethnic identity, a feeling of belonging and pride, and an overall positive adjustment of adolescents (Umaña-Taylor & Rivas-Drake, 2021).

Media depictions carry weight in the development of racial/ethnic attitudes toward the self and others (Ward & Bridgewater, 2023). Media portrayals of racial/ethnic identities are most frequently represented from a White majority perspective. As a result, most media productions revolve around White characters and their complex storylines, while racial/ethnic minoritized groups are less often the center of a story, and their narratives are frequently underdeveloped and misrepresented (Rogers et al., 2021).

Quantity of Racial-Ethnic Minority Representation

Children's programming. Historically, in children's programming, White characters have been overrepresented across all roles, at the expense of characters of color (e.g., Giaccardi et al., 2019; Meyer & Conroy, 2023a). Notably, in line with content models of representation, Klein and Shiffman (2006) demonstrated that the frequency of characters of color in children's cartoons did not linearly increase but fluctuated between the 1930s and 1990s. There was a decrease between the 1930s and 1960s before it improved. These days representation of minoritized ethnic/racial groups varies between 30% and 50% (e.g., Giaccardi et al., 2019; Meyer & Conroy, 2023a). For example, looking at human (leading) characters in US children's programming in 2022, over 50% were human characters of color (Meyer & Conroy, 2023a).

The grouping label "characters of color" encompasses a vast variety of racial/ethnic groups, and the quantity of representation varies per group. In US children's shows released in 2018, the number of Black and Asian characters was mostly in line with the number of Black and Asian US citizens (Giaccardi et al., 2019). Around the same time, a content analysis of programming targeted at 2- to 13-year olds revealed that only 5% of characters with *any* speaking part could be identified as Latinx, while the US youth population comprises 23% Latinx youth (Rogers et al., 2021). A clear case of underrepresentation also holds for Native American and Middle Eastern characters who make up only 1% of characters in children's shows (Giaccardi et al., 2019).

Adolescent programming. Trends in contemporary adolescents programming are similar to those in children's programming. Programming is often characterized by an overrepresentation of White characters, but this seems to diminish in some countries. For example, while in 2018 70% of leading characters in Canadian television shows and movies were White, this decreased to 59% in 2021 (Meyer & Conroy, 2023b). An automated content analysis of US entertainment programs broadcasted between 2010 and 2021 showed a complementary trend for characters of color; screentime for characters with medium and dark skin tones increased from 6.4% to 16.6% (Sabyasachee et al., 2022). This increase was steepest for women with dark skin tones, who were close to absent in 2010. Yet their speaking time remained lowest of all characters. In the Netherlands, fiction programming broadcasted in 2018 to 2020 was still characterized by a striking underrepresentation of characters of color, especially women of color (Crone et al., 2023).

Other racial/ethnic groups, such as Indigenous groups and those from the MENA (Middle Eastern and North African) region remain severely underrepresented in US entertainment content. Among 62,224 speaking characters featured in the most popular US films between 2007 and 2022, a mere 0.2% of the characters were Native Americans and only one had a leading role (Smith et al., 2022), namely Dani Moonstar in the 2022 superhero horror movie *The New Mutants*. The Cheyenne character is played by the Native American actress Blu Hunt. MENA characters—often portrayed as one and the same group—are nearly invisible, reportedly 1% to 2% (e.g., Sabyasachee et al., 2022).

Video games. Compared to TV shows and movies, video games—including those aimed at children—display an even stronger overrepresentation of White leading characters (e.g., Behm-Morawitz & Ta, 2014; Waddell et al., 2022). Over time, there has been little progress in the quantity of characters of color. In 2017, 20% of 8,572 game characters in the UK's best-selling games were of color (Harrisson et al., 2020), compared to 17% in 2009 (Williams et al., 2009). The increase in playable characters was limited to Black characters (Harrisson et al., 2020).

Quality of Ethnic Minority Portrayals

Children's programming. Like the upward—although not always linear—trend observed for quantity of representation of racial/ethnic minoritized groups, the quality of characters has improved over time but leaves room for improvement. For example, there has been a steady decline in overt racism toward characters of color in children's cartoons from the 1930s to the 1990s (Klein & Shiffman, 2006). Simultaneously, cartoon characters of color were still, and continue to be, narrowly presented. For example, Asian characters are shown as socially awkward and the majority of women of color are frequently sexualized (Rogers et al., 2021). In the early 2000s, positive exemplars of racial/ethnic minoritized group portrayals for children were introduced, with the first leading Latinx cartoon character in 2001, *Dora the Explorer*, and one year later, the first Black leading cartoon character on Disney, Penny Proud (Keys, 2016). These characters were no longer one dimensional and the storylines presented their cultural heritage in an authentic manner. Dora shares her Spanish vocabulary and is presented as a unique individual with an adventurous mindset (Keys, 2016).

Adolescent programming. In adolescent programming, tropes reflect a variety of negative and narrow representations. For example, the *White Savior* trope is known to perpetuate racial/ethnic inequality by situating a character of color as subordinate to the White main character (Hunt, 2019). This trope can be found in a range of movies set at high schools, such as the inspirational teacher in *Freedom Writers* (2008), but also in action movies, such as the fighter against slavery in *The Legend of Tarzan* (2016). The status of ethnic/racial groups in society is also reflected in occupation-related characteristics of characters. Characters of color are less often depicted as hardworking, employed, or in a leadership position, and more often as criminals (Giaccardi et al., 2019). Thus, although overt racism toward characters of color decreased, more subtle forms of racism persist and existing inequalities in status or power are reproduced.

The specific types of misrepresentation differ across racial/ethnic groups. For example, in contrast to Latinx and Black characters, Asian characters are often portrayed as hardworking, respectful, and academically successful. This trope is referred to as the "model minority" (Besana et al., 2019). Though this may be perceived as a positive portrayal, it provides a narrow representation that sets high, specific expectations for Asian youth. Moreover, Asian American characters are frequently portrayed as a "perpetual foreigner" distinct from the White majority culture (Mastro et al., 2021). Finally, as Asians are quite often depicted as one group, this denies the unique experiences of specific Asian racial/ethnic groups (e.g., Mastro et al., 2021).

Video games. Stereotypical portrayals of people of color in video games are similar to the media discussed above. For example, Black male characters are often portrayed as violent, criminal, or athletic (Harrisson et al., 2020; St Fleur & DeWinter, 2021). Portrayals are also narrow. For example, Asian men are frequently martial arts fighters (Mastro et al., 2021). The overrepresentation of White ethnic/racial identities in video games is known as "Normative Whiteness" (Dietrich, 2013) which is reflected in customization options that are available. For example, White players have more free default avatar options to choose from that look like them, and thus players of color must spend more money to buy avatar *skins* to have the same opportunity (Reza et al., 2022). Even virtual environments that are frequented by adolescents and allow for *player*-generated avatar options still present as White-dominated spaces. In the educational virtual world of *Whyville*, e.g., young players of color had fewer options for faces matching their skin tones (Kafai et al., 2010). Black game creators working on incorporating Black experiences into The *Sims 4* (2014) indicated that Black representation should go beyond skin color, and so they introduced new hair structures and styles and other forms of cultural expression (St Fleur & DeWinter, 2021).

In Short: Media Representation of Gender, Sexual Orientation, and Race/Ethnicity

Looking back, we can conclude that the youth media landscape more heavily features majority group characters versus minority group characters. As a result, minoritized youth must put in more effort to identify media that supports that part of their identity (Martins et al., 2022). Gender and sexual minority characters are still virtually invisible in children's programming and underrepresented in adolescent programming. Some racial/ethnic identities are now well-represented in quantity, but not yet in quality, while others are fully left behind. The latest content analyses do show positive signs with representations of gender, sexual, and racial/ethnic minoritized group identities becoming more pronounced in TV programming, movies, and, albeit to a lesser extent, also video games. Casts of TV shows are progressively characterized by (cis)gender equality and are increasingly racial/ethnically diverse, and minoritized characters are taking up more leading roles.

Shows for young people that do include minoritized characters in an authentic way are not just popular among minoritized social groups but are received positively by a wide audience, mirroring the social identity gratification needs of minoritized youth (Martins et al., 2022) and the selection preferences of majority audiences (Huber et al., 2022). At the same time, resistance to inclusive media practices remains. For example, the erasure of sexual minority characters in children's programming has often been attributed to being "age inappropriate." Some content creators as well as child protection agencies argue that sexual minority representation is a display of adult sexuality, something they do not find appropriate before children reach adolescence (Vanlee & Kerrigan, 2021). Yet that same argument could apply to a display of heterosexual representation. Research actually shows positive outcomes when parents are exposed to children's programs including sexual minority characters (McAndrew & Bonus, 2022) and prove to be conversation starters for some adolescents with their parents about their sexual identity (Mares et al., 2022).

Looking Ahead: Emergent Themes in Media Representation Research

This final section will focus on three emergent themes to further our understanding of media representation, including the promises and pitfalls of representation in newer (user-generated) technologies, the move toward a more inclusive media research agenda, and incorporating young voices.

New Communication Technologies: The Case of Social Media

First, social media and newer communication technologies (e.g., augmented and virtual reality, AI, and chatbots) hold much promise as alternative sources of media content and experiences for minoritized young people who do not see their identities authentically represented in traditional entertainment media (McInroy & Craig, 2017). Current research underlines the promise of these technologies, but also flags potential inequalities similar to those in more traditional entertainment media.

With social media, for instance, due to their user-generated nature, they potentially provide opportunities for greater diversity and authenticity of identity representations (Miller & Bond, 2022). On the one hand, minoritized group members indeed find positive and authentic representations in social media especially when they actively seek out such content (e.g., Brough et al., 2020; Rollins et al., 2022). For example, YouTube videos viewed by Black young people included a higher proportion of Black characters than White viewers (Rollins et al., 2022). On the other hand, even when actively seeking out authentic minority representation content (e.g., following particular influencers), many minoritized youth still do not see this content in their feeds, such as the "For you-feed" that is based on algorithmic recommendations (Karizat et al., 2021). The continued invisibility of minoritized identities on social media, also referred to as shadow-banning, still persists (Rauchberg, 2022).

Next to a lower visibility, social media also exposes young people to content that negatively portrays minoritized identities. For example, British children, from as early as 8, reported to have seen content containing verbal discrimination such as racism, homophobia, and misogyny (Ofcom, 2024). Rollins et al. (2022) also showed that some of the most popular White YouTubers use discriminatory language, reinforcing inequality as role models for youth. Based on these observations, it is not surprising that members of marginalized groups worry about the inclusivity of new technologies and become more hesitant to adopt them. These worries are not limited to social media but also concern technologies, such as AI. LGBTQ+ young people specifically expressed concerns about inaccuracy and bias in the information provided by generative AI tools; thus, they are more likely than their cisgender and straight peers to say that they did not use this technology (Common Sense Media, 2024), further contributing to digital inequality.

In short, social media and new communication technologies have the potential to serve as an alternative to traditional entertainment media in providing authentic identity representation, but research is needed to ascertain benefits and pitfalls around these developments.

Inclusive Media (Representation) Research Practices

Second, entertainment media researchers are raising awareness that current media theories on youth are scarce and do not include a minority or majority socialization perspective (Ward & Bridgewater, 2023). Relatedly, thus far a mono-categorical approach has been dominant in quantitative research, meaning that media representation content and effects studies focus on one identity aspect glossing over other characteristics of a media character or user (Scharrer et al., 2022). In real life however people have multiple identities that intersect, and the salience of each identity component may vary across individual, time, and context, resulting in unique media experiences (Riles et al., 2022; Ward & Bridgewater, 2023). Theory and research should account for these complexities to optimize our understanding of media experiences (Riles et al., 2022).

Media creators are also slowly making space for characters with intersecting minoritized identities. For example, the acclaimed animated series *Proud Family* was known to provide young viewers with a variety of Black role models, but representation of the LGBTQ+ community was limited. The reboot, *Proud Family 2.0: Louder and Prouder*, includes openly LGBTQ+ characters with well-known queer Black artists as the voice actors.

Incorporate Young Voices

To know how to change the media landscape, we should not only discuss the state of representation, but also include young people who belong to minoritized identity groups in media representation research and media production processes. Now, these young people seem to have resigned themselves to having access to a media landscape that is characterized by under- and misrepresentation (Floegel & Costello, 2019). Young people indicate that they prefer flawed representation over no representation, such as Latinx adolescents mentioning to keep watching "if they only disrespect us a little" (Martins et al., 2022, p. 858) or queer young adults stating that misrepresentation is "literally better than nothing" (Floegel & Costello, 2019, p. 33).

Media researchers as well as media creators should listen more carefully to young people and address their concerns when working toward a media landscape that provides young people with an **identity-empowering environment**. Today's young people, the future media consumers and creators, demand and deserve better content and better representation.

Notes

1 Note. For conciseness, the labels girls/women, boys/men pertain to cisgender identity.
2 The acronym LGBTQIA+ refers to individuals who identify as lesbian, gay, bisexual, transgender, queer, intersex and asexual or other.
3 Screen Australia's report Seeing Ourselves is based on an analysis of 1,961 'main' characters from 199 Australian TV dramas broadcast on public, commercial free-to-air, and subscription television between 2011 and 2015. Children's dramas and comedies were included, but animations were excluded due to the number of non-human characters.
4 https://hollywoodlife.com/2019/12/03/pose-billy-porter-hollywood-trans-inclusive-interview-video/

References

APA (2022). *Gender.* https://apastyle.apa.org/style-grammar-guidelines/bias-free-language/gender

Aubrey, J. S., & Roberts, L. (2020). Effects of media use on development of gender role beliefs. *The International Encyclopedia of Media Psychology*, 1–12. https://doi.org/10.1002/9781119011071.iemp0081

Bandura, A. (1986). *Social foundations of thought and action: A social cognitive theory.* Englewood Cliffs, NJ: Prentice-Hall.

Beasley, B., & Collins Standley, T. (2002). Shirts vs. skins: Clothing as an indicator of gender role stereotyping in video games. *Mass Communication & Society, 5*(3), 279–293. https://doi.org/10.1207/S15327825MCS0503_3

Behm-Morawitz, E., & Ta, D. (2014). Cultivating virtual stereotypes?: The impact of video game play on racial/ethnic stereotypes. *Howard Journal of Communications, 25*(1), 1–15. https://doi.org/10.1080/10646175.2013.835600

Belmonte, J. F. (2017). Teenage heroes and evil deviants: Sexuality and history in JRPGs. *Continuum, 31*(6), 903–911. https://doi.org/10.1080/10304312.2017.1374351

Besana, T., Katsiaficas, D., & Loyd, A. B. (2019). Asian American media representation: A film analysis and implications for identity development. *Research in Human Development, 16*(3-4), 201–225. https://doi.org/10.1080/15427609.2020.1711680

Birchmore, A., & Kettrey, H. H. (2022). Exploring the boundaries of the parasocial contact hypothesis: An experimental analysis of the effects of the "bury your gays" media trope on homophobic and sexist attitudes. *Feminist Media Studies, 22*(6), 1311–1327. https://doi.org/10.1080/14680777.2021.1887919

Bishop, R. S. (1990). Mirrors, windows, and sliding glass doors. *Perspectives: Choosing and Using Books for the Classroom, 6*(3), 9–11. https://scenicregional.org/wp-content/uploads/2017/08/Mirrors-Windows-and-Sliding-Glass-Doors.pdf

Blanco-Fernández, V., & Moreno, J. A. (2023). "Video games were my first safe space": Queer gaming in the animal crossing new horizons LGBTIQA+community. *Games and Culture*, 0(0). https://doi.org/10.1177/15554120231205638

Bond, B. J. (2014). Sex and sexuality in entertainment media popular with lesbian, gay, and bisexual adolescents, *Mass Communication and Society*, 17, 98–120, https://doi.org/10.1080/15205436.2013.816739

Bond, B. J. (2015). Portrayals of sex and sexuality in gay-and lesbian-oriented media: A quantitative content analysis, *Sexuality & Culture*, 19, 37–56, https://doi.org/10.1007/s12119-014-9241-6

Brough, M., Literat, I., & Ikin, A. (2020). "Good social media?": Underrepresented youth perspectives on the ethical and equitable design of social media platforms. *Social Media and Society*, 6(2), 205630512092848. https://doi.org/10.1177/2056305120928488

Clark, C. C. (1969). Television and social control: Some observations on the portrayals of ethnic minorities, *Television Quarterly*, 8, 18–22, https://www.worldradiohistory.com/Archive-Television-Quarterly/TVQ-1969-Spring.pdf

Colliver, B. (2020). Representation of LGBTQ communities in the grand theft auto series. In C. Kelly, A. Lynes, & K. Hoffin (Eds.), *Video games crime and next-gen deviance* (pp. 131–149). Emerald Publishing Limited.

Common Sense Media (2024). *Teen and young adult perspectives on generative AI: Patterns of use, excitements, and concerns*. https://www.commonsensemedia.org/sites/default/files/research/report/teen-and-young-adult-perspectives-on-generative-ai.pdf

Cover, R. (2024). Making queer content visible: Approaches and assumptions of Australian film and television stakeholders working with LGBTQ+ content. *Media International Australia*, 190(1), 116–132. https://doi.org/10.1177/1329878X221077851

Cover, R., & Milne, C. (2023). The "Bury your gays" trope in contemporary television: Generational shifts in production responses to audience dissent. *The Journal of Popular Culture*, 56(5-6), 810–823. https://doi.org/10.1111/jpcu.13255

Coyne, S. M., Linder, J. R., Rasmussen, E. E., Nelson, D. A., & Birkbeck, V. (2016). Pretty as a princess: Longitudinal effects of engagement with Disney princesses on gender stereotypes, body esteem, and prosocial behavior in children. *Child Development*, 87(6), 1909–1925. https://doi.org/10.1111/cdev.12569

Crone, V., Jacobs, J., Nauta, O., Nijboer, R., Pital, V., & Petersen, A. (2023). *Je kunt niet zijn wat je niet kunt zien: Diversiteit en inclusiviteit in de AV-sector*. DSP-groep. https://www.rijksoverheid.nl/documenten/rapporten/2023/03/24/onderzoek-je-kunt-niet-zijn-wat-je-niet-kunt-zien-diversiteit-en-inclusiviteit-in-de-film-en-av-sector

Crookston, S. (2018). Team katniss? Adolescent girls' participation in a voluntary archery after-school program. *Women in Sport and Physical Activity Journal*, 26(2), 99–110. https://doi.org/10.1123/wspaj.2017-0029

Davis, M. M. (2014). From snow to ice: A study of the progression of disney princesses from 1937 to 2014. *Film Matters*, 5(2), 48–52. https://doi.org/10.1386/fm.5.2.48_1

Deerwater, R., Townsend, M., & Hurwitz, A. (2024). *Where We Are On TV 2023-2024*. GLAAD Media Institute. https://assets.glaad.org/m/7c489f209e120a11/original/GLAAD-2023-24-Where-We-Are-on-TV.pdf

Dennis, J. P. (2009). The boy who would be queen: Hints and closets on children's television. *Journal of Homosexuality*, 56(6), 738–756. https://doi.org/10.1080/00918360903054210

Dias, E. V. A., Santos, I. L. S., & Pimentel, C. E. (2023). LGBTQ+ media exposure and attitudes: Measures' development and the moderating role of sexual orientation. *Sexuality Research and Social Policy*, 20(3), 1232–1244. https://doi.org/10.1007/s13178-023-00792-5

Dietrich, D. R. (2013). Avatars of Whiteness: Racial expression in video game characters, *Sociological Inquiry*, 83, 82–105, https://doi.org/10.1111/soin.12001.

Downs, E., & Smith, S. L. (2010). Keeping abreast of hypersexuality: A video game character content analysis, *Sex Roles*, 62, 721–733, https://doi.org/10.1007/s11199-009-9637-1

Elmore, K. C., Scull, T. M., & Kupersmidt, J. B. (2017). Media as a "super peer": How adolescents interpret media messages predicts their perception of alcohol and tobacco use norms. *Journal of Youth and Adolescence*, 46(2), 376–387. https://doi.org/10.1007/s10964-016-0609-9

England, D. E., Descartes, L., & Collier-Meek, M. A. (2011). Gender role portrayal and the Disney princesses, *Sex Roles*, 64, 555–567, https://doi.org/10.1007/s11199-011-9930-7

Floegel, D., & Costello, K. L. (2019). Entertainment media and the information practices of queer individuals. *Library & Information Science Research*, 41(1), 31–38. https://doi.org/10.1016/j.lisr.2019.01.001

Frable, D. E. (1997). Gender, racial, ethnic, sexual, and class identities. *Annual Review of Psychology*, 48(1), 139–162. https://doi.org/10.1146/annurev.psych.48.1.139

GenderGP, (July 2023). *What Netflix's Heartstopper gets right about trans representation.* https://www.gendergp.com/heartstopper-series-review-trans-representation/#:~:text=Elle%2C%20played%20by%20Yasmin%20Finney,much%20her%20friends%20miss%20her.

Gerbner, G. (1969). Toward "Cultural indicators": The analysis of mass mediated public message systems. *AV Communication Review*, 17(2), 137–148. https://doi.org/10.1007/bf02769102

Gerding, A., & Signorielli, N. (2014). Gender roles in tween television programming: A content analysis of two genres, *Sex Roles*, 70, 43–56, https://doi.org/10.1007/s11199-013-0330-z

Giaccardi, S., Heldman, C., Cooper, R., Cooper-Jones, N., Conroy, M., Esparza, P., Breckenridge-Jackson, I., Juliano, L., McTaggart, N., Phillips, H., & Seabrook, R. (2019). See Jane 2019 Report. *The Geena Davis Institute for Gender in Media.* https://geenadavisinstitute.org/research/see-jane-2019/

Gilbert, M., Lynch, T., Burridge, S., & Archipley, L. (2023). Formidability of male video game characters over 45 years. *Information, Communication & Society*, 26(8), 1531–1547. https://doi.org/10.1080/1369118X.2021.2013921

GLAAD. (n.d.). *GLAAD Media Reference Guide*, 11th ed., https://glaad.org/reference/.

Gray, H. (2001). Equity and diversity in media representation: Desiring the network and network desire. *Critical Studies in Media Communication*, 18(1), 103–108. https://doi.org/10.1080/15295030109367127

Gross, L. (2001). Equity and diversity in media representation: The paradoxical politics of media representation. *Critical Studies in Media Communication*, 18(1), 114–119. https://doi.org/10.1080/15295030109367129

Hale, M. L., & Melzer, A. (2022). #LearningGender – Media representations of gender and their effects on gender socialisation. In Kerger, S., Brasseur, L., (Eds.), *Gender and education in Luxembourg and beyond: Local challenges and new perspectives*. Melusina Press.

Harrisson, A., Jones, S., Marchessault, J., Pedraça, S., & Consalvo, M. (2020). The virtual census 2.0: A continued investigation on the representations of gender, race and age in videogames. *AoIR Selected Papers of Internet Research*. https://doi.org/10.5210/spir.v2020i0.11229

Harwood, J. (1999). Age identification, social identity gratifications, and television viewing. *Journal of Broadcasting & Electronic Media*, *43*(1), 123–136. https://doi.org/10.1080/08838159909364479

Ho, X., Perez Escobar, R., & Tran, N. (2022, September). Queer indie games on itch.io, 2013-2022. In *Proceedings of the 17th International Conference on the Foundations of Digital Games* (pp. 1–10). https://doi.org/10.1145/3555858.3555881

Huber, B., Rivas-Lara, S., Karan, M., & Uhls, Y. T. (2022). International audiences want to see more representation on and off the screen. *The Center for Scholars and Storytellers*. https://drive.google.com/file/d/120K1_Px5o9OQ3uUWt_BFIvLBVW3hebp3/view

Hunt, W. (2019). Negotiating new racism: 'It's not racist or sexist. It's just the way it is. *Media, Culture & Society*, *41*(1), 86–103. https://doi.org/10.1177/0163443718798907

Kafai, Y. B., Cook, M. S., & Fields, D. A. (2010). "Blacks deserve bodies too!": Design and discussion about diversity and race in a tween virtual world. *Games and Culture*, *5*(1), 43–63. https://doi.org/10.1177/1555412009351261

Karizat, N., Delmonaco, D., Eslami, M., & Andalibi, N. (2021). Algorithmic folk theories and identity: How TikTok users co-produce knowledge of identity and engage in algorithmic resistance. *Proceedings of the ACM on Human-Computer Interaction*, *5*(CSCW2), 1–44. https://doi.org/10.1145/3476046

Keys, J. (2016). Doc McStuffins and Dora the Explorer: Representations of gender, race, and class in US animation. *Journal of Children and Media*, *10*(3), 355–368. https://doi.org/10.1080/17482798.2015.1127835

Kirsch, A. C., & Murnen, S. K. (2015). "Hot" girls and "cool dudes": Examining the prevalence of the heterosexual script in American children's television media. *Psychology of Popular Media Culture*, *4*(1), 18–30. https://doi.org/10.1037/ppm0000017

Klein, H., & Shiffman, K. S. (2006). Race-related content of animated cartoons. *The Howard Journal of Communications*, *17*(3), 163–182. https://doi.org/10.1080/10646170600829493

Kohlburn, J., Cho, H., & Moore, H. (2023). Players' perceptions of sexuality and gender-inclusive video games a pragmatic content analysis of steam reviews. *Convergence*, *29*(2), 379–399. https://doi.org/10.1177/13548565221137481

Kukshinov, E., & Shaw, A. (2022). Playing with privilege: Examining demographics in choosing player-characters in video games. *Psychology of Popular Media*, *11*(1), 90–101. https://doi.org/10.1037/ppm0000378

LeJacq, Y. (March 2014). Why the gaming industry plans to keep gay characters on the sidelines. *Vice*. https://www.vice.com/en/article/9aky88/ubisoft-explains-why-there-arent-any-gay-video-game-protagonists-yet

Lemish, D., & Elias, N. (2019). Perpetuating gender stereotypes from birth: Analysis of TV programs for viewers in diapers. In Hermansson, C., Zepernick, J. (Eds.) *The palgrave handbook of Children's film and television*. Palgrave Macmillan, Cham. https://doi.org/10.1007/978-3-030-17620-4_27

Lucas, K., & Sherry, J. L. (2004). Sex differences in video game play: A communication-based explanation. *Communication Research*, *31*(5), 499–523. https://doi.org/10.1177/0093650204267930

Lustyik, K. (2013). The protection and promotion of home-grown children's television. In D. Lemish (Ed.), *The Routledge international handbook of children, adolescents, and media* (pp. 378–383). Routledge.

Lynch, T., Tompkins, J. E., Gilbert, M., & Burridge, S. (2024). Evidence of ambivalent sexism in female video game character designs. *Mass Communication and Society*, 1–26. https://doi.org/10.1080/15205436.2024.2311229

Lynch, T., Tompkins, J. E., Van Driel, I. I., & Fritz, N. (2016). Sexy, strong, and secondary: A content analysis of female characters in video games across 31 years. *Journal of Communication*, 66(4), 564–584. https://doi.org/10.1111/jcom.12237

Mares, M. L., Chen, Y. A., & Bond, B. J. (2022). Mutual influence in LGBTQ teens' use of media to socialize their parents. *Media Psychology*, 25(3), 441–468. https://doi.org/10.1080/15213269.2021.1969950

Marshall, D. (2010). Popular culture, the 'victim' trope and queer youth analytics. *International Journal of Qualitative Studies in Education*, 23(1), 65–85. https://doi.org/10.1080/09518390903447176

Martinez, R. A. M., Andrabi, N., Goodwin, A. N., Wilbur, R. E., Smith, N. R., & Zivich, P. N. (2023). Conceptualization, operationalization, and utilization of race and ethnicity in major epidemiology journals, 1995–2018: A systematic review. *American Journal of Epidemiology*, 192(3), 483–496. https://doi.org/10.1093/aje/kwac146

Martin, K. A., & Kazyak, E. (2009). Hetero-romantic love and heterosexiness in children's G-rated films. *Gender & Society*, 23(3), 315–336. https://doi.org/10.1177/0891243209335635

Martins, N., Gonzales, A. L., & Mastro, D. (2022). If they only disrespect us a little, and the story is interesting, I keep watching: Navigation of ethnic media gratifications by Latino teens. *Journal of Adolescent Research*, 37(6), 841–870. https://doi.org/10.1177/07435584211062109

Masanet, M. J., Ventura, R., & Ballesté, E. (2022). Beyond the "trans fact"? Trans representation in the teen series Euphoria: Complexity, recognition, and comfort. *Social Inclusion*, 10(2), 143–155. https://doi.org/10.17645/si.v10i2.4926

Mastro, D., Peebles, A., Rogers, O., & Robb, M. B. (2021). *Ethnic-racial representation in screen media*. Common Sense.

Mazières, A., Menezes, T., & Roth, C. (2021). Computational appraisal of gender representativeness in popular movies. *Humanities and Social Sciences Communications*, 8(1), 1–9. https://doi.org/10.1057/s41599-021-00815-9

McAndrew, J., & Bonus, J. A. (2022). I've got a girl crush: Parents' responses to stories about sexuality in children's television. *Journal of Homosexuality*, 69(9), 1524–1548. https://doi.org/10.1080/00918369.2021.1917222

McDade-Montez, E., Wallander, J., & Cameron, L. (2017). Sexualization in US Latina and white girls' preferred children's television programs. *Sex Roles*, 77, 1–15. https://doi.org/10.1007/s11199-016-0692-0

McInroy, L. B., & Craig, S. L. (2017). Perspectives of LGBTQ emerging adults on the depiction and impact of LGBTQ media representation. *Journal of Youth Studies*, 20(1), 32–46. https://doi.org/10.1080/13676261.2016.1184243

McLaren, J. T., Bryant, S., & Brown, B. (2021). "See me! Recognize me!" An analysis of transgender media representation. *Communication Quarterly*, 69(2), 172–191. https://doi.org/10.1080/01463373.2021.1901759

Meyer, M., & Conroy, M. (2023a). *See Jane 2023: How has on-screen representation in children's television changed from 2018 to 2022?* The Geena Davis Institute on Gender in Media. https://geenadavisinstitute.org/wp-content/uploads/2024/01/GDI-See-Jane-2023-TV-Report.pdf

Meyer, M., & Conroy, M. (2023b). *Representation and inclusion in film and television produced in British Columbia*. The Union of British Columbia Performers and The Geena Davis Institute on Gender in Media.

Miller, B., & Bond, B. J. (2022). Broadcasting yourself: Perspectives of LGBTQ YouTube microcelebrities. *Western Journal of Communication*, 86(4), 541–560. https://doi.org/10.1080/10570314.2022.2087894

Molina-Guzmán, I. (2018). #OscarsSoWhite: How Stuart Hall explains why nothing changes in Hollywood and everything is changing. In P. Decherney, & K. Sender (Eds.), *Stuart Hall lives: Cultural studies in an age of digital media* (pp. 86–102). Routledge.

Morgan, E. M. (2019). Same-sex relationships and LGBTQ youth. In S. Hupp & J. D. Jewell (Eds.), *The encyclopedia of child and adolescent development* (pp. 1–10). Wiley. https://doi.org/10.1002/9781119171492.wecad488

Nielsen. (January, 2024). *Streaming unwrapped: Streaming viewership goes to the library in 2023*. https://www.nielsen.com/insights/2024/streaming-unwrapped-streaming-viewership-goes-to-the-library-in-2023/

Ofcom. (2024). Understanding pathways to online violent content among children. Qualitative research report March 2024. https://www.ofcom.org.uk/online-safety/protecting-children/pathways-to-online-violent-content/

Park, S. Y. (2012). Mediated intergroup contact: Concept explication, synthesis, and application. *Mass Communication and Society*, *15*(1), 136–159. https://doi.org/10.1080/15205436.2011.558804

Pinsof, D., & Haselton, M. G. (2017). The effect of the promiscuity stereotype on opposition to gay rights. *PloS One*, *12*(7), e0178534. https://doi.org/10.1371/journal.pone.0178534

Prommer, E., Stüwe, J., & Wegner, J. (2021). *Sichtbarkeit und vielfalt: Fortschrittstudie zur audiovisuellen diversität* [Visibility of variety: Progress report on audiovisual diversity]. Unpublished manuscript. https://tinyurl.com/PrommerDiversity

Raley, A. B., & Lucas, J. L. (2006). Stereotype or success? Prime-time television's portrayals of gay male, lesbian, and bisexual characters. *Journal of Homosexuality*, *51*(2), 19–38. https://doi.org/10.1300/J082v51n02_02

Rauchberg, J. S. (2022). # shadowbanned: Queer, trans, and disabled creator responses to algorithmic oppression on TikTok. In P. Pain (Ed.), *LGBTQ digital cultures* (pp. 196–209). Routledge.

Reza, A., Chu, S., Nedd, A., & Gardner, D. (2022). Having skin in the game: How players purchase representation in games. *Convergence*, *28*(6), 1621–1642. https://doi.org/10.1177/13548565221099713

Riles, J. M., Ramasubramanian, S., & Behm-Morawitz, E. (2022). Theory development and evaluation within a critical media effects framework. *Journal of Media Psychology*. https://doi.org/10.1027/1864-1105/a000339

Rogers, O., Mastro, D., Robb, M. B., & Peebles, A. (2021). *The inclusion imperative: Why media representation matters for kids' ethnic-racial development*. Common Sense.

Rollins, D., Bridgewater, E., Munzer, T., Weeks, H. M., Schaller, A., Yancich, M., Gipson, W., Drogos, K., Robb, M. B., & Radesky, J. S. (2022). *Who is the "you" in YouTube? Missed opportunities in race and representation in children's YouTube videos, 2022*. Common Sense. https://www.commonsensemedia.org/sites/default/files/research/report/2022-youtube-report-final-web.pdf

Sabyasachee, B., Bose, D., Conroy, D., Narayanan, S. S., Ricco, S., Singh, K., & Somandepalli, K. (2022). *#SeeItBeIt: What Families Are Seeing on TV*. The Geena Davis Institute on Gender in Media. https://geenadavisinstitute.org/research/see-jane-2022-tv-see-it-be-it-what-children-are-seeing-on-tv/

Santoniccolo, F., Trombetta, T., Paradiso, M. N., & Rollè, L. (2023). Gender and media representations: A review of the literature on gender stereotypes, objectification and sexualization. *International Journal of Environmental Research and Public Health*, *20*(10), 5770. https://doi.org/10.3390/ijerph20105770

Scharrer, E. (2013). Representations of gender in the media. In *The Oxford handbook of media psychology* (pp. 267–273). Oxford University Press.

Scharrer, E., Ramasubramanian, S., & Banjo, O. (2022). Media, diversity, and representation in the US: A review of the quantitative research literature on media content and effects. *Journal of Broadcasting & Electronic Media*, 66(4), 723–749. https://doi.org/10.1080/08838151.2022.2138890

Screen Australia. (2016). *Seeing ourselves: Reflections on diversity in Australian TV drama*. www.screenaustralia.gov.au/getmedia/157b05b4-255a-47b4-bd8b9 f715555fb44/TV-Drama-Diversity.pdf

Shaw, A., & Friesem, E. (2016). Where is the queerness in games?: Types of lesbian, gay, bisexual, transgender, and queer content in digital games, *International Journal of Communication*, 10, 3877–3889. Retrieved from http://ijoc.org/index.php/ijoc/article/viewFile/5449/1743.

Shaw, A., Lauteria, E. W., Yang, H., Persaud, C. J., & Cole, A. M. (2019). Counting queerness in games: Trends in LGBTQ digital game representation, 1985–2005. *International Journal of Communication*, 13, 26.

Smith, S. L., Pieper, K., & Wheeler, S. (2022). *Inequality in 1,600 popular films: Examining portrayals of gender, race/ethnicity, LGBTQ+ & disability from 2007 to 2022*. https://assets.uscannenberg.org/docs/aii-inequality-1600-films-20230216.pdf

Snyder, A. L., Bonus, J. A., & Cingel, D. P. (2023). Representations of LGBQ+ families in young children's media, *Journal of Children and Media*, 17, 154–160. https://doi.org/10.1080/17482798.2023.2173856

St Fleur, A., & DeWinter, J. (2021). "Unfiltered and true to itself": How content creators represent the Black community in The Sims 4. *American Journal of Play*, 13, 297–319. https://files.eric.ed.gov/fulltext/EJ1333256.pdf

Steinke, J. (2017). Adolescent girls' STEM identity formation and media images of STEM professionals: Considering the influence of contextual cues, *Frontiers in Psychology*, 8, 716. https://doi.org/10.3389/fpsyg.2017.00716

Steyer, I. (2014). Gender representations in children's media and their influence. *Campus-Wide Information Systems*, 31(2/3), 171–180. https://doi.org/10.1108/CWIS-11-2013-0065

Tajfel, H., & Turner, J. C. (1979). An integrative theory of intergroup conflict. In W. G. Austin, & S. Worchel (Eds.), *The social psychology of intergroup relations* (pp. 33–47). Brooks/Cole.

Thorfinnsdottir, D., & Jensen, H. S. (2017). Laugh away, he is gay! Heteronormativity and children's television in Denmark. *Journal of Children and Media*, 11(4), 399–416. https://doi.org/10.1080/17482798.2017.1312470

Tompkins, J. E., Lynch, T., Van Driel, I. I., & Fritz, N. (2020). Kawaii killers and femme fatales: A textual analysis of female characters signifying benevolent and hostile sexism in video games. *Journal of Broadcasting & Electronic Media*, 64(2), 236–254. https://doi.org/10.1080/08838151.2020.1718960

Towbin, M. A., Haddock, S. A., Zimmerman, T. S., Lund, L. K., & Tanner, L. R. (2004). Images of gender, race, age, and sexual orientation in Disney feature-length animated films. *Journal of Feminist Family Therapy*, 15(4), 19–44. https://doi.org/10.1300/J086v15n04_02

Townsend, M., & Deerwater, R. (2022). *Where Are We On TV 2021-2022*. GLAAD Media Institute. https://assets.glaad.org/m/49c8b636b1ee99eb/original/GLAAD-2021-22-Where-We-Are-on-TV.pdf

Umaña-Taylor, A. J., & Rivas-Drake, D. (2021). Ethnic-racial identity and adolescents' positive development in the context of ethnic-racial marginalization: Unpacking risk and resilience. *Human Development*, 65(5-6), 293–310. https://doi.org/10.1159/000519631

Utsch, S., Bragança, L. C., Ramos, P., Caldeira, P., & Tenorio, J. (2017). Queer identities in video games: Data visualization for a quantitative analysis of representation. *Proceedings of SBGames*, 850–851. https://sbgames.org/sbgames2017/papers/CulturaFull/175360.pdf

Valkenburg, P. M., & Peter, J. (2013). The differential susceptibility to media effects model. *Journal of Communication*, *63*(2), 221–243. https://doi.org/10.1111/jcom.12024

Van Wichelen, T., & Dhoest, A. (2023). Pink-wearing hairdressers to manly gay men: LGBT+ in Flemish children's fiction. *Communications*, *48*(1), 112–129. https://doi.org/10.1515/commun-2021-0013

Vanlee, F., & Kerrigan, P. (2021). Un/fit for young viewers: LGBT+ representation in Flemish and Irish children's television. In C. M. Scarcelli, D. Chronaki, S. De Vuyst & S. Villanueva Baselga (Eds.), *Gender and sexuality in the European media: Exploring different contexts through conceptualisations of age* (Vol. 16, pp. 24–40). Routledge.

Vivian. (2024, July 16). Mariowiki.com, https://www.mariowiki.com/Vivian

Waddell, T. F., Moss, C., Holz, A., & Ivory, J. D. (2022). Character portrayals in digital games: A systematic review of more than three decades of existing research. *Journal of Broadcasting & Electronic Media*, *66*(4), 647–673. https://doi.org/10.1080/08838151.2022.2100376

Walsh, A., & Leaper, C. (2020). A content analysis of gender representations in preschool children's television. *Mass Communication & Society*, *23*(3), 331–355. https://doi.org/10.1080/15205436.2019.1664593

Ward, L. M., & Bridgewater, E. (2023). Media use and the development of racial attitudes among US youth. *Child Development Perspectives*, *17*(2), 83–89. https://doi.org/10.1111/cdep.12480

Ward, L. M., & Grower, P. (2020). Media and the development of gender role stereotypes, *Annual Review of Developmental Psychology*, *2*, 177–199 https://doi.org/10.1146/annurev-devpsych-051120-010630

Ward, L. M., Reed, L., Trinh, S. L., & Foust, M. (2014). Sexuality and entertainment media. In D. L. Tolman, L. M. Diamond, J. A. Bauermeister, W. H. George, J. G. Pfaus, & L. M. Ward (Eds.), *APA handbook of sexuality and psychology, vol. 2. Contextual approaches* (pp. 373–423). American Psychological Association. https://doi.org/10.1037/14194-012

Whitehouse, K., Hitchens, M., & Matthews, N. (2023). Trans* and gender diverse players: Avatars and gender-alignment, *Entertainment Computing*, *47*, 100584. https://doi.org/10.1016/j.entcom.2023.100584

Williams, D., Martins, N., Consalvo, M., & Ivory, J. D. (2009). The virtual census: Representations of gender, race and age in video games. *New Media & Society*, *11*(5), 815–834. https://doi.org/10.1177/1461444809105354

Wingrove-Haugland, E., & McLeod, J. (2021). Not "minority" but "minoritized. *Teaching Ethics*, *21*(1), 1–11. https://doi.org/10.5840/tej20221799

Yan, H. Y. (2019). "The rippled perceptions": The effects of LGBT-inclusive TV on own attitudes and perceived attitudes of peers toward lesbians and gays. *Journalism & Mass Communication Quarterly*, *96*(3), 848–871. https://doi.org/10.1177/1077699018821327

4 Parents/Caregivers

Wonsun Shin

As children grow, they develop a wide range of knowledge, attitudes, and skills. This process is known as socialization. *Socialization* refers to how a learner, such as a child, acquires knowledge, motivations, values, and behaviors essential for functioning as a competent member of society (Grusec, 2002). Children's socialization does not happen in isolation but through interactions with various agents, including parents, peers, media, and cultural and social institutions. Although various agents influence children's socialization process and its outcomes, parents have been the prime focus of research as the key socialization agents (Shin & Lwin, 2019), serving as internal and primary socialization agents within the home—the ground zero for media education.

Parents as Primary Socialization Agents

Then, what makes parents crucial socialization agents for children? Firstly, parents are among the first socialization agents that children encounter and interact with before they expand their social boundaries to schools and peers. These early interactions and influences play a crucial role in a child's socialization process and outcomes, leaving a profound and lasting impact throughout their lives (Godleski et al., 2020). Secondly, parents and children form a biosocial system, maintaining close physical and emotional proximity. This closeness necessitates a shared understanding of acceptable behaviors, prompting parents to instill in their children the values and conduct deemed appropriate within the home boundary and society at large (Grusec & Davidov, 2007). Lastly, most societies place an expectation on parents to assume responsibility for the care, well-being, and intellectual development of their children. This expectation, as articulated in the United Nations Convention on the Rights of the Child (Article 18), emphasizes that parents and guardians bear the primary responsibility for the upbringing and development of their children. Such expectations are echoed by various organizations and institutions, including the American

DOI: 10.4324/9781003453123-5

Psychological Association and the Australian Human Rights Commission, and are also enshrined in the form of law, regulations, and codes of conduct in many countries.

Laible and Thompson (2007) explained several ways in which parents directly affect children's socialization processes and outcomes: Parents interact and communicate with their children to convey social norms, values, and principles. This refers to *social interaction*. Parents also use rewards and punishments to control and regulate their children's behaviors, providing incentives when children meet parental expectations and imposing restrictions in opposite situations. This reward-punishment mechanism is known as *reinforcement*. Lastly, parents serve as children's role models, as children tend to mimic the behaviors and actions of their parents. This is called *modeling*. In addition to the direct influences that parents exert on their children through social interaction, reinforcement, and modeling, parents also act as 'gatekeepers,' influencing how children interact with and are affected by other external socialization agents (Tannen et al., 2007). This is closely related to the role of parents as primary socialization agents who manage the surroundings of their children, including their media environment, to ensure children are protected from undesirable social influences.

Taking an inclusive approach, this chapter defines 'parent' as the primary caregiver with legal responsibility for the upbringing, development, and well-being of a child. This definition includes not only natural parents but also various types of legal guardians, such as adoptive, de facto, and stepparents. The term 'child' is also broadly defined to encompass anyone who has not reached adulthood (minor). It includes both young children and adolescents under 18 who tend to be more susceptible to diverse social influences, including media effects, as compared to their adult counterparts, due to their relatively lower levels of cognitive skills and lack of life experiences.

Parental Mediation: Origin and Types

Media is one of the most important external socialization agents and social surroundings for children, affecting their views of self, others, and the world in general, as detailed in other chapters of this book. As the primary agents of socialization, parents are expected or motivated to manage and control the influence of media on their children by implementing various intervention and supervision strategies. The role of parents in children's media use as supervisors and gatekeepers has been well recognized in the field of *parental mediation*.

Parental mediation refers to the strategies and techniques that parents/caregivers implement to supervise and regulate their children's media use, with the aim of enhancing positive media impacts on children while mitigating the negative aspects pertinent to media consumption (Shin & Lwin, 2019). The root of modern parental mediation research can be traced back to the early 1980s, primarily in the United States, when scholars began to pay increased attention to the impact of deregulation on the quality of children's television programs (Mendoza, 2009). With the loosening of regulations, children's television programs became more commercialized and less educational, raising concerns about the low quality of children's programming and its negative impacts on youths (Kunkel, 1999). As societal systems like regulations failed to provide sufficient protection for young people, researchers shifted their focus to the home front and the role of parenting in shaping children's television viewing behaviors.

Early research on parental mediation (e.g., Bybee et al., 1982; Desmond et al., 1985; Dorr et al., 1989; Nathanson, 1999) focused predominantly on children's television viewing, as television was the primary media for children at that time. These studies acknowledged the multifaceted nature of parental mediation, identifying several key strategies that parents employ to moderate their children's television viewing. The three broad parental mediation strategies identified from this body of research are active mediation, restrictive mediation, and co-viewing. *Active mediation*, also known as instructive mediation and evaluative mediation, refers to parents actively engaging in critical discussions and conversations with their children about the proper ways to use and understand media and its content. An example of active mediation includes parents explaining to their children the negative aspects of violent television programs. *Restrictive mediation* involves parents making efforts to control and limit their children's access to and use of media. In the context of television viewing, this can include parents setting limits on when and how much their children can watch TV, as well as preventing them from viewing certain programs or genres. *Co-viewing*, also known as co-use, entails parents using media alongside their children, e.g., watching the same television programs with the child in the same room. However, unlike active mediation, there may not be purposeful discussions or specific rules set by the parents during the co-viewing experience.

These three mediation types represent the three aforementioned ways in which parents socialize their children: *Social interaction* involving parent-child communication (active mediation), *reinforcement* through rules and control (restrictive mediation), and *modeling* where parents serve as role models of media use (co-viewing). In this sense, parental mediation can be understood as a socialization process in which parents shape their children's media use and its outcomes through social interaction, reinforcement, and modeling.

With the emergence and growth of the Web and digital media in the late 1990s and early 2000s, the media landscape has become significantly diversified. In response to that, scholars have identified additional types of parental mediation relevant to digital media. Examples are *technical mediation*, e.g., installing software and utilizing other technological means to filter media content (Eastin et al., 2006); *monitoring*, e.g., checking children's email messages and social media posts (Shin & Lwin, 2022); and *investigative mediation*, e.g., searching for information online to better understand media trends and children's media use (Jiow et al., 2016). Nonetheless, the three parental mediation strategies identified before the digital era—active mediation, restrictive mediation, and co-use—remain important parental mediation strategies across varying media contexts (Chen & Shi, 2019). Thus, these three strategies have been examined in diverse scenarios involving children's use of digital media, including their involvement in or vulnerability to cyberbullying (Chen et al., 2023), internet addiction (Liu, 2020), and exposure to content (e.g., watching child-inappropriate online videos) and contact risks online (e.g., adding strangers to friend lists on social media) (Kirwil, 2009; Shin & Kang, 2016). Thus, this chapter focuses on these three parental mediation strategies and their effects.

How Does Parental Mediation Work?

When considering the effects and effectiveness of parental mediation, the first question to ask is whether parental mediation influences children's media use and/or the outcomes associated with that use. The short answer is yes, as indicated by meta-analyses of parental mediation studies.[1] In a meta-analysis encompassing 57 parental mediation studies, focusing specifically on associations with negative outcomes of child media use (excessive media use, aggression, substance use, and sexual behaviors), Collier et al. (2016) discovered that both active and restrictive mediation were negatively associated with adverse media outcomes. However, co-use had the opposite effect, being positively related to child aggression and time spent on media. In another meta-analysis examining 52 studies on the effects of parental mediation on the amount of media use and incidence of media-related risks among children, Chen and Shi (2019) found that while restrictive mediation was more effective than active mediation in decreasing the amount of media use, active mediation and co-use were more effective than restrictive mediation in protecting children from media-related risks. Despite some discrepancies between the two meta-analyses (e.g., co-use being positively associated with adverse media outcomes in Collier et al. (2016) but negatively related to undesirable outcomes in Chen and Shi (2019)), both studies clearly show that parental mediation does have discernable impacts on children's media use and its consequences.

Recognizing the importance of parenting in children's media socialization, the subsequent crucial inquiry to address is precisely how each form of parental mediation functions in shaping children's media socialization. The general consensus from parental mediation research underscores that different types of parental mediation yield differing outcomes in children. Regarding active mediation, research has consistently demonstrated its effectiveness in decreasing negative media effects for *both* young children and older youths in a wide range of media contexts. To illustrate, active mediation has been found to diminish undesirable television advertising effects on children aged 8 to 12 (Buijzen & Valkenburg, 2005), cultivate critical orientation toward mobile advertising practices among teen smartphone users (Shin et al., 2020), enhance privacy management skills among adolescent social media users (Kang et al., 2022), and instill positive attitudes toward healthy food consumption among youth aged 10 to 16 (Yee et al., 2019).

Shin and Lwin (2019) outlined key reasons that render active mediation an effective parental intervention, even for older children like teenagers with an increasing pursuit of autonomy: Active mediation involves fostering communication between parents and children. This communication-based parental mediation enables parents to articulate the reasons behind their media intervention efforts. Simultaneously, it provides children with the opportunity to pose questions about the rationales for parental mediation and engage in further discussions on media-related issues with their parents. This dyadic communication process is likely to enhance children's critical thinking skills, making them less vulnerable to harmful media effects. It can also instill in children the belief that their ideas are acknowledged and respected by their parents, and consequently, their decision to adhere to parental expectations is self-determined rather than externally forced. Drawing on *self-determination theory* (Ryan & Deci, 2000), the sense of self-determination fostered by supportive parenting practices is expected to result in moral internalization, which, in turn, leads children to adopt desirable media behaviors even in the absence of direct parental supervision. This explains why active mediation has often been found to be more effective in eliciting positive media outcomes among older children like adolescents when compared to control-based restrictive mediation which can cause *psychological reactance* (i.e., motivation to resist rules or authority when personal freedoms are perceived threatened) (Brehm, 1966), leading teenagers to be more actively engaged in restricted/prohibited behaviors such as divulging personal information to online strangers (Lwin et al., 2008; Sasson & Mesch, 2014; Shin & Kang, 2016).

However, this does not mean that active mediation is always superior to restrictive mediation. Although restrictive mediation's top-down, one-way-street approach may cause unintended effects, it is still considered an effective parental mediation strategy if the goal is to limit children's exposure to specific types of media and associated risks (Chen & Shi, 2019; Collier et al., 2016; Livingstone & Helsper, 2008). As long as children follow the rules set by their parents, restrictive mediation serves as a safeguard against unwanted media effects. Moreover, from the perspective of children, a set of rules and restrictions directly governing their behaviors may be more noticeable and deemed important as compared to general and broad discussions on media-related issues (Lwin et al., 2017). From the parent's point of view, restrictive mediation may also be considered easier and more straightforward to implement, as it does not require extensive knowledge of media, unlike active mediation involving discussions and explanations of specific media issues (Shin, 2015).

Interestingly, the comparison between restrictive versus active mediation also reveals a flip side of active mediation. While discussion-based active mediation can cultivate critical thinking skills in both young and old children without triggering psychological reactance, engaging in media-related conversations is presumed to demand more effort. Parents need to possess a good understanding of media to have meaningful and impactful conversations with their tech-savvy children. They also need to find time to capture their children's attention and actively participate in these discussions. However, considering the constantly changing mediascape with emerging and evolving technologies, coupled with the busy lifestyles of both parents and children, implementing effective active mediation is easier said than done. Specifically, research indicates that parents tend to hold more positive attitudes toward active mediation than restrictive mediation (Shin, 2015; Shin & Kim, 2019). However, when it comes to actual implementation, parents are less likely to undertake proactive forms of active mediation that demand extensive knowledge and effort, such as suggesting specific ways to use the internet safely or recommending specific mobile apps, as compared to other socialization agents like peers and school teachers (Shin & Lwin, 2017).

When active and restrictive mediation may not be the most viable option, co-use can serve as a useful alternative for parents. Co-use allows parents to implicitly exercise parental mediation by serving as role models for media users, exemplifying proper media usage (Nikken, 2018). Unlike active mediation, co-use does not necessarily involve purposeful and instructive remarks from parents, making it less burdensome for them. In contrast to restrictive mediation, co-use does not impose specific rules that limit children's access to and use of media, thereby avoiding unintended boomerang effects. As co-use implies parent-child co-presence for shared media experience, it also provides an opportunity for parents to observe and understand how their children use media, possibly facilitating meaningful conversations about media use later on. Another advantage of co-use is that shared media experience can enhance family relationships.

Wang et al. (2018) found that video game co-playing among family members positively correlated with family satisfaction and closeness. Similarly, Padilla-Walker et al. (2012) demonstrated that adolescents' watching television and movies and playing video games with their parents was positively associated with higher levels of family connection. Given that co-use involves time spent together between youth and parents, it can also provide an opportunity for children and teenagers to influence their parents, e.g., teaching parents how to play a new game, thereby making youth an agent in parental media socialization.

Despite the potentially positive roles of media co-use, studies examining its effects have produced mixed insights (Shin & Lwin, 2019). To illustrate, while Chen and Shi's meta-analysis (2019) revealed a negative association between co-use and risky media behaviors, Collier et al.'s (2016) meta-analysis showed a positive association between co-use and undesirable media outcomes (e.g., aggression). Examining co-use effects across various media contexts, Padilla-Walker et al. (2012) found that while television co-viewing and game co-playing positively affected family connection, social media co-use had the opposite effect. Some studies in television contexts (An & Lee, 2010; Nathanson, 1999) suggested that co-use is less effective than active and restrictive mediation in influencing children's television viewing behaviors.

A plausible explanation for the inconsistent findings on co-use is that its effectiveness depends on how parents share media experiences with children and how children perceive co-use. Simply watching the same television program in the same room without any accompanying critical comments can be seen by children as a parental endorsement of the program rather than a purposeful media intervention (Nathanson, 1999). While playing games with parents can be enjoyable and strengthen parent-child bonding, it may not necessarily improve media literacy in children unless it involves critical discussions about the games and gaming (Nikken, 2018). Furthermore, children may find the co-use of personal peer-to-peer media, such as social and mobile media, more intrusive and inappropriate compared to the co-use of more shareable media, like television and game consoles in the living room (Padilla-Walker et al., 2012). Altogether, the effectiveness of co-use seems contingent upon various factors, including media usage contexts, types of media involved, and how children view parental involvement in media co-use.

Table 4.1 presents the definitions and examples of the three parental mediation strategies and summarizes how each mediation works.

Before discussing the determinants of parental mediation in the next section, it is important to stress that the three types of parental mediation are not mutually exclusive. For instance, if a parent reports high engagement in active mediation, it does not mean that the parent abandons other

Table 4.1 Overview of active mediation, restrictive mediation, and co-use.

Type	Active mediation	Restrictive mediation	Co-use
Definition	Parental engagement in explaining and discussing media-related issues with children	Parental control and limitation of children's access to and use of media	Parent and child using media together
Examples	• Explaining why certain mobile apps are inappropriate for children. • Suggesting ways to behave toward other people online. • Discussing how to protect personal information on social media.	• Restricting the amount of time the child can spend on digital media. • Limiting the types of apps that the child can download. • Setting rules regarding the types of personal information the child can share on social media.	• Watching the same television program in the same room. • Playing a video game together. • Using the same social media site with the child and 'friending' the child on SNS.
Pros	• Effective for both young and old children. • Affording the parent-child interactive discussions on media issues and risks. • Fostering critical thinking skills in children. • Facilitating children's internalization of parental media expectations without causing much reactance.	• Effective in limiting children's exposure to media that may have harmful effects. • More salient (easy for children to note) and straightforward than other forms of mediation. • Not requiring parents to possess extensive media knowledge and skills. • May work well for younger children receptive to parental authority.	• Less intrusive and burdensome. • Enhancing parents' understanding of children's media usage. • May lead to reverse socialization (i.e., children teaching their parents how to use media).

(Continued)

Table 4.1 (Continued)

Type	Active mediation	Restrictive mediation	Co-use
Cons	• Demanding time and effort. • Requiring parents to possess advanced knowledge and understanding of media trends and issues relevant to children.	• Less likely to instill a critical orientation toward media-related issues and risks. • May trigger psychological reactance in older children when growing need for autonomy.	• Unclear effects and effectiveness. • May be viewed as parental endorsement of media content rather than purposeful media intervention. • Difficult to implement for more personal, peer-to-peer communication.

Source: Author.

types of mediation. In reality, parents often employ a combination of different mediation approaches, integrating various strategies to maximize their influence on children's media usage (Chen et al., 2023; Lwin et al., 2008; Steinfeld, 2021).

Lwin et al. (2008) shed light on the synergetic effects of active and restrictive mediation by introducing a fourfold parental mediation typology: ***selective*** (high on both active and restrictive mediation), ***promotive*** (high on active mediation and low on restrictive mediation), ***restrictive*** (high on restrictive mediation and low on active mediation), and ***laissez-faire*** (low on both active and restrictive mediation). Their research explored the impacts of these typologies on children's exposure to online privacy risks, revealing that selective mediation was the most effective, while laissez-faire was the least effective in managing pre-teens' disclosure of personal information online. In a more recent study, Chen et al. (2023) investigated the combined effects of active mediation, restrictive mediation, and non-intrusive mediation (i.e., parents adding their children as social media friends to monitor activities) on teenagers' susceptibility to cyberbullying. Their findings showed that a combination of high active mediation, low restrictive mediation, and high non-intrusive inspection significantly reduced teens' likelihood of experiencing or perpetrating cyberbullying.

What Affects Parental Mediation?

Parenting styles vary widely. Some may prefer rule-based restrictive mediation, whereas others are more inclined to engage in discussion-based active mediation. Proactivity in parental mediation also differs, with some parents actively participating while others are less involved. What accounts for these variations in parental mediation practices?

Two consistent factors influencing parental mediation are the ages of children and parents' views on media (Wang et al., 2023; Warren, 2017). Specifically, parents of older children are less likely to engage in parental mediation compared to parents of younger children. This decline is attributed to the diminishing role of parents as socialization agents as children grow older and spend more time with external influences like peers, teachers, and media (Shin & Lwin, 2019). As children age, their knowledge and experience relating to media technologies also increase, reducing the need for close parental media supervision. The negative association between children's age and parental mediation tends to be more pronounced in restrictive mediation (Livingstone et al., 2011; Wang et al., 2023), which can be explained by older children's inclination to seek autonomy and their tendency to react to controlling parenting approaches.

Studies have also indicated that those who are concerned about the potential harmful impacts of media on their children are more likely to engage in media education and supervision. This holds true across diverse media contexts, including television (Nathanson, 1999), electronic games (Nikken & Jansz, 2006), internet (Warren, 2017), smartphones (Shin, 2018), and overall digital technologies (Shin & Lwin, 2022). Wang et al.'s (2023) meta-analysis of factors predicting parental mediation offers a nuanced insight into this matter. It shows that active mediation is predicted by *both* positive and negative attitudes toward media. However, restrictive mediation is associated only with negative media attitudes. The findings seem to imply that while active mediation is driven by parental intention to foster balanced discussions on media issues, considering both positive and negative aspects, restrictive mediation is likely motivated by a desire to shield children from harmful media content and associated risks, leading them to focus more on the negative aspects.

In contrast to the ages of children and parental perceptions of media effects, the role of broader societal and cultural factors has received less research attention. Research exploring the role of culture, e.g., is relatively scarce. Moreover, little is known about how differing socioeconomic status and other situational factors affect parental mediation. This gap may be due to the fact that most existing studies on parental mediation, predominantly based on national or regional surveys, examine 'general' populations within a single country or cultural context. Nonetheless, given that macro societal factors like culture and socioeconomic status can exert significant impacts on a family's access to and perceptions of media technologies, this chapter draws the reader's attention to the role of these understudied but crucial factors as potential determinants of parental mediation.

The first factor to examine is *culture*. Culture is important because it shapes social norms, values, and beliefs, thereby influencing family conduct and parenting practices. For instance, there is a well-established contrast between Asian and Western parenting styles. Specifically, Asian parenting often prioritizes family conformity and deference, while Western parenting places a greater emphasis on individual character development (Shin & Lwin, 2019). In multicultural societies like the United States, cultural-ethnic minorities exhibit diverse parenting attitudes as well. According to a Pew Research Center survey (Minjin & Horowitz, 2023), Hispanic parents in the United States tend to praise their children more than criticize them, when compared to their White, Black, and Asian counterparts in the same country; Black parents often see themselves as overprotective rather than providing children with too much freedom; Asian parents place higher importance on their children's college education and marriages. Of course, this does not mean that *all* White, Asian, Black, or Hispanic parents do these things; it simply reflects general norms identified in research. In addition to comparing parenting styles or parental mediation strategies *across* different social groups, further research should be conducted to understand these processes *within* a particular social group, as well, how even under particular cultural conditions and norms, variations in approaches are likely to exist.

Given that parental mediation is a form of parenting practice bound to social and cultural contexts, cultural differences are likely to manifest in parental mediation, as demonstrated by several cross-cultural studies. Kirwil (2009) found in European countries that co-use is preferred in individualistic cultures, whereas collectivistic cultures favor restrictive mediation. Shin and Lwin (2022) compared parental digital media mediation practices in two high digital penetration countries in the Asia Pacific: Australia (representing Western, individualistic culture) and Singapore (non-Western, collectivistic culture). They found that Australian parents were more proactively engaged in varying types of parental mediation to supervise and manage their children's digital device use. The authors argued that the finding reflected the cultural emphasis on holistic child upbringing and authoritative parenting in Australia that places great value on both responsiveness and demandingness. On the other hand, Singaporean parents, focusing heavily on academic success and technology as an academic aid, appeared less concerned and more relaxed about children's digital media use. Regarding the impact of culture on parental mediation *outcomes*, Chen and Shi's (2019) meta-analysis comparing Eastern and Western countries showed that active mediation was more effective in Eastern countries, likely due to the pervasive collectivism in these societies. The authors argued that in Eastern cultures, active mediation is more likely to align with subjective norms, where parental influence is deemed normative. Overall, although limited in quantity, existing studies suggest that national culture (or sub-culture within a country) plays an important role in understanding how and why parents engage in different forms and levels of parental mediation.

In addition to culture, the *socioeconomic status* (SES) of individuals within a cultural and societal context is presumed to have significant impacts on their knowledge of, access to, and competencies in various media platforms and content (Koch et al., 2024; Sun et al., 2021). In today's diverse and intricate media environment, effective parental mediation—especially discussion-based active mediation—demands considerable time and effort, making parental SES a crucial factor influencing the quality of home media education. For instance, Nikken and Opree (2018) demonstrated that low-income families tend to have fewer media devices at home, and due to these experiences of inequities in access, parents in lower-income, lower-education, and single-caregiver families often lack basic technical skills in digital media usage. Several studies have also documented a meaningful association between parental SES and active mediation. Specifically, Sun et al. (2021) found that affluent parents were more likely to engage in higher levels of active mediation, resulting in reduced levels of social network site addiction in children. Similarly, Koch et al. (2024) revealed that parents with high SES were more actively involved in active mediation, leading to increased youth digital maturity characterized by self-determined use of digital technologies for psychological growth and well-being.

Notably, these findings on SES also underscore the disadvantaged position of low SES families, highlighting inequities in home-based media education. Given these inequities in opportunities and access, parents in low SES are less likely to have the opportunity to acquire and develop media/digital literacy, rendering their mediation effort less effective and reducing children's chances of obtaining media-related knowledge and skills in the home context.

Macro and situational factors, such as national and global *crises*, can also affect parental mediation. A recent illustration of this phenomenon is COVID-19. This unprecedented global pandemic impacted various aspects of our lives, markedly altering children's use of media. With the extended lockdowns and social distancing measures, children in many societies had to forgo their usual social and outdoor activities. They spent prolonged periods at home, heavily relying on screen media to compensate for the lost social engagement opportunities (Nolan et al., 2022). The increase in screen time was observed across age groups globally, spanning North America (McClain, 2022), Europe (Trott et al., 2022), and Oceania (Rhodes, 2020). In terms of specific types of screen media, a national survey of Australian

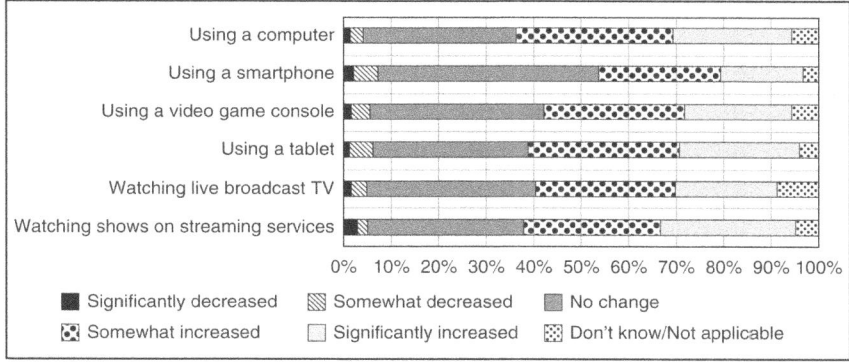

Figure 4.1 Changes in children's screen media use during COVID lockdowns.
Source: Child and Family Mediascape Research Group

parents, conducted by the Child and Family Mediascape Research Group at the University of Melbourne,[2] demonstrated that more than half of parents noticed increases rather than decreases in their children's use of multiple screen media during lockdowns (see Figure 4.1).

The transformed mediascape for children introduced new challenges for parents, who found it difficult to limit screen time due to its necessity for schoolwork and other activities.

Simultaneously, with parents also spending more time at home, they had to adjust their media intervention strategies to adapt to the new situation. Several surveys conducted during the pandemic provide empirical evidence for these adjustments: Australian parents relaxed their rules about children's screen time (Rhodes, 2020) and increased their engagement in media co-use during the lockdowns (Baxter et al., 2020). Parents in the United States were also less likely to limit their children's screen time (McClain, 2022). Similarly, parents in the UK struggled to control screen time, leading many to relax some of their media rules (Ofcom, 2021). Interestingly, Day et al. (2024) found that while parents in Australia increased their engagement in active mediation and co-use during the pandemic, the types of parental mediation employed returned closely to the patterns observed before the pandemic once the pandemic lockdowns concluded. In other words, parents reverted to their pre-pandemic strategies after the conclusion of COVID lockdowns. Taken together, prior studies suggest that parental mediation is not a static but a dynamic process, entailing active adaptation to social changes. This underscores the importance of understanding the overall media ecosystem surrounding children and their families, which may differ among families (Iqbal et al., 2021).

Conclusion and Future Agenda

Parental mediation research initially focused on how media intervention at home protects children from harmful television impacts. Over the last five decades, this field of study has expanded substantially, providing valuable insights into the crucial role that families and caregivers play in shaping children's media socialization across diverse platforms, including the internet, video games, social and mobile media, and smart technologies. The primary finding from this extensive research is that parents indeed influence children's acquisition and development of media-related knowledge, attitudes, skills, and behaviors. However, it is important to recognize that the effects of parental mediation are not uniform; they do not consistently result in the intended positive outcomes in children.

The impact and effectiveness of parental mediation, or how receptive children are to it, depend on various factors. It hinges on how parents implement media intervention strategies, the types of media involved, and parent-child characteristics. For instance, while restrictive mediation can be effective in reducing younger children's exposure to online harm, it can trigger psychological resistance in adolescents. Active mediation, on the other hand, may more effectively shape older children's media consumption attitudes and behaviors through two-way communication and social interaction, but it demands significant time, knowledge, and effort from parents. Co-use promotes family bonding and enhances parental understanding of media use without necessitating close regulations and purposeful discussions. However, it may not be particularly effective in developing children's media literacy, especially in more personal, peer-to-peer media contexts. The next chapter in this book will focus on media literacy in school and community settings.

Given that each strategy has its own set of pros and cons, and recognizing that the 'one-size-fits-all' approach is unlikely to achieve desired parenting outcomes, parents often combine different strategies or alter their tactics based on specific situations to enhance their influence on children's media use. The decision to implement varying mediation strategies is shaped not only by internal parent-child factors but also by cultural, societal, and environmental factors. In essence, parental mediation is a dynamic process, reflecting parents' adaptive strategies in response to intricate and ever-changing child mediascapes. While this chapter focused primarily on the three most traditional and widely known types of mediation—active mediation, restrictive, and co-use, it also noted that scholars in this field have proposed additional or hybrid dimensions of parental mediation such as technical mediation, selective mediation, and social co-use. This underscores the ongoing evolution of parental mediation, necessitating more nuanced approaches to both research and practical applications in the field.

Altogether, while parental mediation stands as a well-established field offering rich insights into the impact of homes on youth media socialization, there remain underexplored areas. First, parental mediation research has focused more on traditional and established media forms such as television and the internet than emerging technologies like short-form video, smart devices, algorithm-based or data-driven personalized media content, and generative AI. Additionally, most studies have centered on children's use of a single type of media, despite the reality that children often engage in media multitasking. Investigating evolving and emerging technologies and media trends warrants further research attention.

Second, even though parents commonly employ various mediation methods, limited research has delved into the combined or synergetic effects of these parental mediation strategies. This presents a significant gap in our understanding of real-world parental mediation practices, thereby offering an avenue for future research in this domain.

Third, much of the existing parental mediation research has been based on the views reflecting general populations or those with easy access to technologies in developed countries. There is a notable absence of research focusing specifically on disadvantaged populations or those in developing countries. Detailed investigations into marginalized segments with low income and limited access to media technology will provide a more comprehensive understanding of the role of families in youth media education. This, in turn, will contribute meaningfully to media policymaking centered on diversity, equity, and inclusion.

Lastly, while parents often teach and manage their children on media usage, they also learn from their youngsters about new media trends. This bottom-up child-to-parent socialization, commonly known as reverse socialization, is occurring, but academic research into reverse socialization in media remains scant. Given that one's knowledge and understanding of media affects their media practices, including parental mediation, the role of reverse socialization in parental mediation practice and its effect deserves further research attention.

Notes

1 Meta-analysis research involves the analysis of results from multiple empirical studies addressing the same topic to determine the overall trends of the examined research domain. For an overview of meta-analytic methodology, see Mikolajewicz and Komarova (2019).
2 https://arts.unimelb.edu.au/school-of-culture-and-communication/our-research/child-family-mediascape

References

An, S.-K., & Lee, D. (2010). An integrated model of parental mediation: The effect of family communication on children's perception of television reality and negative viewing effects. *Asian Journal of Communication, 20*(4), 389–403. https://doi.org/10.1080/01292986.2010.496864

Baxter, J., Budinski, M., Carolle, M., & Hand, K. (2020). *Life during COVID-19: Dads spend more quality time with kids.* https://aifs.gov.au/sites/default/files/publication-documents/covid-19-survey-report_4_dads_spend_more_quality_time_with_kids_0.pdf

Brehm, J. W. (1966). *A theory of psychological reactance.* Academic Press.

Buijzen, M., & Valkenburg, P. M. (2005). Parental mediation of undesired advertising effects. *Journal of Broadcasting & Electronic Media, 49*(2), 153–165. https://doi.org/10.1207/s15506878jobem4902_1

Bybee, C. R., Robinson, D., & Turow, J. (1982). Determinants of parental guidance of children's television viewing for a special subgroup: Mass media scholars. *Journal of Broadcasting, 26*(3), 697–710. https://doi.org/10.1080/08838158209364038

Chen, L., Liu, X., & Tang, H. (2023). The interactive effects of parental mediation strategies in preventing cyberbullying on social media. *Psychology Research and Behavior Management, 16*, 1009–1022. https://doi.org/10.2147/prbm.S386968

Chen, L., & Shi, J. (2019). Reducing harm from media: A meta-analysis of parental mediation. *Journalism & Mass Communication Quarterly, 96*(1), 173–193. https://doi.org/10.1177/1077699018754908

Collier, K. M., Coyne, S. M., Hawkins, A. J., Padilla-Walker, L. M., Erickson, S. E., Memmott-Elison, M. K., & Rasmussen, E. E. (2016). Does parental mediation of media influence child outcomes? A meta-analysis on media time, aggression, substance use, and sexual behavior. *Developmental Psychology, 52*(5), 798–812. https://doi.org/10.1037/dev0000108

Day, K., Shin, W., & Nolan, S. (2024). Children's reading and screen media use before, during and after the pandemic: Australian parent perspectives. *Communication Research and Practice, 10*(1), 45–59. https://doi.org/10.1080/22041451.2024.2322810

Desmond, R. J., Singer, J. L., Singer, D. G., Calam, R., & Colimore, K. (1985). Family mediation patterns and television viewing. *Human Communication Research, 11*(4), 461–480. https://doi.org/10.1111/j.1468-2958.1985.tb00056.x

Dorr, A., Kovaric, P., & Doubleday, C. (1989). Parent-child coviewing of television. *Journal of Broadcasting & Electronic Media, 33*(1), 35–51. https://doi.org/10.1080/08838158909364060

Eastin, M. S., Greenberg, B. S., & Hofschire, L. (2006). Parenting the internet. *Journal of Communication, 56*(3), 486–504. https://doi.org/10.1111/j.1460-2466.2006.00297.x

Godleski, S. A., Eiden, R. D., Shisler, S., & Livingston, J. A. (2020). Parent socialization of emotion in a high-risk sample. *Developmental Psychology, 56*(3), 489–502.

Grusec, J. E. (2002). Parental socialization and children's acquisition of values. In M. H. Bornstein (Ed.), *Handbook of parenting* (2nd ed., Vol. 5: Practical Issues in Parenting, pp. 143–167). Psychology Press.

Grusec, J. E., & Davidov, M. (2007). Socialization in the family: The roles of parents. In J. E. Grusec, & P. D. Hastings (Eds.), *Handbook of socialization: Theory and research* (pp. 287–308). The Guilford Press.

Iqbal, S., Zakar, R., & Fischer, F. (2021). Extended theoretical framework of parental internet mediation: Use of multiple theoretical stances for understanding socio-ecological predictors [conceptual analysis]. *Frontiers in Psychology, 12*. https://doi.org/10.3389/fpsyg.2021.620838

Jiow, H. J., Lim, S. S., & Lin, J. (2016). Level up! Refreshing parental mediation theory for our digital media landscape. *Communication Theory, 27*(3), 309–328. https://doi.org/10.1111/comt.12109

Kang, H., Shin, W., & Huang, J. (2022). Teens' privacy management on video-sharing social media: The roles of perceived privacy risk and parental mediation. *Internet Research, 32*(1), 312–334. https://doi.org/10.1108/INTR-01-2021-0005

Kirwil, L. (2009). Parental mediation of children's internet use in different European countries. *Journal of Children and Media, 3*(4), 394–409. https://doi.org/10.1080/17482790903233440

Koch, T., Laaber, F., & Florack, A. (2024). Socioeconomic status and young people's digital maturity: The role of parental mediation. *Computers in Human Behavior, 154*, 108157. https://doi.org/10.1016/j.chb.2024.108157

Kunkel, D. (1999). Children's television policy in the United States: An ongoing legacy of change. *Media International Australia, Incorporating Culture and Policy, 93*, 51–63. https://research.ebsco.com/linkprocessor/plink?id=15f8634a-8954-338d-b82e-20b240dbf2c4

Laible, D., & Thompson, R. A. (2007). Early socialization: A relationship perspective. In J. E. Grusec, & P. D. Hastings (Eds.), *Handbook of socialization: Theory and research* (pp. 181–207). The Guilford Press.

Liu, Y.-L. (2020). Maternal mediation as an act of privacy invasion: The association with internet addiction, *Computers in Human Behavior, 112*, 106474. https://doi.org/10.1016/j.chb.2020.106474

Livingstone, S., Haddon, L., Görzig, A., & Ólafsson, K. (2011) Risks and safety on the internet: the perspective of European children: full findings and policy implications from the EU Kids Online survey of 9-16 year olds and their parents in 25 countries. *EU Kids Online*, Deliverable D4. EU Kids Online Network, London, UK.

Livingstone, S., & Helsper, E. J. (2008). Parental mediation of children's internet use. *Journal of Broadcasting & Electronic Media, 52*(4), 581–599. https://doi.org/10.1080/08838150802437396

Lwin, M. O., Shin, W., Yee, A. Z. H., & Wardoyo, R. J. (2017). A parental health education model of children's food consumption: Influence on children's attitudes, intention, and consumption of healthy and unhealthy foods. *Journal of Health Communication, 22*(5), 403–412. https://doi.org/10.1080/10810730.2017.1302523

Lwin, M. O., Stanaland, A. J. S., & Miyazaki, A. D. (2008). Protecting children's privacy online: How parental mediation strategies affect website safeguard effectiveness. *Journal of Retailing, 84*(2), 205–217. https://doi.org/10.1016/j.jretai.2008.04.004

McClain, C. (2022). *How parents' views of their kids' screen time, social media use changed during COVID-19*. Pew Research Center. https://www.pewresearch.org/short-reads/2022/04/28/how-parents-views-of-their-kids-screen-time-social-media-use-changed-during-covid-19/

Mendoza, K. (2009). Surveying parental mediation: Connections, challenges and questions for media literacy. *Journal of Media Literacy Education, 1*, 28–41.

Mikolajewicz, N., & Komarova, S. V. (2019). Meta-analytic methodology for basic research: A practical guide [methods]. *Frontiers in Physiology, 10*. https://doi.org/10.3389/fphys.2019.00203

Minjin, R., & Horowitz, J. (2023). *Parenting in America today.* https://www.pewresearch.org/social-trends/2023/01/24/race-ethnicity-and-parenting/

Nathanson, A. I. (1999). Identifying and explaining the relationship between parental mediation and children's aggression. *Communication Research*, 26(2), 124–143. https://doi.org/10.1177/009365099026002002

Nikken, P. (2018). Do (pre)adolescents mind about healthy media use: Relationships with parental mediation, demographics and use of devices. *Cyberpsychology*, 12(2), 1–13. https://doi.org/10.5817/CP2018-2-1

Nikken, P., & Jansz, J. (2006). Parental mediation of children's videogame playing: A comparison of the reports by parents and children. *Learning, Media and Technology*, 31(2), 181–202. https://doi.org/10.1080/17439880600756803

Nikken, P., & Opree, S. J. (2018). Guiding young children's digital media use: SES-differences in mediation concerns and competence. *Journal of Child and Family Studies*, 27(6), 1844–1857. https://doi.org/10.1007/s10826-018-1018-3

Nolan, S., Day, K., Shin, W., & Wang, W. Y. (2022). Books versus screens: A study of Australian children's media use during the COVID pandemic. *Publishing Research Quarterly*, 38(4), 749–759. https://doi.org/10.1007/s12109-022-09899-w

Ofcom. (2021). *Children and parents: Media use and attitudes report 2020/2021.* https://www.ofcom.org.uk/__data/assets/pdf_file/0025/217825/children-and-parents-media-use-and-attitudes-report-2020-21.pdf

Padilla-Walker, L. M., Coyne, S. M., & Fraser, A. M. (2012). Getting a high-speed family connection: Associations between family media use and family connection. *Family Relations*, 61(3), 426–440. https://doi.org/10.1111/j.1741-3729.2012.00710.x

Rhodes, A. (2020). *COVID-19 pandemic: Effects on the lives of Australian children and families.* https://rchpoll.org.au/wp-content/uploads/2020/07/nchp-poll18-report-covid.pdf

Ryan, R. M., & Deci, E. L. (2000). Self-determination theory and the facilitation of intrinsic motivation, social development, and well-being. *American Psychologist*, 55(1), 68–78. https://doi.org/10.1037//0003-066x.55.1.68

Sasson, H., & Mesch, G. (2014). Parental mediation, peer norms and risky online behavior among adolescents. *Computers in Human Behavior*, 33, 32–38. https://doi.org/10.1016/j.chb.2013.12.025

Shin, W. (2015). Parental socialization of children's internet use: A qualitative approach. *New Media & Society*, 17(5), 649–665. https://doi.org/10.1177/1461444813516833

Shin, W. (2018). Empowered parents: The role of self-efficacy in parental mediation of children's smartphone use in the United States. *Journal of Children and Media*, 12(4), 465–477. https://doi.org/10.1080/17482798.2018.1486331

Shin, W., & Kang, H. (2016). Adolescents' privacy concerns and information disclosure online: The role of parents and the internet. *Computers in Human Behavior*, 54, 114–123. https://doi.org/10.1016/j.chb.2015.07.062

Shin, W., & Kim, H. K. (2019). What motivates parents to mediate children's use of smartphones? An application of the theory of planned behavior. *Journal of Broadcasting & Electronic Media*, 63(1), 144–159. https://doi.org/10.1080/08838151.2019.1576263

Shin, W., & Lwin, M. O. (2017). How does "talking about the internet with others" affect teenagers' experience of online risks? The role of active mediation by parents, peers, and school teachers. *New Media & Society*, 19(7), 1109–1126. https://doi.org/10.1177/1461444815626612

Shin, W., & Lwin, O. M. (2019). *Screen obsessed: Parenting in the digital age.* World Scientific.

Shin, W., & Lwin, M. O. (2022). Parental mediation of children's digital media use in high digital penetration countries: Perspectives from Singapore and Australia. *Asian Journal of Communication, 32*(4), 309–326. https://doi.org/10.1080/01292986.2022.2026992

Shin, W., Lwin, M. O., Yee, A. Z. H., & Kee, K. M. (2020). The role of socialization agents in adolescents' responses to app-based mobile advertising. *International Journal of Advertising, 39*(3), 365–386. https://doi.org/10.1080/02650487.2019.1648138

Steinfeld, N. (2021). Parental mediation of adolescent internet use: Combining strategies to promote awareness, autonomy and self-regulation in preparing youth for life on the web. *Education and Information Technologies, 26*(2), 1897–1920.

Sun, X., Duan, C., Yao, L., Zhang, Y., Chinyani, T., & Niu, G. (2021). Socioeconomic status and social networking site addiction among children and adolescents: Examining the roles of parents' active mediation and ICT attitudes. *Computers & Education, 173,* 104292. https://doi.org/10.1016/j.compedu.2021.104292

Tannen, D., Kendall, S., Gordon, C., Tannen, D., Kendall, S., & Gordon, C. (2007). Gatekeeping in the family: How family members position one another as decision makers. In D. Tannen, S. Kendall, & C. Gordon (Eds.), *Family talk: Discourse and identity in four American families* (pp. 165–194). Oxford University Press. https://doi.org/10.1093/acprof:oso/9780195313895.003.0007

Trott, M., Driscoll, R., Irlado, E., & Pardhan, S. (2022). Changes and correlates of screen time in adults and children during the COVID-19 pandemic: A systematic review and meta-analysis. *EClinicalMedicine, 48,* 101452. https://doi.org/10.1016/j.eclinm.2022.101452

Wang, M., Lwin, M. O., Cayabyab, Y. M. T. M., Hou, G., & You, Z. (2023). A meta-analysis of factors predicting parental mediation of children's media use based on studies published between 1992–2019. *Journal of Child and Family Studies, 32*(5), 1249–1260. https://doi.org/10.1007/s10826-022-02459-y

Wang, B., Taylor, L., & Sun, Q. (2018). Families that play together stay together: Investigating family bonding through video games. *New Media and Society, 20*(11), 4074–4094. https://doi.org/10.1177/1461444818767667

Warren, R. (2017). Multi-platform mediation: U.S. mothers' and fathers' mediation of teens' media use. *Journal of Children and Media, 11*(4), 485–500. https://doi.org/10.1080/17482798.2017.1349685

Yee, A. Z. H., Lwin, M. O., & Lau, J. (2019). Parental guidance and children's healthy food consumption: Integrating the theory of planned behavior with interpersonal communication antecedents. *Journal of Health Communication, 24*(2), 183–194. https://doi.org/10.1080/10810730.2019.1593552

5 Media Literacy Education

Srividya Ramasubramanian, Shannon Burth, and Patrick R. Johnson

This chapter covers definitions, examples, and contemporary debates about media literacy education through the lens of access, diversity, inclusion, and equity. We consider how media literacy enriches the lives of children and teens while also empowering them, with positive implications for their knowledge of and social interactions in the world around them and about themselves. We share up-to-date theory and research findings relevant to media literacy education, especially for diverse young media users, while drawing connections with larger questions of access, equity, diversity, and inclusion. We also look at how media literacy education could sometimes, ironically, exclude minoritized youth, thus reinforcing rather than challenging power, status quo, hierarchies, and inequalities. This chapter explores how media literacy education can reflect or challenge wider hierarchies of societal power and privilege.

Media Literacy Education: Definitions and Conceptualization

Definitions of media literacy are varying, contested, and evolving. In 2007, the National Association of Media Literacy Education (NAMLE) defined media literacy as the ability to "access, analyze, evaluate, create, and act using all forms of communication" (National Association for Media Literacy Education, 2007, para 1). This definition has been recently updated to encompass our changing media landscape and social world. As of 2023, the definition has been expanded to include more forms of media (electronic, visual, and digital) and more applications of these skills (hands-on experiences and media production) (National Association for Media Literacy Education, 2023, para. 3-4). To increase clarity, the National Association for Media Literacy Education (n.d.) offers the following definition of media literacy, in addition to their original description from 2007:

> Media refers to all electronic or digital means and print or artistic visuals used to transmit messages. Literacy is the ability to encode

and decode symbols and to synthesize and analyze messages. Media literacy is the ability to encode and decode the symbols transmitted via media and synthesize, analyze and produce mediated messages.

Media education is the study of media, including 'hands-on' experiences and media production. Media literacy education is the educational field dedicated to teaching the skills associated with media literacy.

Broadly, *literacy* refers to learning in ways where learners gain competencies to use their skills to participate within society. That is, learners must be able to use the competencies they attain within specific contexts of their everyday lives. Media and communication involve the ability to access, make sense of, and create texts. With the advent of Internet technologies and other new media systems, traditional print literacies relating to the ability to read and write have now evolved into multimedia literacies and digital literacies. While books and print literacies remain important in education, teachers, parents, and other educators have also had to restructure education to accommodate new media literacies into their curriculum. Therefore, media literacy is closely related to digital literacy, new media literacy, multimedia literacy, news literacy, advertising literacy, entertainment literacy, and information literacy. However, these terms also have slightly different meanings. For instance, *news literacy* only relates to the ability to access, interpret, and produce news messages. *Information literacy* refers to accessing, evaluating, and interpreting information, including from but not limited to media sources. More recently, with the increasing relevance of algorithms, digital platforms, and datafication within the larger generative AI context, we also need to consider including *data and algorithmic literacy* within the overall umbrella of media literacy.

While it is typically believed that there are two main approaches to media literacy education—protectionism and empowerment—these two are often intertwined, and such broad classifications oversimplify the complexity of media literacy education. *Protectionist perspectives* were initially developed to address and focus primarily on the negative effects of media that were seen as harmful, especially to children (Hobbs & Jensen, 2009). Critics of this perspective shifted the conversation to an *empowerment perspective*, focusing less on media's negative influence and more on users' agency. This approach to media literacy education focuses more on how students use, produce, and engage with media (Hobbs, 2011). In reality, most media literacy interventions combine the protectionist and empowerment perspectives to encourage critical reflection on media content, including understanding how media affects individuals and society. Instead of seeing this as a dichotomy or an "either-or" situation, protection *and* empowerment are necessary in media literacy education (Hobbs, 2010). These approaches are deeply linked, especially if the goal is to embrace digital media for social change while also being candid about the inherent risks associated with youth and adolescents interacting online (Hobbs, 2010).

While reviewing different types of media literacy education and its impact, we will continue to refer back to NAMLE's core principles (access, analyze, evaluate, create, and act) and move past a simplistic dichotomy of protectionist versus empowerment approaches in ways that further a more nuanced understanding of contemporary media literacy education.

Critical Media Literacy for Understanding Diversity, Equity, and Inclusion

Media literacy education connects with diversity, equity, and inclusion (DEI) in many different ways. Using NAMLE's definition of media literacy as "access, analyze, evaluate, create, and act using all forms of communication" (see Figure 5.1), we can consider how issues of equity and inclusion influence each step of this process.

COMPETENCIES OF DIGITAL AND MEDIA LITERACY

Competency	DESCRIPTION
Access	Finding and using media and technology tools skillfully, while sharing appropriate and relevant information with others.
Analyze	Decoding, interpreting, and making sense of media messages and their representations, including thinking about the media industries/creators behind the messages.
Evaluate	Making judgments about media messages and their accuracy, credibility, and quality. This also includes critiquing or challenging these messages and considering their potential effects.
Create	Composing or generating content using creativity and confidence in self expression, with purpose, audience, and composition techniques in mind.
Act	Using media individually or collaboratively to share knowledge with your communities. This also includes participating at local, national, and international levels to contribute to change making.

Sources: *Digital and media literacy: a plan of action*, Renee Hobbs (https://www.aspeninstitute.org/wp-content/uploads/2010/11/Digital_and_Media_Literacy.pdf); *Critically analyzing the meanings of "critical" media literacy*, W. James Potter (https://doi.org/10.23860/JMLE-2023-15-3-9); *Core principles of media literacy education*, National Association for Media Literacy Education (https://namle.org/wp-content/uploads/2023/05/NAMLE-Principles-Final-2.1.pdf)

Figure 5.1 Competencies of media and digital literacy.
Source: Authors

Regarding *"access,"* research on the digital divide reminds us that material access to media is not universal but disparate due to location, socioeconomic status, etc. (Ragnedda & Muschert, 2013; Van Dijk, 1999, see Chapter 2). The participation gap refers to the uneven distribution of skills and knowledge needed for online participation, even after fulfilling material access (Jenkins, 2006). Next, we can consider the skills associated with *"analyze"* in terms of how learners have the literacies to make sense of, interpret, and analyze media representations. Here, inclusion and diversity are important considerations regarding how various social groups are represented, underrepresented, and misrepresented within the media.

Then, we consider *evaluation* of media content regarding the message's veracity, credibility, and quality. This could be a more technical evaluation of the media message's syntax, grammar, aesthetics, and technical aspects. It could also include evaluating the quality of the message in terms of critical thinking to consider biases, stereotypes, and ideological considerations (see Chapters 3 and 7). Next, media literacy education can include *creation*. Curricula and activities that embody "create" can range from podcast production (Montgomery, 2014) to poetry (Call-Cummings et al., 2020). Creation-based media literacy education is hands-on and student-centric. Creation also presents opportunities to develop and share a more diverse set of stories, voices, and experiences, which can ultimately lead to a more inclusive media environment. Finally, media literacy education can include *action.* Act is the final principle from NAMLE's definition and includes active digital citizenship, including civic participation (voting, attending rallies, donating to advocacy groups; Berger, 2009; see Chapter 10) and media activism.

The core principles of media literacy were put forth by Len Masterman (2001) and the Center for Media Literacy (http://www.medialit.org/bp_mlk.html) They are as follows:

1 All media are socially constructed
2 Media messages are constructed with their syntax and grammar
3 The same media message can be experienced differently by different people
4 All media messages have values, beliefs, worldviews, and biases embedded in them
5 Media messages are created to gain power or profit

These core principles are foundational to connecting media literacy education and DEI. By stating that all media are constructed, we challenge simplistic assumptions that media are a mirror of society that presents reality as it is. Therefore, the starting point of connecting media literacy with DEI is to understand that media are created, shaped, organized, and positioned in specific ways within the larger symbol systems within society. Media are not windows into the world but instead constructions of meanings using coded signs and symbols within a culture.

Media are part of symbol systems within society. These symbols and signifiers are not arbitrary but are connected with ideology and hegemony. In other words, dominant groups' culture, values, preferences, worldviews, and beliefs are typically privileged within mainstream media messages. Therefore, media often serve as cultural tools for constructing dominant groups as "naturally" superior, normal, ideal, and preferred.

This aspect of connecting media literacy with larger societal structures, power, authority, and dominant groups is called *critical media literacy*. Critical media literacy involves a critical analysis of media to interrogate structures of power and systems of oppression (Kellner & Share, 2005). It helps develop critical consciousness with media users to use their agency and voice to consider media in the broader societal context and challenge dominant ideologies (Kellner & Share, 2007; Potter, 2023).

Notably, the National Association for Media Literacy Education (2023) has now included critical media literacy within its recently revised core principles, emphasizing that media literacy should present diverse perspectives and amplify historically marginalized voices, including voices from the Global South and geographic areas without much digital access. Indeed, it centers on inclusion and social justice by emphasizing critical inquiry about systems of power, oppression, and inequities within media industries.

In the rest of this chapter, we use critical media literacy as the foundation to elaborate on existing gaps and potential areas for improvement within media literacy education to make it more inclusive and equitable. Although not numerous, some organizations and institutes provide instructional resources such as lesson plans, guides, activities, and toolkits focusing on diversity, inclusion, and equity. We share these as case studies and examples for those interested in accessing these materials, such as teachers, youth organizers, educators, scholars, parents, content creators, and media users.

Access and Media Literacy Education

As noted, access is the first consideration for media literacy education. When implementing MLE, it is important to ask: Who has access to media? To media literacy? To media literacy education? Access can be linked to individual (i.e., income, gender, language literacy, tech access, race, age, sexuality, ability) and institutional (i.e., policies, priorities, government/ state, space, time, support for teachers) factors.

Schools are the most common institutions associated with media literacy, often providing access to spaces, programs, and resources for students, teachers, and parents. Schools are the most likely place to build a sustainable educational infrastructure for media literacy education. At the time of writing, three states in USA (Delaware, New Jersey, and Texas) require K-12 media literacy instruction; five (Colorado, Connecticut, Illinois, Nebraska, and Rhode Island) require limited media literacy instruction; and six require media literacy standards across K-12 (Delaware, Florida, New Jersey, and Ohio) or in some grade levels (Minnesota and Nebraska) (McNeill & Duff, 2024). This leaves many students without required access to media literacy and media literacy education in their schools. Although media literacy education is more widely available in some global locations (such as Canada, Australia, and the United Kingdom), such sporadic access is frequently the case around the world.

In most of the United States, media literacy is not mandatory in the curriculum. This means that much of media literacy instruction is done by teachers and librarians who actively want to address media literacy in their education spaces. Non-profit organizations and after-school programs are increasingly important in providing educators with resources to teach their students how to become more media literate. Leaving the teaching of media literacy to individuals could also mean not guaranteeing equitable access to media literacy education for all students.

We highlight two media literacy organizations as examples of how to address access issues. *Project Look Sharp* tackles access through institutional levels, particularly targeting students' needs and providing teachers with instructional resources to aid media literacy and access to media literacy in schools. The second, *Common Sense Media*, addresses access at an individual level, especially for parents. They seek to identify ways to improve parents' access to media literacy and topics emerging within it, like gender, race, and sexuality.

Media literacy organizations like **Project Look Sharp** (PLS) (https://www.projectlooksharp.org/) seek to address access for students and teachers in their work. PLS utilizes "critical thinking, metacognition, and civic engagement" to enhance K-16 students' media literacy. PLS has created hundreds of lesson plans—over 500 free, and hosted professional development experiences worldwide to bring media literacy to all communities. They do this thanks to external funders, which allow these materials to be accessible beyond Ithaca, New York, where they are located. The PLS team designed the materials (i.e., lesson plans, handouts, and guides) to be usable across grade levels, disciplines, and topics. In doing so, PLS believes they are making media literacy easier to build into curricula and more accessible to students of all demographics. One of the defining features of their media literacy programming is what they call their "way of thinking," which is the "***constructivist media decoding method.***" The approach helps students to (1) decode a message, (2) be reflective through inquiry-based thinking, and (3) build a deeper understanding of "students' mediated reality." The organization shares that this approach is "highly successful with traditionally disenfranchised students" (Project Look Sharp, 2024). By giving students and teachers a shared way of thinking, their method emphasizes an approach to media literacy education where addressing inequitable access is a priority for building more inclusive and equitable futures.

Another organization, *Common Sense Media* (https://www.commonsensemedia.org/), aims to give parents/caregivers more authority over access to media. By providing tips and reviews of various media, *Common Sense Media* highlights what parents should expect from their children's media choices. It provides recommendations based on the child's age, the media's content, and other parent recommendations. This creates an information ecosystem that not only gives parents what they "Need to Know" but also is a space for parents to articulate their understanding of the media texts critically. Built on a mission to "protect privacy and support community," *Common Sense Media* aims to enhance "advocacy efforts around digital equity and tech accountability" through media literacy practices focused on parents (Common Sense Media, 2024). Therefore, parents who might not be familiar with media literacy can still access such educational resources, including if they belong to traditionally marginalized communities without access to such materials and resources.

Diversity and Media Literacy Education

Diversity intersects with media literacy education by 1) looking at representations in media texts and 2) working with diverse populations to increase media literacy skills. Diversity, in both cases, refers to race, ethnicity, social class, gender, ability status, and sexual identity, among other identities. Likewise, diverse media representations can sit at the intersection of several of these identities, representing, say, women of color or queer disabled individuals.

To address diverse media representation in media literacy education, we can revisit NAMLE's core principles of "analyze" and "evaluate," as well as inquiry-based critical media literacy. Analyzing and evaluating means thinking critically about the media messages we create and receive. By remembering that all media messages are "constructed" and have embedded ideologies, we can approach each message through this lens (NAMLE, n.d.). To focus on the diversity of representation in media, we can ask: Who made this media text? Who does this media text privilege? What values, ideologies, and points of view are represented (or missing) from this text? (Kellner & Share, 2019). In practice, media literacy education encourages us to ask these questions, in and out of the classroom, with peer, teachers and other educators, and at home with family and friends (Kellner & Share, 2019).

Scholarly work on diversity of media representation reveals a significant need for media literacy education to encourage these conversations. For example, content analyses such as the study conducted by Bond (2014) reveal an overrepresentation of heterosexuality and an underrepresentation of LGBTQ identities in media. Similarly, scholars consistently and across time note disproportionate and inaccurate media representations of racial and ethnic minorities (Mastro, 2015; Mastro & Stern, 2003; Scharrer et al., 2022; Tukachinsky et al., 2015). Botha and Harvey (2024) also point out how physical disabilities are often misrepresented in entertainment media. Media literacy education can teach the skills to interrogate how diverse media representations are, considering misrepresentation or lack of representation. Scharrer and Ramasubramanian (2015) point out how, though understudied, this link between diverse media representation and media literacy education holds great potential.

Also, we see media literacy organizations that address and serve diverse populations. This can address elements of "access" that are discussed above. Access to media literacy skills is the first step and is often not as readily available to minoritized populations. This section will highlight organizations offering media literacy education to diverse and minoritized populations. This includes organizations that work with diverse racial and ethnic minorities, social classes, genders, disabilities, and sexual identities. Many also take an intersectional approach, engaging with multiple minoritized identities, and often with youth populations.

Several media literacy organizations are devoted to promoting diversity, especially the voices of minoritized youth from marginalized communities. One such organization that works with marginalized youth is the *Narratio Fellowship* (https://narratio.org/), a U.S.-based program dedicated to working with resettled refugee youth to foster storytelling and leadership skills while receiving media training and networking support. The fellows use multiple media to share their experiences with immigration, displacement, and resettlement through films, poetry, and photography.

Similarly, at the intersection of race/ethnicity and gender, organizations such as *Latinitas* (https://latinitasonline.org/) and the *Black Girls' Literacy Collective* (https://www.barrettrosser.com/bglp) teach women of color to challenge stereotypical representations with alternative storytelling. By telling alternative stories of representation, women center their lived experiences and disrupt stereotypical media representations of women of color (McArthur, 2016; Sousa & Ramasubramanian, 2017). Likewise, organizations such as *Girls Who Code* (https://girlswhocode.com/) teach important digital literacy skills to young women from historically underrepresented groups in computer science, a typically male-dominated field. *ZUMIX* (www.zumix.org) is also dedicated to developing digital skills, specifically those associated with music production. Located in Boston, ZUMIX is designed to offer the tools and skills needed to develop award-winning music for low-income youth.

Organizations such as *Ability Media* (www.abilitymediagroup.com) and *Visions & Voices* (https://visions-voices.org/) were created to address the lack of representation for disabled individuals in media. *It Gets Better* (https://itgetsbetter.org/) and *Global Action Project* (https://global-action.org/) harness the power of storytelling to empower LGBTQ+ youth. Both also provide a wide range of resources for workshops and curricula.

These organizations provide materials, resources, workshops, and fellowship opportunities for diverse and often minoritized populations to increase media literacy skills.

Equity and Media Literacy Education

Although media literacy education emphasizes the diversity of representation in the media, equity is not achieved automatically. *Equity* is about challenging and responding to historic inequities in access, opportunity, and participation in media and education. The recent glossary of terms shared by NAMLE defines equity as "justice and fairness in creating equal outcomes for all, especially for minoritized, marginalized, and underserved groups" (National Association of Media Literacy Education, 2023).

An equitable media literacy education should address systemic inequities by ensuring all young people have the necessary access and resources to engage with media critically. This involves rethinking K-12 education systems to integrate equity and social justice into media literacy education, moving beyond individualistic approaches to foster collective action and civic engagement (Ramasubramanian & Darzabi, 2020). Moreover, addressing issues of difference requires going beyond multiculturalist perspectives that celebrate cultural diversity without tackling deeper issues of colonialism, racial hierarchies, and white supremacy (Ramasubramanian & Miles, 2018). This extends to other forms of inequities as well.

The digital divide starkly illustrates inequitable access to media (see Chapter 2). Communities of color, tribal reservations, and economically disadvantaged areas often face significant barriers to technological and media infrastructure, exacerbated by historical practices like redlining and the neoliberal media market (Ibrahim, 2023; Korostelina & Barrett, 2023). This divide extends to educational settings, where public schools in wealthier, typically White neighborhoods enjoy better access to broadband internet and media resources. This leaves children from lower-income families at a significant disadvantage, especially during the COVID-19 pandemic (Berners-Lee, 2020; Vogels, 2021).

Media literacy, traditionally focused on individual skills such as critical thinking and comprehension, often overlooks broader societal and community-level concerns such as access. Media literacy education is crucial for empowering youth to navigate the complex digital landscape they inherit. This educational process is integral to fostering equitable civic participation, yet disparities in access and opportunities present significant challenges.

Media literacy education requires attending to the multifaceted relationship between media literacy education and equity, particularly regarding community-level factors and a model for *equitable media literacy practice* (EMLP) (Johnson et al., 2024). The EMLP model emphasizes the need for media literacy practices to be deeply intertwined with equity and social justice issues, something several scholars have acknowledged previously (see also Frechette, 2019; Hobbs, 2010; Mihailidis et al., 2021b). According to EMLP, equity in media literacy education refers to fair access, opportunity, and advancement for all, striving to eliminate barriers that hinder the participation of marginalized groups. This approach underscores the interconnectedness of individual agency, community empowerment, and democratic support within media literacy education (Mihailidis et al., 2021a). Furthermore, media literacy education must extend beyond the classroom to involve community organizations, media professionals, and families in collaborative efforts to promote civic participation and engagement with diverse perspectives (Jenkins et al., 2018; Martens & Hobbs, 2015). This collaborative approach is crucial for developing a more just and equitable society where media literacy empowers individuals as critical media consumers and active participants in democracy.

Equitable media literacy education is pivotal for fostering informed, engaged, and critically thinking citizens. By addressing structural inequities, promoting collaboration, empowering community change agents, and creating inclusive spaces for dialogue and action, media literacy education can contribute to a more equitable and democratic society. To achieve this, the EMLP framework proposes four components: *addressing inequitable access, fostering collaboration, empowering change agents*, and *making space for marginalized voices*. These components emphasize systemic improvement, action-oriented collaboration, community empowerment, and creating inclusive spaces for critical engagement with media. For instance, technological infrastructure improvements and educational initiatives must be prioritized to bridge the digital divide and ensure equitable access to media literacy resources. This model fosters a relational, communal, and collaborative environment, addressing the often-neglected aspects of traditional media literacy education. Through heightened civic engagement and democratic participation, EMLP positions equity at the core of media literacy, urging practitioners to confront and mitigate structural barriers. EMLP aims to illuminate and tackle the inherent challenges of achieving equity amidst diverse individual, community, and societal concerns (Johnson et al., 2024).

Inclusion and Media Literacy Education

While diversity is the presence of difference, inclusion is about valuing diversity through the lens of historical inequities to bring about intentional changes to practice and policies. *Inclusion* is about creating a welcoming environment and a sense of belonging, especially for those who might have been historically marginalized. As the examples and case studies discussed above illustrate, media and education can be sites where societal inequalities, exclusions, and marginalization are experienced based on a range of identities such as gender, race, ethnicity, citizenship status, religion, sexual orientation, ability, and so on. For instance, mainstream media and public education systems tend to replicate and reinforce dominant ideologies rather than challenge them (Ramasubramanian et al., 2021). Building on the EMLP framework that centers equity, collaboration, empowerment of changemakers, and centering of marginalized voices (Johnson et al., 2024), we ask what it takes to move from recognizing historic inequities toward deliberate steps for a culture of inclusion and belongingness within media literacy education.

Indeed, recognizing the need for greater inclusion within media literacy practice and research, NAMLE notes that historically marginalized groups and communities are those "that have been and may continue to be relegated to the periphery of society and denied full participation in society because of unequal power dynamics in social, political, and cultural systems." Such conversations about equity, inclusion, and social justice have traditionally not been central to media literacy education. In the last decade, there has been an increased consciousness about issues such as systemic racism, gender bias, and environmental injustices, leading to greater self-reflection among media literacy education practitioners considering questions of equity within media literacy education.

Mainstream media and platforms play an important role in what types of media stories are being created. Given that ownership of media corporations continues to be extremely biased by a few powerful elites, with only half a dozen digital corporations monopolizing almost the entire digital media infrastructure, the diversity of content, perspectives, and voices is also limited (Pickard, 2020). Furthermore, media corporations are skewed to represent socio-political elites and are focused on commercial interests rather than serving the citizenry for democratic purposes. Because of this concentration of ownership and consolidation of various media formats and organizations, there has been very little original, innovative, and creative entertainment media (Hendrickx & Ranaivoson, 2021; Stanton et al., 2020; Wargo & Clayton, 2018; Yosso, 2000, 2002). With the advent and popularity of social media such as Facebook and Instagram and digital technological platforms such as Google, there are concerns about rampant misinformation within media platforms, which often benefit these companies in generating audience interactions. Due to their profit orientation, there is little interest in public discourse or digital citizenship for dialogue and civic engagement in these platforms.

When considering who is excluded from media literacy education, one must contend that millions of children worldwide continue not to have basic access to media and education. Even frameworks such as EMLP remain within the larger knowledge production and media industry largely centered in the Global North, the West, and Eurocentrism. There are many taken-for-granted ways in which media literacy education is structured that continue to privilege dominant ideas of democracy, whiteness, and Anglocentric privilege that will take concerted efforts to correct. Thus, they must be adapted, tested, and expanded to be relevant and meaningful to contexts beyond Western, educated, democratic, and rich nations. To achieve this vision, we must build our capacity to adapt media literacy to serve a more inclusive future, actively making space for marginalized voices and ensuring that democracy becomes an equitable domain for all citizens.

A Trauma-Informed Equity-Minded Asset-Based Model (TEAM) for Media Literacy Education

Media literacy's evolution calls for a forward-looking, equitable, and democratic approach that promises a more inclusive community engagement. We must take action-oriented, multi-pronged, collaborative approaches to achieve the shared ideal of inclusive and just futures within media literacy education, the media industry, and educational systems. In this section, we share a *Trauma-informed, Equity-minded Asset-based Model* (*TEAM*) as a framework to move us closer to this shared collective goal of greater inclusion within media literacy education.

The *trauma-informed approach* recognizes that social institutions, including education and media, can serve as sites of long-term generational and cultural trauma. Here, trauma is to be understood not as physical or even emotional distress but as chronic trauma that affects multiple generations and is related to marginalization, trivialization, and erasures of people, practices, and perspectives that are deemed as the Other. Such othering within the context of media and education is evident in ways that curricula, syllabi, excellence, merit, beauty, intelligence, and other moral judgments are associated with cultural hegemony and dominant group values. For instance, within the United States, education systems, including media literacy education, are embedded within deeply ingrained principles of normative whiteness (Ramasubramanian et al., 2021). For dominant group members within these educational systems, how whiteness is enmeshed with education through values, beliefs, unstated norms, and expectations within and outside the classroom are often not immediately apparent because of their privilege. However, minoritized communities excluded from policies, practices, and power networks might experience these systems, including educational systems, as sites of generational oppression and cultural trauma that is replicated through the centuries. Similarly, media systems could serve as spaces where social groups are marginalized, erased, ridiculed, or trivialized.

One needs to take an *equity-minded approach* to address these structural and systemic traumas. That is, it is not enough to make sure that all students and teachers within media literacy education are treated equally. They need to be treated *equitably* in ways that correct the imbalances and inequalities that they have experienced historically and contemporaneously. Such an equity-oriented approach is one we have discussed at length already above through multiple case studies and examples.

Additionally, the TEAM approach advocates for an "*asset-based framing*" of learners and media users from marginalized groups. Here, the researchers caution scholars, educators, and media literacy practitioners from framing learners merely as victims who are vulnerable, passive, and lacking agency. Instead, they recommend that in addressing systemic inequalities and cultural trauma through education and media, one has to intentionally include those who are othered through a lens of agency and voice. Instead of seeing their culture, ways of being, and values as burdens or deficits to be fixed by the educational system, it is important to see them as assets to organizations and society. That is, people from marginalized groups are much more than victims of trauma. The deficit-based framing places the onus on individual learners from marginalized groups to assimilate into mainstream education, just like those within the media industry, who are also expected to fit into mainstream media. An asset-based approach places responsibility on structures, systems, and society for marginalization and exclusions. This shift in responsibility means we must address deeper systemic problems through structural analysis and solutions.

The TEAM approach thus pushes media literacy educators and practitioners working with children and media to be self-reflexive in their positionality and complicity within the classroom, media spaces, and elsewhere in the world with powerful elite and dominant cultures. The ethics of care, active listening, openness, peer learning networks, collaboration, agency, and voice in shared storytelling are all key aspects of this approach to recognizing and addressing inequities in media, education, and media literacy interventions.

References

Berger, B. (2009). Political theory, political science, and the end of civic engagement. *Perspectives on Politics*, 7(2), 335–350. https://www.jstor.org/stable/40406934

Berners-Lee, T. (2020). Covid-19 makes it clearer than ever: access to the internet should be a universal right. *The Guardian*. https://www.theguardian.com/commentisfree/2020/jun/04/covid-19-internet-universal-right-lockdown-online

Bond, B. (2014). Sex and sexuality in entertainment media popular with lesbian, gay and bisexual adolescents. *Mass Communication and Society*, 17, 98–120. https://doi.org/10.1080/15205436.2013.816739

Botha, S., & Harvey, C. (2024). Disabling discourses: Contemporary cinematic representations of acquired physical disability. *Disability & Society*, 39(1), 62–84. https://doi.org/10.1080/09687599.2022.2060801

Call-Cummings, M., Hauber-Özer, M., LePelch, V., DeSenti, K. L., Colandene, M., Sultana, K., & Scicli, E. (2020). "Hopefully this motivates a bout of realization": Spoken word poetry as critical literacy. *Journal of Adolescent & Adult Literacy*, 64(2), 191–199. https://doi.org/10.1002/jaal.1082.

Common Sense Media. (2024). Growing up with Common Sense: How tech is changing childhood. *Common Sense Media*. https://www.commonsense.org/20-years-of-impact/.

Frechette, J. (2019). Keeping media literacy critical during the post-truth crisis over fake news. *The International Journal of Critical Media Literacy*, 1(1), 51–65.

Hendrickx, J., & Ranaivoson, H. (2021). Why and how higher media concentration equals lower news diversity–The Mediahuis case. *Journalism*, 22(11), 2300–2815.

Hobbs, R. (2010). *Digital and media literacy: A plan of action*. Aspen Institute.

Hobbs, R. (2011). What a difference ten years can make: Research possibilities for the future of media literacy, *Journal of Media Literacy Education*. 3, 29–31. https://digitalcommons.uri.edu/jmle/vol3/iss1/11/

Hobbs, R., & Jensen, A. (2009). The past, present, and future of media literacy education. *Journal of Media Literacy Education*, 1, 1–11.

Ibrahim, Y. (2023). *Digital racial: Algorithmic violence and digital platforms*. Rowman & Littlefield.

Jenkins, H. (2006). *Convergence culture: Where old and new media collide*. NYU Press.

Jenkins, H., Shresthova, S., Gamber-Thompson, L., Kligler-Vilenchik, N., & Zimmerman, A. (2018). *By any media necessary: The new youth activism* (Vol. 3). NYU Press.

Johnson, P. R., Tully, M., Foster, B., Mihailidis, P., Ramasubramanian, S., Burth, S. K., & Riewestahl, E. (2024). Developing a framework for equitable media literacy practice: Voices from the field. *Communication, Culture and Critique*, 0(0), 1–18. https://doi.org/10.1093/ccc/tcae023

Kellner, D., & Share, J. (2005). Towards critical media literacy: Core concepts, debates, organizations, and policy. *Discourse: Studies in the Cultural Politics of Education*, 26, 369–386. https://doi.org/10.1080/01596300500200169

Kellner, D., & Share, J. (2007). Critical media literacy, democracy, and the reconstruction of education. In D. Macedo, & S. R. Steinberg (Eds.), *Media literacy: A reader* (pp. 3–23). Peter Lang Publishing.

Kellner, D., & Share, J. (2019). *The critical media literacy guide: Engaging media and transforming education*. Brill.

Korostelina, K. V., & Barrett, J. (2023). Bridging the digital divide for native American tribes: Roadblocks to broadband and community resilience. *Policy & Internet, 15*, 306–326. https://doi.org/10.1002/poi3.339

Martens, H., & Hobbs, R. (2015). How media literacy supports civic engagement in a digital age. *Atlantic Journal of Communication, 23*(2), 120–137. https://doi.org/10.1080/15456870.2014.961636

Masterman, L. (2001). A rationale for media education. In Kubey, R. (Ed.). *Information & behaviour*. Transaction.

Mastro, D. (2015). Why the media's role in issues of race and ethnicity should be in the spotlight. *Journal of Social Issues, 71*(1), 1–16.

Mastro, S. E., & Stern, S. R. (2003). Representations of race in television commercials: A content analysis of prime-time advertising. *Journal of Broadcasting & Electronic Media, 47*(4), 638–647.

McArthur, S. (2016). Black girls and critical media literacy for social activism. *National Council of Teachers of English, 48*(4), 362–379. https://www.jstor.org/stable/26492574

McNeill, E., & Duff, A. J. (2024). *The U.S. media literacy policy report*. Media Now. https://medialiteracynow.org/wp-content/uploads/2024/02/MediaLiteracyNowPolicyReport2023_publishedFeb2024b.pdf.

Mihailidis, P., Ramasubramanian, S., Tully, M., Foster, B., Riewestahl, E., Johnson, P., & Angove, S. (2021a). Do media literacies approach equity and justice? *Journal of Media Literacy Education, 13*(2), 1–14. https://doi.org/10.23860/JMLE-2021-13-2-1

Mihailidis, P., Ramasubramanian, S., Tully, M., Foster, B., Johnson, P. R., Riewestahl, E., & Angove, S. (2021b). *Equity and impact in media literacy practice: Mapping the field in the United States*. National Association for Media Literacy Education. https://elabhome.blob.core.windows.net/downloads/617af5ab4165df1aed89b4b5-Report.PDF_FINAL.pdf.

Montgomery, S. E. (2014). Critical democracy through digital media production in a third-grade classroom. *Theory & Research in Social Education, 42*(2), 197–227. https://doi.org/10.1080/00933104.2014.908755

National Association for Media Literacy Education. (n.d.). *What is media literacy? Media literacy defined*. NAMLE. https://namle.org/resources/media-literacy-defined/

National Association for Media Literacy Education (2007). *Core principles of media literacy education in the United States*. http://namle.net.

National Association for Media Literacy Education (2023). *Core principles of media literacy education*. https://namle.org/wp-content/uploads/2023/05/NAMLE-Principles-Final-2.1.pdf

Pickard, V. (2020). Restructuring democratic infrastructures: A policy approach to the journalism crisis. *Digital Journalism, 8*(6), 704–719.

Potter, J. (2023). Critical analysis of critical thinking. *Journal of Media Literacy Education, 14*(1), 108–123. https://doi.org/10.23860/JMLE-2022-14-1-8

Project Look Sharp. (2024). *Our approach*. https://www.projectlooksharp.org/our-approach.php

Ragnedda, M., & Muschert, G. W. (2013). *The digital divide: The internet and social inequality in international perspective*. Routledge.

Ramasubramanian, S., & Darzabi, R. (2020). Civic engagement, social justice, and media literacy. In B. Christ, & B. De Abreu (Eds.), *Media literacy in a disruptive media environment* (pp. 272–282). Routledge.

Ramasubramanian, S., & Miles, C. (2018). White nationalist rhetoric, neoliberal multiculturalism, and color-blind racism: Decolonial critique of Richard Spencer's campus visit. *Javnost-The Public*, *25*(4), 426–440. https://doi.org/10.1080/13183222.2018.1463352.

Ramasubramanian, S., Riewestahl, E., & Landmark, S. (2021). The trauma-informed equity-minded asset-based model (TEAM): The six R's for social justice-oriented educators. *Journal of Media Literacy Education*, *13*(2), 29–42. https://doi.org/10.23860/JMLE-2021-13-2-3

Scharrer, E., & Ramasubramanian, S. (2015). Intervening in the media's influence on stereotypes of race and ethnicity: The role of media literacy education. *Journal of Social Issues*, *71*(1), 171–185. https://doi.org/10.1111/josi.12103

Scharrer, E., Ramasubramanian, S., & Banjo, O. (2022). Media, diversity, and representation in the U.S.: A review of the quantitative research literature on media content and effects. *Journal of Broadcasting & Electronic Media*, *66*(4), 723–749. https://doi.org/10.1080/08838151.2022.2138890

Sousa, A., & Ramasubramanian, S. (2017). Challenging gender and racial stereotypes in online spaces: Alternative storytelling among Latino/a youth in the U.S. In D. Lemish & M. Götz (Eds.), *Beyond the stereotypes? Images of boys and girls, and their consequences*. Nordicom.

Stanton, C. R., Hall, B., & DeCrane, V. W. (2020). "keep it sacred!": Indigenous youth-led filmmaking to advance critical race media literacy. *International Journal of Multicultural Education*, *22*(2), 46–65.

Tukachinsky, R., Mastro, D., & Yarchi, M. (2015). Documenting portrayals of race/ethnicity on primetime television over a 2-year span and their association with national-level racial/ethnic attitudes. *Journal of Social Issues*, *71*(1), 17–38. https://doi.org/10.1111/josi.12094

Van Dijk, J. (1999). *The network society, social aspects of new media*. Sage.

Vogels, E. A. (2021). *Digital divide persists even as lower-income Americans make gains in tech adoption*. Pew Research Center. https://www.pewresearch.org/fact-tank/2021/06/22/digital-divide-persists-even-as-americans-with-lower-incomes-make-gains-in-tech-adoption/

Wargo, J. M., & Clayton, K. (2018). From PSAs to reel communities: Exploring the sounds and silences of urban youth mobilizing digital media production. *Learning, Media and Technology*, *43*(4), 469–484.

Yosso, T. J. (2000). *A critical race and LatCrit approach to media literacy: Chicana/o resistance to visual microaggressions*. University of California.

Yosso, T. J. (2002). Critical race media literacy: Challenging deficit discourse about Chicanas/os. *Journal of Popular Film and Television*, *30*(1), 52–62.

6 Policies

Sun Sun Lim and Becky Pham

In the rapidly evolving digital landscape where our reliance on digital media continues to grow, ensuring the rights of children has become a crucial societal concern. The United Nations defines "children" as any persons under the age of 14, and "youth" as those between the ages of 15 and 24 (United Nations, n.d.). Digital media has become a necessary lifeline for children and youth to socialize and be connected to the world, but online activity across diverse realms can also expose them to risk. One in three Internet users are children and 95% of American adolescents use at least one social media platform, yet major social media companies have not been created in consideration of the needs and interests of children (Ito et al., 2021; Jang et al., 2023). Apart from being vulnerable, children are highly dependent on their parents and other adults to advocate for them while they are subject to various forms of economic, structural, and educational inequality. Addressing the digital rights of children involves safeguarding their privacy and misuse of their personal data, protecting them from harm, and having them participate actively in the design of digital products and services tailored to their specific needs such as social media, educational technologies, and online games. Several pieces of legislation across the world aim to advance these rights, each reflecting the unique challenges and perspectives of their regions.

Building on this drive to productively shape and reshape digital media for children, this book chapter offers a multi-faceted, international, and nuanced synthesis of recent academic literature and regulatory initiatives. Organized under three main themes of "privacy," "protection," and "participation," the diverse perspectives and examples covered in this chapter can serve as key points of discussion for future conversations on regulation and children's digital rights, even as digital policies remain constantly in flux and technological innovation proceeds unabated.

DOI: 10.4324/9781003453123-7

Privacy

The concept of privacy has become more multi-faceted and complex in our networked, digitalized society, and perhaps even more so for children as they often lack the awareness and experience to navigate potential risks. Nevertheless, UNICEF (2018) offers helpful guidance by laying out key dimensions of children's online privacy—physical, communication, informational, and decisional privacy. The breach of *physical* privacy happens when technologies such as tracking, monitoring, or live broadcasting expose a child's image, activities, or location. Privacy concerns in *communication* arise from unauthorized access to posts, chats, and messages. *Information* privacy infringement occurs through the unauthorized collection, storage, and processing of children's personal data, particularly when done without their comprehension or consent. Lastly, children's *decisional* privacy is undermined by restrictions on their access to essential information, which can hinder their independent decision-making or subvert their evolving developmental capacities.

Childhood is a period of rapid development that needs the right support from adults, without compromising children's agency, independent views, and growing media literacy. Indeed, children need appropriate assistance in accordance with their age and maturity, and guidance to understand and engage with the Internet and media content (UNICEF, 2018). As a result, the report specifically focuses on upholding children's entitlement to privacy and safeguarding of personal data, ensuring the right to freedom of expression and access to information, protecting against reputational harm, providing developmentally appropriate protection, and guaranteeing access to remedies for infringements and abuses of their rights, in accordance with the stipulations of the UN Convention on the Rights of the Child (United Nations, 1989).

Building on these dimensions enunciated by UNICEF (2018), Livingstone et al. (2019) propose a more constructive framework for understanding children's online privacy. They take a pragmatic approach, focusing on the nature of relationships and contexts in which children operate in digital environments and how they perceive the implications for their privacy, referred to as the "appropriate flow of personal information" (Nissenbaum, 2010, p. 3). Specifically, they identify three main types of relationships (or contexts) where privacy is crucial—interactions between an individual and: (i) other individuals or groups ("interpersonal privacy"), (ii) a public or third-sector (not-for-profit) organization ("institutional privacy"), or (iii) a commercial (for-profit) organization ("commercial privacy") (Livingstone et al., 2019). Interpersonal, institutional, and commercial privacy thus helpfully demarcate the realms in which children's online privacy must be honored and the actors involved whose duty of care can be specified and ensured through public education and/or regulation. We can thus assess the coverage and efficacy of policy and regulation using this framework.

It is critical to note that with children, a key privacy conundrum lies in the simultaneous impetus to share personal information online which is crucial for children's empowerment, and the concurrent safeguarding of their privacy which is vital for safety (Livingstone et al., 2019). Fundamentally, despite children appreciating their need for privacy and employing protective measures, they also value opportunities for online engagement. Although a high degree of individual autonomy comes with online exploration, decisions, and practices regarding individual privacy are also shaped by the social environment. In other words, as children determine how much personal information to share or withhold, they are influenced by networked communication and sharing norms that impact their choices; they need to have the wherewithal to balance privacy concerns with the desire for participation, self-expression, and a sense of belonging (Livingstone et al., 2019). However, negotiating such tradeoffs is challenging even for adults, let alone children. This is where policy and regulation can play a critical role in mandating how children's online privacy can be safeguarded and indeed promoted.

In our increasingly datafied society, policies and safeguards for children's online privacy must preserve informational privacy and address the salient dimension of data—its collection, use, misuse, and abuse (Lupton & Williamson, 2017). Children are increasingly subject to datafication through technologies such as mobile media, wearable devices, social media platforms, educational software, and even toys (Holloway & Green, 2016; Lupton & Williamson, 2017). The data produced by these technologies are frequently employed for *dataveillance*, encompassing the monitoring and assessment of children by themselves or others. This may involve recording and evaluating various aspects such as appearance, growth, development, health, social relationships, moods, behavior, educational accomplishments, and other features. Through this process, the details in children's lives become so-called "objective" digital data collected in massive quantities for retrieval and use by actors and corporations in ways often unknown to children themselves or that differ from their original intentions. Exploitative tactics include tracking children's online behavior and selling such data to marketers who use it to target advertising at children, generate algorithmic predictions of children's future needs and wants, and leverage such predictions for future policies and interventions in children's lives—without incorporating their voices or seeking their initial consent (Lupton & Williamson, 2017). Indeed, engaging in online activities has distinct consequences for the informational privacy of children, and optimal protection is ensured when children, or their parents or guardians, provide voluntary and well-informed consent for the processing of their personal data (UNICEF, 2018). Furthermore, the processing of children's data must be conducted in a fair, lawful, and transparent manner, aligning with the original purpose for which the data was collected (Third et al., 2014). As well, the data pertaining to children should ideally be kept to the minimal necessary extent, ensuring accuracy and regular updates (UNICEF, 2018). Last but not least, children must be educated, informed, and empowered to actively safeguard their personal data (Third et al., 2014).

Establishing regulatory levers for ensuring children's physical, communication, informational, and decisional privacy across interpersonal, institutional, and commercial interactions should thus be an urgent imperative of governments worldwide. Several jurisdictions have launched various initiatives that have helped set the benchmark in terms of such regulations. The *Children's Online Privacy Protection Act (COPPA)* in the United States sets strict guidelines for online platforms and services directed toward children under 13 (Anderson, 2024). Enacted in 2000, COPPA has had a significant impact on addressing concerns about children's online privacy. It serves as a guardian by imposing strict regulations to protect children's personal information in the digital realm and has been successful in reducing the collection and dissemination of children's data by websites. It requires obtaining parental consent before collecting, using, or disclosing personal information of young users.

For example, in June 2023 the Federal Trade Commission (FTC) enacted COPPA and levied a $20 million fine. Microsoft was found to have violated COPPA regulation by retaining children's personal information far longer than it should have when the users signed up for Xbox accounts. Instead of being deleted, the children's personal data were stored up to years even when parents of under-13 players did not finish the required signup process (Peters, 2023). As a result of COPPA, platforms for children have implemented age verification and parental consent mechanisms, fostering responsible data handling. Businesses and advertisers have adjusted their strategies, adopting more transparent and responsible approaches in compliance with COPPA. COPPA's influence also extends beyond immediate compliance efforts, prompting educational initiatives and raising awareness about online privacy (Anderson, 2024). Despite its notable improvements, challenges persist, especially for smaller online entities. The evolving nature of technology continually tests COPPA's adaptability. Overall, COPPA has helped forge a more conscientious and privacy-oriented digital landscape for children, fostering a culture of responsibility and ethical consideration within the online ecosystem (Anderson, 2024). However, COPPA has also been critiqued for considerable deficiencies and limitations.

In the European Union, the *General Data Protection Regulation (GDPR)* empowers individuals, including children, with control over their personal data. It mandates clear information about data processing and requires parental consent for children under 16. Member states can lower this age limit, but not below 13. Preventing the misuse of children's personal data is a global concern. COPPA in the U.S. and GDPR in the EU, as mentioned earlier, play pivotal roles in regulating the collection and use of personal data of children. Both legislations emphasize the importance of explicit consent and transparent data practices. Australia's *Privacy Act* includes a set of principles to regulate the handling of personal information, applicable to both adults and children. It emphasizes the importance of obtaining informed consent and ensuring the security of children's personal data. In Australia, the Office of the eSafety Commissioner works toward protecting the privacy of children online by providing resources and guidelines for parents, educators, and industry stakeholders. The Privacy Act serves as a legal framework to address data protection concerns. Singapore's *Personal Data Protection Act (PDPA)* also addresses the protection of children's personal information, emphasizing the need for organizations to obtain parental consent when collecting data from minors. Singapore's PDPA establishes principles for the fair and responsible handling of personal data, including that of children. The law requires organizations to have reasonable security arrangements to protect against unauthorized access, disclosure, and misuse of personal information.

Protection from Harm

Children derive considerable benefits from their online opportunities, especially with regard to peer interactions, and even more so for those from marginalized groups, for example, LGBTQ teens, who find the online realm a safe space to seek peers encountering similar challenges of marginalization (Lim, 2022). However, these benefits can also be undermined by the risks and harms they may face including exposure to violent, sexual, or other age-inappropriate content, online predators, hate speech, and cyberbullying, and other forms of online harassment. Online environments that afford anonymity and connectivity can also be conducive to spreading hateful ideologies that often target minoritized or racialized communities. Such hateful content can connect individuals sharing the same prejudice, create a false sense of normalcy about hate speech, and instigate intergroup violence. In response to moral panics but also legitimate public concern about the threats that the online world can pose to children, governments around the world have sought to introduce regulations that impose on tech companies and online content providers a greater burden of responsibility to shield children from these dangers.

A widely known example is the United States which promulgated the ***Children's Internet Protection Act (CIPA)*** that requires schools and libraries that receive federal funding for internet access to implement measures ensuring internet safety, including filtering content that may be harmful to minors. Yet, regulation of social media companies to protect minors in the United States has been unevenly pursued by both individual states and the federal government, resulting in fragmented directives and contentious debates and lawsuits (Jang et al., 2023). For instance, states such as Arkansas, California, Louisiana, Utah, and Texas have enacted new legislation in 2022 to 2023 to curb social media use through provisions such as verifying users' legal age, requiring parents' or guardians' consent for minors, providing a parent or guardian access to the content and interactions from a minor's account, adjusting the default settings to a high level of privacy, and clarifying liability for failure to perform age verification and illegal retention of data. Companies such as Amazon, Google, Meta, Yahoo, and TikTok have fought against such state legislation (Jang et al., 2023).

At the federal level, Congress is close to passing two bills to "childproof" the Internet, namely, the ***Kids Online Safety Act (KOSA)*** and ***COPPA 2.0*** (Kelly, 2023). KOSA would allow the Federal Trade Commission to police companies that fail to prevent minors from seeing harmful content on their platforms, such as eating disorders, suicidal thoughts, substance abuse, and gambling. KOSA would ban minors aged 13 and below from using social media and require minors under 17 to obtain parental consent before using a social media platform. At the same time, KOSA has proposed a clearer definition for a social media platform's "design feature" to come under law enforcement, rather than focusing merely on the content that the platform hosts. Design features that constitute the company's business model are those that would encourage minors to spend more time and attention on the platform, such as infinite scrolling and rewards for staying online. If it becomes law, KOSA will be among the most significant online child safety statutes since COPPA went into effect in 2000 (Feiner, 2024; Kelly, 2023). On the other hand, COPPA 2.0 has proposed to raise the age of protection from 13 to 16 years of age, and to ban platforms from targeting minors with ads (Kelly, 2023).

In the European Union, the ***Safer Internet Programme*** aims to promote a safer online environment for children. It includes initiatives to raise awareness, provide educational resources, and encourage cooperation between stakeholders to combat online risks. The EU's ***Digital Services Act (DSA)*** that went into effect in August 2023 demands tech companies rethink their policies on transparency, moderation, and advertising. In a bid to protect democracy and children's online safety, DSA bans targeted advertising to children, or that based on a user's sexual orientation, religion, ethnicity, or political beliefs. DSA requires social media platforms to provide more transparency on their algorithms and to provide their users with the right to opt out of recommendation systems and profiling, while sharing key data with authorities and researchers (Roth, 2023).

The UK's *Online Safety Act* became law in October 2023 to handle legal but harmful content online, especially to protect children. Such content includes materials that are not explicitly against the law but can pose risks, such as health-care disinformation, political disinformation, and encouraging suicide or eating disorders. Besides age verification, social media companies will also have to prevent younger users from seeing age-inappropriate content such as pornography, cyberbullying, harassment, and offers parents easy access to report concerns (Guest, 2023). Australia's eSafety Commissioner plays a crucial role in protecting children from online harms. The commissioner oversees a range of functions, including the removal of cyberbullying material and empowering parents and educators with resources to enhance online safety.

Asian jurisdictions have also witnessed state efforts to shore up the protection of children from online harms. China's Cyberspace Administration published draft rules in August 2023 to expand control over minors' content and time spent on smart devices, rather than on smartphone apps whose settings were argued by parents to be too easy for children to bypass. Under these draft rules, a "minor mode" would limit a user's time spent online per day in accordance with their age. Minors aged under 8 would be limited to 40 minutes, those aged 8 to 15 to an hour, and users aged 16 to 18 to two hours. Minors would also be prohibited from using smart devices between 10 p.m. and 6 a.m. unless their parents/caregivers override these settings. Online platforms would be required to promote educational and popular science to minors under 16, and motivational content to those approaching 18 years old (Li, 2023).

Singapore, among the most digitally connected countries in the world, has also been actively addressing online safety through initiatives like the Media Literacy Council and the Singapore Children's Society, which provide educational programs and resources to equip children with digital literacy skills. Besides these public education efforts, Singapore's Infocomm Media Development Authority (IMDA) has also established the *Code of Practice for Online Safety* in 2023 to pave the way toward a safer digital environment (Ocampo, 2023). Its primary goal is to mitigate the perils associated with harmful content circulating on social media platforms, especially for vulnerable demographics such as children. This initiative mandates that social media platforms elevate online safety standards in Singapore by controlling the dissemination of harmful content. Additionally, Singapore also passed the *Online Safety (Miscellaneous Amendments) Act* in the same year to buttress efforts to combat hazardous content on online platforms. Under this Act, IMDA is empowered to designate social media platforms with significant reach or impact in Singapore as compliant with the *Online Safety Code*, ensuring that major social media platforms actively contribute to shielding users from potentially harmful content.

The Online Safety Code stipulates that social media platforms must prioritize user safety, particularly that of minors, by minimizing their exposure to harmful content. To achieve this, platforms are required to establish robust systems and mechanisms for effectively addressing harmful material. These efforts encompass establishing clear community standards and implementing advanced content filtering techniques, ensuring a safer online environment for all users. Moreover, the Online Safety Code equips Singaporean users with tools to manage their safety on social media platforms. These tools empower users to conceal potentially harmful content, restrict location sharing, and manage the visibility of their accounts to other users. Furthermore, social media platforms are mandated to provide user-friendly reporting mechanisms for hazardous content or unwanted interactions, encouraging users to actively contribute to a safer digital community. These reports are crucial for maintaining accountability and transparency, offering insights into platforms' security measures and efficacy in combating unsafe content. Publicly accessible online, these reports enable users to make informed decisions regarding the safety of different social media platforms. The IMDA plans to publish the first set of annual online safety reports on its website in the latter half of 2024.

Participation of Children

Given the enormity of the online safety challenge, it is imperative that a multi-stakeholder approach be adopted for any meaningful change to be effected. But it is equally vital that one key stakeholder group to be included is young people themselves. Inviting children to participate in research, policy, and consultation takes into account children's access to resources and knowledge and ensures a commitment to inclusivity for children given the power hierarchies between children and adults, as well as between policymakers and lay people. Digital technology does not just evolve rapidly, but is made more complex by children's changing needs as they grow older, while children today are exposed to more geographically diverse ideas and an unprecedented pace of change. Moreover, adults tend to fail to recognize children's unique social and moral perspectives, seeing children as "becomings" rather than "beings" (Ito et al., 2021). Article 12 of the Convention on the Rights of the Child states that children capable of forming their own views should have the right to express those views freely, in all matters affecting them, in accordance with their age and maturity (United Nations, 2005). Rather than having groups of adults from diverse public and private sectors talk over children's heads about online safety, young people's views on this critical issue that affects them directly must be actively solicited, effectively distilled and purposefully disseminated. To address equity and inclusivity concerns, this approach must be sustainable, socio-culturally relevant, and inclusive from the perspectives of participating children. Empowering children to actively participate in the design of digital products and services ensures that these technologies cater to their needs, preferences, and safety.

Across the world, various countries have made encouraging attempts to reflect the importance of children's agency in managing their online activity, although they tend to have been more symbolic than concrete. COPPA in the United States encourages the development of kid-friendly platforms and features, thereby encouraging the notion of involving children in shaping their digital experiences. The EU's GDPR acknowledges the importance of considering the interests and rights of children when designing services. Notably, it encourages the use of clear and plain language that children can easily understand, fostering a user-centric approach. Australia's Digital Platforms Inquiry, although not specific to children, emphasizes the need for digital platforms to consult with stakeholders, including children, when designing and implementing changes that may impact user experiences.

Singapore's Smart Nation initiative encourages the active involvement of citizens, including children, in shaping the digital landscape. The government collaborates with various sectors to ensure that digital innovations align with the diverse needs of the population. In fact, a commendable collective effort to tackle online harms against women and girls was undertaken in Singapore. In July 2021, the *Sunlight Alliance for Action (AfA)*, under the stewardship of Singapore's Ministry of Communication and Information, brought together 48 representatives from key relevant sectors including academia, industry, civil society, government, and youths themselves (Ministry of Communications and Information, 2022). Sunlight AfA prefaced its work by conducting a survey to assess the scale and scope of the problem, uncovering useful pointers for priority issues to address. A key finding was that three in ten of the 1,049 survey respondents reported being personally affected by or having borne witness to gender-based online harms such as cyberstalking or receiving unwelcome and unwanted images.

The public-private alliance was given a period of one year to accomplish several objectives that comprised charting a research roadmap for critical research priorities, establishing a support center and online resource portal for individuals affected by online harms, and launching public education and volunteerism programs. The strict timeline facilitated the delivery of concrete initiatives and productive collaborations emerged from the interactions of the cross-sector networks that drove the alliance forward. This successful experiment in private-public-youth partnership demonstrated the significant benefits of community efforts that transcended sector divides, especially for an issue that affects people across the board. It proves the adage that if the Internet is made safer for the vulnerable, it is safer for everyone.

In this regard, one especially laudable effort in mobilizing children's participation in online safety has been by the Association of Southeast Asian Nations (ASEAN), which organized its first-ever ASEAN ICT Forum on Child Online Protection in November 2022 in Phnom Penh, Cambodia (Galvin, 2022). This event illuminated the virtues of having children at the table and articulating their opinions in their own words—a significant advancement considering that young people's views are not always accorded their requisite weight. The report arising from the consultation process outlines a very clear set of directives exhorting industry players to place the digital rights of children front and center. Titled "Call to Action from Children and Young People to the Private Sector on Child Online Protection," this landmark document is the culmination of consultations with young people across eight ASEAN Member States—Cambodia, Indonesia, Lao PDR, Malaysia, Myanmar, the Philippines, Thailand, and Vietnam. It underlines four key areas where children and young people seek improvements for a safer and more welcoming digital environment: child-centered features and functions; effective reporting and feedback mechanisms; digital literacy and online digital safety guidance; and data protection and respect for privacy (UNICEF, 2022).

The fact that many children participated in the forum which brought together a diverse spectrum of private and public sector representatives, as well as from academia, underlines the import and genuine intent of this effort. Many children recounted personal experiences of online harms in their daily lives that made their advocacy even more persuasive. For instance, one Indonesian boy in the 12 to 14 age group shared that losing his data online meant losing his gaming data, which could cause him to be "really emotional." Other adolescents and late adolescents from Myanmar and Vietnam bemoaned a sore dearth of public education on cybersecurity and the real-life consequences of using the Internet at a young age (UNICEF, 2022). Organizations present at the event included Zoom, Meta, and LEGO, start-ups Hekate and VRapeutic, and relevant industry bodies including Fair Play Alliance and Tech Coalition. This welcome progress could also help allay previous public concerns about ASEAN's unsystematic approach to regulating online child safety thus far, largely due to wide gaps in economic and technological advancements among its member countries and ASEAN being an interstate body rather than a supranational entity like the EU (Bland, 2021; Mubarak, 2015).

As the above discussion evinces, channeling young people's views to industry and government representatives is paramount for improving young people's online safety. Indeed, multiple leading humanitarian organizations have also released valuable toolkits with clear, detailed guidelines on how to directly consult children and youth for their inputs, and involve them as part of the solution rather than as part of the problem. The UN's "Making Commitments Matter: A Toolkit for Young People to Evaluate National Youth Policy" in 2005 (United Nations, 2005) provides practical tools for youth representatives and organizations to evaluate community-level and national policies that directly impact them, and for relevant civil societies to determine the extent to which they have bettered the lives of young people. The toolkit lists 15 priority areas for youth that included concerns as important for today as in 2005 such as education, leisure-time activities, information and communication technologies, and globalization. Providing concrete checklists for actionable items and criteria to monitor the process of involving young people, the toolkit recommends consulting methods such as individual interviews with young people, focus group discussions with young people, highlighting case studies of good practices, and examples of achievements. Besides listening to young people, the toolkit further promotes the development of youth skills through conducting thorough analyses of youth activities in relation to their communities and structural constraints, before spotting potential opportunities for cooperation toward pragmatic causes such as employment, food security, and awareness of healthy lifestyles.

The UK-based Save the Children also launched "So you want to consult with children? A toolkit of good practice" in 2003 (Save the Children International, 2003). Straightforward, easy-to-follow, and comprehensive, the toolkit breaks down the process of consulting children into seven steps: Getting started, organizing a consultation with children, planning a preparatory meeting with and for children, having children on the delegation, creating an enabling environment, ensuring that children are safe, and ensuring quality follow-up. The toolkit especially emphasizes the participatory nature of this process, through which children are free to express their views outside of their usual home or community environment, and are welcome to be consulted and to debate, but not to achieve tangible learning goals.

More recently, General Comment No.26—or guidelines by the UN's Committee on the Rights of the Child to deal with our current environmental crisis—published the "Children and Young People's Second Consultation Toolkit" (General Comment, 2022). A series of both online and offline consultations at local, regional, and global levels across 103 countries took place to inform the creation of the General Comment's first draft, before the second consultation round sought further feedback on the first draft. Remarkably, these consultations and the toolkit were designed by a Children's Advisory Team that included 13 children aged 11 to 17 from all over the world, and not by adults. The toolkit suggests methods and tips to involve children and young people that include workshops as well as creative consulting activities such as drawing maps, creating

3D models and posters, and writing short messages on postcards. Child-friendly, fun, and insightful, this handy planning aid underscores the need to be flexible in adapting consulting activities for children with different needs and abilities without shying away from the realities of environmental harm and risks that children are encountering.

Similarly, academic research in education, child development, and media studies has increasingly involved children and young people in their research methodologies. This approach has been referred to as "co-participatory research" (Green et al., 2022; Kumpulainen et al., 2014; Purdy & Spears, 2020) or "co-design" (Green et al., 2022; Milkaite & Lievens, 2020) or "participatory co-design" (Ey & Spears, 2020). The paradigm has shifted from where research is *done to* children and young people, to something that is conducted *with* them and thus, disrupting the traditional power relationship between researchers and participants. Children and young people are not only co-constructors of knowledge, but also co-designers and co-facilitators of research (Kumpulainen et al., 2014; Purdy & Spears, 2020). The research process foregrounds children and young people as active agents in documenting, explaining, and reflecting their own experiences, in relation to their own socio-cultural settings. The emphasis is on the children's own voices and initiatives. Instead of only using the researcher's interview questions as the stimulus, the children can produce and select their own research stimuli such as a photo or a drawing of their own to speak about (Kumpulainen et al., 2014).

In one such study that explored how children aged 4 to 8 in Australia understood bullying in early childhood settings, the children were provided with a set of simple cartoon scenarios to verbalize which scenario represented bullying, aggression, or play. The children were reportedly highly confused, or named almost every form of aggression as bullying, or did not differentiate between tumble play and bullying. Using the data through the lens of the children's evolving understanding of bullying, the researchers and educators were able to identify and define the nature and magnitude of bullying problems in the classroom (Ey & Spears, 2020). Thus, through participatory research, children are ideally empowered to both acquire critical thinking skills and design preventative measures directly relevant to their context and authentic experiences (Green et al., 2022).

Insights from children's participation in policy and academic research, however, should not be separated from our understanding of how children engage in learning within other contexts such as at home, at school, and online. Academic research findings have repeatedly reminded us that children are interconnected in multiple media contexts with parents, peers, teachers, and strangers where they receive immediate feedback and help build shared values (Ito et al., 2013; Livingstone & Blum-Ross, 2020). An approach that assumes a disconnect between these different contexts can undermine existing opportunities and promising pathways for

112 *Children, Media, and Technology*

collaboration. For example, it can cause policymakers and educators to feel that they must "make up for" the limitations of children's home environment and further burden children to work on connecting their different learning identities by themselves, rather than build up positive connections between regulatory initiatives and the learning that children have already gained at home by enlisting the parents' help and guidance where applicable, while still successfully prioritizing and honoring children's agency (Livingstone & Blum-Ross, 2020).

Ultimately, with technology reaching right into the palm of every child, it is absolutely vital that we take an all-hands-on-deck approach to enhance online safety. Above all, we must ensure that companies developing digital products for children and young people are first, actively consulting them on what they deem important for a secure and edifying online environment; and second, referencing relevant academic literature to stay up-to-date with the latest research findings on children's digital media experiences and ecology (Figure 6.1).

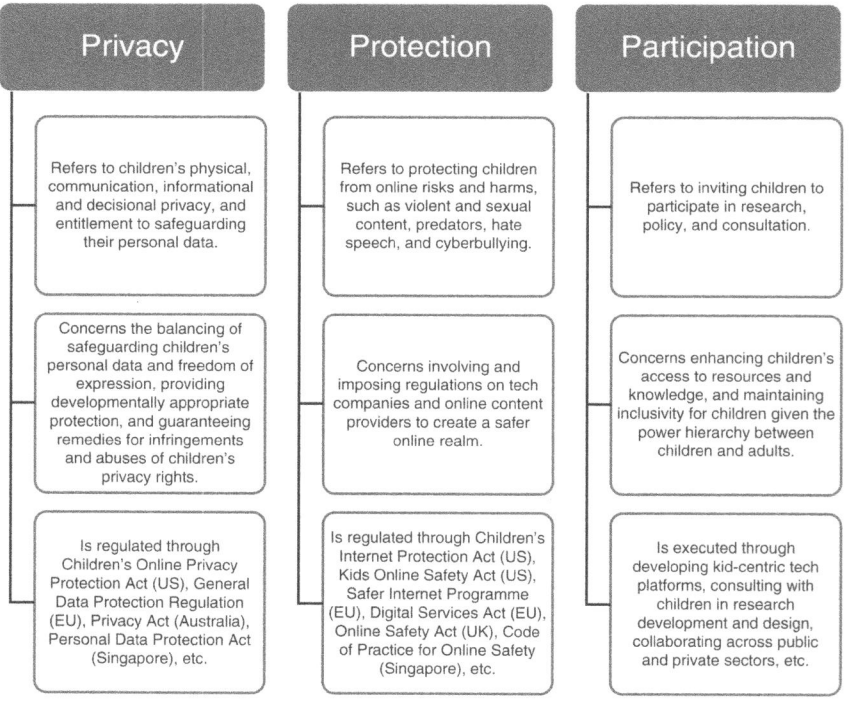

Figure 6.1 Defining, managing, and enacting children-centric policies for privacy, protection, and participation.

Source: Authors.

Conclusion

In conclusion, safeguarding the digital rights of children requires a comprehensive approach that addresses privacy, protection from harm, prevention of data misuse, and active involvement in design. Legislations in the United States, EU, ASEAN, Australia, China, and Singapore reflect the global commitment to creating a secure and empowering digital environment for the youngest members of society. As the digital landscape continues to evolve, ongoing efforts and international cooperation are essential to adapt and strengthen these safeguards for the benefit of children worldwide. Through these shared goals and collaborative experiences, children and youth are able to garner socio-cultural capital and resources, transform themselves to be catalysts for change, and cultivate even more diversity of viewpoints, equity, and community connections.

References

Anderson, H. (2024). The guardian of the digital era: Assessing the impact and challenges of the Children's online privacy protection act. *Law and Economy, 3*(2), 6–10.

Bland, B. (2021, August 24). Weak and inadequate, ASEAN yet remains indispensable. *Nikkei Asia.* https://asia.nikkei.com/Opinion/Weak-and-inadequate-ASEAN-yet-remains-indispensable#

Ey, L. A., & Spears, B. (2020). Engaging early childhood teachers in participatory co-design workshops to educate young children about bullying. *Pastoral Care in Education, 38*(3), 230–253.

Feiner, L. (2024, February 15). Kids Online Safety Act gains enough supporters to pass the Senate. *The Verge.* https://www.theverge.com/2024/2/15/24073878/kids-online-safety-act-new-senate-support

Galvin, J. M. (2022, November 24). The private sector's role in keeping children and young people safe online in ASEAN. *UNICEF Blog.* https://www.unicef.org/eap/blog/private-sectors-role-keeping-children-and-young-people-safe-online-asean

General Comment. (2022, November). *Children and young people's second consultation toolkit.* https://childrightsenvironment.org/wp-content/uploads/2022/11/Childrens-Second-Consultation-Toolkit.pdf

Green, D. M., Taddeo, C. M., Price, D. A., Pasenidou, F., & Spears, B. A. (2022). A qualitative meta-study of youth voice and co-participatory research practices: Informing cyber/bullying research methodologies. *International Journal of Bullying Prevention, 4*(3), 190–208.

Guest, P. (2023, October 26). The UK's controversial online safety act is now law. *WIRED.* https://www.wired.com/story/the-uks-controversial-online-safety-act-is-now-law/?_sp=5fee23f2-07e3-4141-8b98-66bd7e5287cb.1710213555833&redirectURL=%2Fstory%2Fthe-uks-controversial-online-safety-act-is-now-law%2F%3F_sp%3D5fee23f2-07e3-4141-8b98-66bd7e5287cb.1710213555833

Holloway, D., & Green, L. (2016). The internet of toys. *Communication Research and Practice, 2*(4), 506–519.

Ito, M., Cross, R., Dinakar, K., & Odgers, C. (2021). Introduction: Algorithmic rights and protections for children. *MIT Open.* https://wip.mitpress.mit.edu/pub/intro-algorithmic-rights-and-protections/release/1?readingCollection=646d0673

Ito, M., Gutiérrez, K., Livingstone, S., Penuel, B., Rhodes, J., Salen, K., Schor, J., Sefton-Green, J., & Watkins, S. C. (2013). *Connected learning: An agenda for research and design*. Digital Media and Learning Research Hub. https://dmlhub.net/publications/connected-learning-agenda-for-research-and-design/index.html

Jang, K., Pan, L., & Turner, N. (2023, August 14). Commentary: The fragmentation of online child safety regulations. *Brookings Institution*. https://www.brookings.edu/articles/patchwork-protection-of-minors/

Kelly, M. (2023, July 27). Senate panel advances bills to childproof the Internet. *The Verge*. https://www.theverge.com/2023/7/27/23809876/kosa-coppa-2-child-safety-privacy-protection-social-media

Kumpulainen, K., Lipponen, L., Hilppö, J., & Mikkola, A. (2014). Building on the positive in children's lives: A co-participatory study on the social construction of children's sense of agency. *Early Child Development and Care, 184*(2), 211–229.

Li, X. (2023, August 4). China proposes even stricter restrictions on children's screen time. *Sixth Tone*. https://www.sixthtone.com/news/1013463

Lim, S. S. (2022). Media and peer culture: Young people sharing norms and collective identities with and through media. In D. Lemish (Ed.), *Routledge handbook of children, adolescents and media* (2nd ed., pp. 347–354). Routledge.

Livingstone, S., & Blum-Ross, A. (2020). *Parenting for a digital future*. Oxford University Press.

Livingstone, S., Stoilova, M., & Nandagiri, R. (2019). *Children's data and privacy online: Growing up in a digital age: An evidence review*. London School of Economics and Political Science.

Lupton, D., & Williamson, B. (2017). The datafied child: The dataveillance of children and implications for their rights. *New Media & Society, 19*(5), 780–794.

Milkaite, I., & Lievens, E. (2020). Child-friendly transparency of data processing in the EU: From legal requirements to platform policies. *Journal of Children and Media, 14*(1), 5–21.

Ministry of Communications and Information. (2022, August). *SUNLIGHT Alliance for Action: Tackling online harms, especially those targeted at women and girls*. https://www.mci.gov.sg/files/Press%20Releases%202022/mci%20sunlight%20report%20fa-ed-compressed.pdf

Mubarak, A. R. (2015). Child safety issues in cyberspace: A critical theory on trends and challenges in the ASEAN region. *International Journal of Computer Applications, 129*(1), 48–55.

Nissenbaum, H. (2010). *Privacy in context. Technology, policy, and the integrity of social life*. Stanford University Press.

Ocampo, Y. (2023, 25 July). Singapore's code of practice for online safety. *OpenGov*. https://opengovasia.com/2023/07/25/singapores-code-of-practice-for-online-safety/

Peters, J. (2023, June 5). Microsoft to pay $20 million FTC settlement over improperly storing Xbox account data for kids. *The Verge*. https://www.theverge.com/2023/6/5/23750320/microsoft-xbox-ftc-settlement-account-data-kids-coppa

Purdy, N., & Spears, B. (2020). Co-participatory approaches to research with children and young people. *Pastoral Care in Education, 38*(3), 187–190.

Roth, E. (2023, August 25). The EU's Digital Services Act goes into effect today: here's what that means. *The Verge*. https://www.theverge.com/23845672/eu-digital-services-act-explained

Save the Children International. (2003). *So you want to consult with children? A toolkit of good practice*. https://resourcecentre.savethechildren.net/pdf/2553.pdf/

Third, A., Bellerose, D., Dawkins, U., Keltie, E., & Pihl, K. (2014). *Children's rights in the digital age: A download from children around the world*. Young and Well Cooperative Research Centre.

UNICEF. (2018) *Children's online privacy and freedom of expression: Industry toolkit*. New York: UNICEF. https://issuu.com/unicefusa/docs/unicef_toolkit_privacy_expression?e=29613278/60947364

UNICEF. (2022). *A call to action from children and young people to the private sector on child online protection*. https://www.unicef.org/eap/documents/call-action-children-and-young-people

United Nations. (n.d.). *Global issues: Youth*. https://www.un.org/en/global-issues/youth

United Nations. (1989). *Convention on the rights of the child*. UN, Office of the High Commissioner for Human Rights.

United Nations. (2005, October 2). *Making commitments matter toolkit*. https://www.un.org/development/desa/youth/publications/2005/10/8414/

Part II
Interpretations/Implications

7 Social Identity

L. Monique Ward, Jasmine Banks, Enrica Bridgewater, and Miranda Reynaga

A central developmental task of adolescence is identity consolidation, developing a firmer sense of who you are in the world and what kind of person you want to be. Completing this task involves testing out interests and activities, contemplating choices, prioritizing individual identities, and confirming belief systems. This is not a solitary endeavor and involves interacting with other people such as family members, friends, and teammates, and with institutions such as schools, religious institutions, and the media.

Indeed, the media can play a significant role in this identity work by providing models to emulate or reject and by offering a platform to test out one's beliefs. In this chapter, we examine the contributions of social identities to adolescents' media choices and media effects, with a particular emphasis on racial and gender identities. Drawing on specific communication and psychological theories, we discuss how these identities shape our media choices and perceptions. We also discuss how media use shapes our beliefs about race and gender and our corresponding identities. We include discussions of the roles both of traditional screen media, such as television programs, films, and music videos, and social media, such as social networking sites and chat spaces. We recognize that other identities, such as religious identity and sexual identity, also drive and are affected by media content, but leave the discussion of sexual identity to Chapter 3.

Dominant Theoretical Perspectives Linking Media Consumption and Identity Work

Several theories have been developed to explain how our identities and feelings about our memberships in specific societal groups shape and are shaped by our media consumption. Some theories focus on how exposure to media content contributes to our beliefs about our group and other groups. For example, ***Cultivation Theory*** argues that in consuming mainstream media, youth are exposed to specific messaging about race or gender, and, over time, will come to see the content as normative and will come to cultivate or adopt comparable beliefs (Gerbner, 1998). Therefore, with heavy television consumption, youth are more likely to adopt beliefs that align with the content viewed. According to **Social Cognitive Theory** (Bandura, 2001), individuals can learn behaviors and assumptions through observing media representations. The strength of this learning is influenced by personal characteristics (e.g., age, gender, race) and the viewers' ability to relate to the portrayed characters (Ward & Grower, 2020). In this way, youth are more likely to learn from media models they identify with and are therefore more likely affected by same-gender and same-race characters (Terán et al., 2023).

Other theories focus more on the individual characteristics of viewers that shape their attention to specific media content. One such theory is the **Media Practice Model** (Steele & Brown, 1995). According to this approach, adolescents' selections, interpretations, and uses of media are strongly influenced by social group factors such as race and gender, by adolescents' emerging identities, and by conditions in their lives, labeled "lived experience," that include friendships and peer culture experiences, family life, religious backgrounds and beliefs, and neighborhood influences. Adolescents are believed to carry their particular life histories with them and to filter their perceptions of media content through these experiences. This model also emphasizes that engagement with media is an iterative and reciprocal process: youths' choice to engage with certain media over others is due, in part, to their social identities, and the strength of their identification with these identities may also be shaped by their media use patterns (Steele & Brown, 1995). For example, findings indicate that having a stronger ethnic/racial identity and more awareness of ethnic/racial stereotypes makes it more likely that youth will select a program featuring a character from their ethnic/racial group (Archer et al., 2022).

Similarly, according to the **Differential Susceptibility to Media Effects Model** (Valkenburg & Peter, 2013), individuals seek out media that align with their existing dispositions, developmental level, and social group norms. Many specific dispositional variables factor in, including personality, race, gender, social class, and existing cognitions and attitudes. This model argues that repeated media use may shape adolescents' beliefs in certain areas and also that teens who are already predisposed to embrace certain beliefs may be attracted to media content that conforms with those notions.

Traditional Media and Gender Identity and Beliefs

Nature of Gender Portrayals

As we have seen in Chapter 3, mainstream media in the United States, including television and film, often reflect and reinforce narrow representations of gender (Aubrey & Roberts, 2020; Scharrer & Warren, 2022; Ward

& Grower, 2020). Most analyses have focused on portrayals on television, where women remain underrepresented across genres, although the numbers have been increasing (Aubrey & Roberts, 2020). Girls and women are frequently depicted as objects for male consumption, emphasizing physical appearance, romantic appeal, and selflessness (Ward & Grower, 2020). On television, women more often than men are dressed provocatively, portrayed as emotionally dependent on men, and defined by their relationship status (Sink & Mastro, 2017; Smith et al., 2012). For example, in one analysis of tween programs, female characters were more likely than men to conform to idealized beauty norms, spend more time grooming on screen, and receive comments about their looks (Gerding & Signorielli, 2014). In contrast, boys and men are often portrayed as embodying dominance, aggression, and intelligence (Ward & Grower, 2020). Boys and men are often depicted as emotionally detached, objectifying towards women, tough, physically strong, and avoiding of characteristics associated with femininity (Aubrey & Roberts, 2020; Scharrer & Warren, 2022).

Regarding occupational roles, men are shown working outside the home more frequently than women; when women are depicted in the workforce, they often occupy gender-stereotypical roles such as secretarial work or nursing (Aladé et al., 2022; Hermann et al., 2022; Hopper-Losenicky, 2017; Sink & Mastro, 2017; Smith et al., 2012). Highly intelligent women on television often downplay their femininity and adopt non-traditional appearances to be perceived as independent (Wiest, 2016). These portrayals reinforce narrow gender stereotypes, particularly for women of color, who face stigma from multiple systems of oppression based on their gender and race (Aladé et al., 2022). Differences also persist in portrayals of Science, Technology, Engineering, and Mathematics or STEM. Disproportionately, television depicts scientists as White, socially awkward men (Steinke, 2017). In one analysis of educational television, Aladé et al. (2022) found that women, especially women of color, were portrayed as scientists far less than White men and, when included, were given far less screen time. When women are represented in STEM, they are often hypersexualized and referenced as potential distractions to the men they work with (Long et al., 2010; Steinke & Tavarez, 2017).

Scholars have also noted traditional gender portrayals in media featuring Disney princesses (e.g., *Snow White, Beauty and the Beast*) and superheroes (e.g., *Spiderman*). In the first systematic, quantitative content analysis of the first nine Disney princess films, England et al. (2011) coded the behavior and actions of the prince and princess characters for the prevalence of 13 traditionally masculine characteristics (e.g., athletic, brave) and 16 traditionally feminine characteristics (e.g., helpful, nurturing). Findings indicated that princes were portrayed with more physical strength than princesses, and princesses were more likely than princes to display affection, fear, submission, nurturing behaviors, grooming behaviors, and crying. The mix of attributes portrayed has changed over time, with princesses starting out very passive and "feminine" initially, but gaining in more "masculine" attributes. Recent princesses are more well-rounded, determined, independent characters who are insistent on being true to themselves (Hine et al., 2018). Indeed, in more recent Disney Princess films (e.g., *Tangled, Brave, Frozen*), princesses exhibited more "masculine" characteristics than princes did.

Empirical Evidence of Exposure Effects

Is there any evidence that regular consumption of this media content shapes young people's beliefs and perceptions about women's and men's capabilities and roles? Empirical studies demonstrate that heavier television consumption among *adults* predicts greater endorsement of traditional gender beliefs (e.g., Giaccardi et al., 2016; Giaccardi et al., 2017; Mustafaj & Dal Cin, 2023; Ward & Grower, 2020). However, less is known about media contributions to gender beliefs among youth (Bond, 2016; Dohnt & Tiggemann, 2006; Terán et al., 2023).

Despite the fact that younger populations are less often studied, several studies suggest that television exposure may shape youths' gendered beliefs, reinforcing gender stereotypes and impacting their self-concept, beliefs, and aspirations (Bond, 2016; Dohnt & Tiggemann, 2006; Terán et al., 2023). We see effects for multiple domains. First, we see media contributions to **traditional gender role attitudes, to beliefs about how women and men should look and behave**. Via both survey and experimental designs, exposure to media content has been associated with stronger support of more traditional or stereotypical beliefs about gender roles and attributions (for review, see Ward & Grower, 2020). For example, Coyne et al. (2016) investigated whether young children's engagement with Disney princess culture was associated with greater stereotypical behavior years later. At Time 1, parents reported on their children's engagement with princess culture, defined as children's frequency of viewing princess culture media, playing with princess culture toys, and identifying with individual princesses. Children also noted their preferences for certain gender-typed toys. For both girls and boys, princess culture engagement was associated with greater levels of female gender-stereotypical behavior (e.g., playing with dolls or tea sets) but not male gender-stereotypical behavior (e.g., playing with construction toys). In addition, for girls and boys, princess culture engagement at Time 1 was associated with higher female gender-stereotypical behavior one year later, even controlling for initial levels of stereotypical behavior. These effects were most prominent among children whose parents actively talk with them about media content. Looking at superhero media, Coyne et al. (2014) assessed 3- to 6-year-olds' exposure to superhero media content and toy play and preferences years later. For boys but not girls, exposure to superhero media content predicted greater play fighting, sports play, and playing of ball games. In addition, exposure to superhero content predicted girls' weapon play.

A second domain concerns *assumptions and preferences about careers and academic achievement*. First, exposure to traditional media content that highlights women's appearance or sexual appeal has been linked to diminished academic performance or weaker interest in certain careers among adolescent girls (Pacilli et al., 2016; Slater et al., 2017). Second, exposure to traditional gender stereotypes via the media has been linked to less interest in STEM fields for girls, although findings do not appear for all variables studied (for review, see Ward & Grower, 2020). In one experimental study with elementary school-aged children, Bond (2016) identified that young girls exposed to characters on television that represented gender-stereotypical professions reported greater interest in gender-stereotypical occupations than girls exposed to neutral or non-gender-stereotypical occupations, specifically women in STEM. Identifying the contributions of media use to occupational attitudes is crucial, as adolescence is critical for career exploration and forming academic and occupational identities (Gehrau et al., 2016; Uka, 2015).

Transgender and Gender Diverse Media Experiences

Scholars have also examined the contributions of media use to gender beliefs among transgender and gender diverse (TGD) youth, which is a term that encompasses youth whose gender is different from the sex they were assigned at birth (Aubrey & Roberts, 2020). TGD youth can identify within the gender binary (transgender women and transgender men) or beyond it (non-binary, transfeminine, transmasculine, genderqueer, agender, and two-spirit). Approximately 1.6 million youth aged 13 and older in the United States identify as TGD, double the number since 2017 (Hermann et al., 2022).

Findings suggest that being exposed to other TGD folks on television can help TGD youth accept their TGD identity, aiding them with a greater sense of belonging while also promoting acceptance among their cisgender peers (Capuzza & Spencer, 2017; McLaren et al., 2021). In an experimental study, Tompkins et al. (2015) found that participants who viewed videos that humanize transgender people expressed decreased anti-transgender beliefs between the pre- and post-test. However, not all representations of TGD individuals are positive. Whereas positive portrayals have the power to inspire young, impressionable TGD youth, negative or stereotypical portrayals of TGD people risk reinforcing harmful narratives (Pang et al., 2022). For example, in one study, greater exposure to negative TGD portrayals was associated with reduced engagement with gender-affirming care among Swedish TGD youth (Indremo et al., 2022). Moreover, in interviews, several TGD adolescents noted that exposure to negative portrayals and news stories about TGD people increased their stress, whereas positive portrayals led to greater self-acceptance and feelings of belonging (Indremo et al., 2022; Pang et al., 2022). Continued exploration is needed of the benefits for both cis-gender and TGD youth of gender diversity in media representations.

Social Media and Gender Identity and Beliefs

Social media offer numerous opportunities to both observe gender norms and expectations of others and to offer presentations of oneself. Gender norms and assumptions are conveyed via images and videos, selfies, comments about others' content, and comments and hashtags included with one's own content. It is possible this content could reflect and support traditional gender roles or could challenge them.

One approach to studying gender portrayals on social media has been via formal content analyses, whereby scholars amass a large segment of social media content, such as hundreds of photographs, vlog comments, or online advertisements, and then systematically code and analyze them for dominant themes. Most current analyses highlight the prominence of traditional gender norms and expectations in this social media content (see also Chapter 8). One common pattern noted is gender differences in self-presentation in photographs and selfies (Döring et al., 2016; Kapidzic & Herring, 2011; 2014; Rose et al., 2012; Tortajada et al., 2013). Photos of teen girls and young women are more likely than photos of boys/men to present the user in sexualized ways, perhaps with a tilted head, seductive gaze, a pout, showing more skin, or lying down. The focus is on women's beauty, attractiveness, and seductiveness. By contrast, photographs of boys/men are more likely to feature them as active and dominant, to show them in active poses that emphasize strength (e.g., flexing), and to show them staring directly at the camera or looking casually away. In their analysis of gender portrayals within 500 Instagram selfies, Döring et al. (2016) found significant gender differences for 11 of the 12 comparisons and found that selfies were actually more gender-stereotypical than magazine advertisements. In these and other ways, teens are believed to enact idealized forms of masculinity and femininity and to align their self-presentation with dominant gender norms and with gender presentation in mainstream media (Van Oosten et al., 2017).

Gender norms and expectations are also conveyed by the nature of advertising on YouTube programming that focuses more on youthfulness and ideal bodies for women than for men (Roth-Cohen et al., 2022) and in the comments posted. Zhou (2020) analyzed the comments written on 200 most-watched vlogs produced by female vloggers on two, large user-generated content platforms: YouTube and Bilibili, a video platform based in China. Three dominant themes emerged within these comments, including a focus on women's physical appearance, expressions of sexual desire toward the vlogger, and a prizing of traditional gender roles for women, such as motherhood and homemaking. Some appearance comments were positive, rewarding women for being thin, and others were negative, criticizing specific features of women's appearance; together these comments set up a rigid scrutiny that treated female bodies as objects to be evaluated.

Findings also highlight that user motives and approaches often differ by gender (Zheng et al., 2016). Surveying California high school students (53% White, 19% Latinx), Manago et al. (2023) found that girls reported using social media more than boys for emotion bonding, appearance validation, and social compensation (the latter defined as using social media to compensate for face-to-face challenges). Boys reported using social media more than girls for activity bonding.

It is often expected that regular consumption and use of this social media content, which often reflects and reproduces traditional gender norms in the larger culture, should lead users to be more stereotypical in their own approach to gender. Currently, there has been little testing of this dynamic among youth, and the limited data suggest that social media use is related to both greater and weaker support of traditional gender beliefs among teens. Examining associations within two national datasets of US 12th graders, Turiel (2022) found that greater time spent using social media was associated with *weaker* sexist attitudes concerning workplace equality. However, surveying US adolescents ages 13 to 18, Scharrer and Warren (2022) found that heavier use of YouTube was associated with *stronger* endorsement of masculine norms reflecting an emotionally detached dominance. Further study is needed of potential associations between diverse forms of social media use and gender beliefs among youth.

Emerging data suggest that sexual and gender minority youth (SGMY), including gay youth and TGD youth, may face unique risks online (see also Chapter 9). Data indicate that 74% of SGMY "often" or "sometimes" encounter homophobic comments on social media (Rideout et al., 2021). SGMY also report frequent online bullying victimization and digital microaggressions (Humphries et al., 2021; McInroy et al., 2024; Webb et al., 2021; Ybarra et al., 2015). Furthermore, SGMY describe navigating complex identity-related experiences, including identity disclosure (e.g., "coming out" to some social media audiences or being unintentionally outed; Bates et al., 2020; Berger et al., 2022; Craig & McInroy, 2014; Escobar-Viera et al., 2018) and exposure to limited, stereotypical, or dehumanizing portrayals of SGM people in media (McInroy & Craig, 2015).

Despite these challenges, social media provides opportunities that may be uniquely beneficial to SGMY. Relative to their heterosexual, cisgender peers, SGMY report that social media are more important for their well-being, in terms of creative expression, inspiration, and social support (Rideout et al., 2021). Digital contexts can provide SGMY with community spaces where they can access support and resources (Craig et al., 2021; McInroy et al., 2019), find romantic partners (Korchmaros et al., 2015), engage in identity exploration and negotiation (Berger et al., 2022), and view affirming images of and stories from SGM role models (Selkie et al., 2020). Surveying 1,231 US youth 10 to 17, Coyne et al. (2023) found that gender identity affected the ways in which social media use connected to user mental health. Being an active social media user was associated with *lower* rates of mental health problems, especially for TGD youth. It is believed that on social media, TGD youth can use photos, pronouns, and other content to actively present and be themselves in a way that aligns with their identity. For example, Herrmann et al. (2024) collected data in Germany from 114 TGD adolescents aged 11 to 18 with a diagnosis of gender dysphoria. They found that the majority (60%) had experimented with their gender identity online before they did so in everyday life, and 31% came out online before telling their friends or parents. They reported feeling significantly more understood and accepted online than by their parents, classmates/peers, and teachers. Sexual and gender minority interviewees in one study reported that seeing others receive positive feedback on LGBTQ-related posts, such as high "like" counts, was insightful and inspiring, and encouraged them to feel comfortable engaging in the identify-related behaviors that drew such comments (Fox & Ralston, 2016). Thus, for marginalized and stigmatized populations such as sexual and gender minority youth, social media may provide unique and beneficial opportunities.

Traditional Media and Ethnic/Racial Identity

During adolescence, youth often begin to reflect on what being a member of their particular ethnic/racial group means to their identity. Youth are presented with several messages about their ethnic/racial group from various sources including media. White people are the most well-represented group in television and film in terms of quantity and quality of portrayals (Scharrer et al., 2022). Ethnic/racial minorities tend to be underrepresented and/or misrepresented in traditional media. Despite making up 40.2% of the

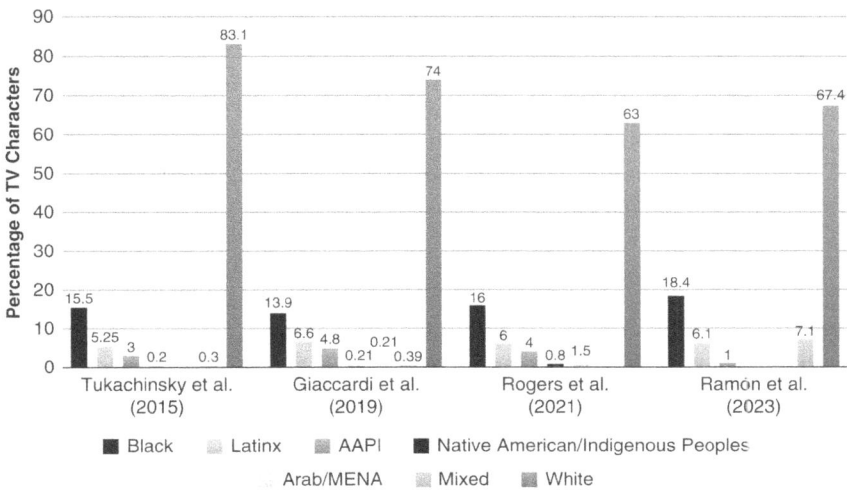

Figure 7.1 Lead characters by Ethnic/Racial group in broadcast scripted shows.
Source: Authors.
Note: This figure includes percentages of TV characters by ethnic/racial group from four content analyses and reports across eight years: Tukachinsky et al. (2015), primetime TV characters; Giaccardi et al. (2019), lead characters on children's TV programs; Rogers et al. (2021), primetime TV characters; Ramón et al. (2023), lead characters in broadcast scripted TV shows. Percentages for Arab/MENA people were not mentioned in the Tukachinsky et al. (2015) article. Percentages for mixed people were not mentioned in the Rogers et al. (2021) article. Native American/Indigenous Peoples and Arab/MENA people made up 0% of lead characters in broadcast scripted TV shows in the Ramón et al. (2023) article.

US population, people of color usually represent a much smaller proportion of lead characters on mainstream television programs (see Figure 7.1). Additionally, people of color make up only a little over a quarter (26.1%) of leading characters in children's television programs and children's films (28.8%) (Giaccardi et al., 2019).

Although progress has been made related to portrayals of ethnic/racial minorities over the past few decades, youth are still more likely to see Black characters portrayed as loud and angry; hypersexualized Latinx characters; Asian American and Pacific Islander (AAPI) characters as high academic achievers with few social skills; Native American/Indigenous Peoples as "savages" or overtly spiritual; and Arab/Middle Eastern and North African (MENA) characters as terrorists (Castañeda, 2018; Dixon, 2019; Hawkins et al., 2024; Lacroix, 2011; Zhang, 2010). A key question that has emerged for scholars who study media use among ethnic/racial minorities is: How might watching these and other kinds of media content affect youth of color's ethnic/racial beliefs and their feelings about their ethnic/racial group membership (also known as their ethnic/racial identity)? Scholars have found that there is no "one size fits all" answer to this question; findings differ depending on the ethnic/racial group in question and on whether the media content targets mainstream audiences or ethnic/racial minorities (Ramasubramanian et al., 2017).

Black Youth. Research studies focusing on Black children have mostly explored how media may be impacting their perceptions of their ethnic/racial group. For example, Jordan and Hernandez-Reif (2009) assigned Black and White preschoolers (aged 3–5) to either a moral story condition (where they heard a story about a Black child saving a baby duck) or a nonmoral story condition (where they heard a story about a child and a baby duck but were not told of the character's skin tone). The preschoolers were also shown Black and White cartoon characters and asked questions including "Who looks nice?" and "Who looks bad?" The researchers found that after hearing the story featuring a Black child as the hero, Black preschoolers were less likely to say that the Black cartoon child "looks bad" as compared to Black preschoolers who did not know the skin tone of the hero in the story.

Research focusing on Black adolescents has investigated how exposure to traditional media impacts the ways that Black youth think about their ethnic/racial group and specific stereotypes associated with their ethnic/racial group. Generally, scholars have found that watching different types of media content may impact Black youths' perceptions of themselves and their ethnic/racial group differently (Ward, 2004), with exposure to Black-oriented media often having a stronger and even a more positive effect than exposure to mainstream media. For example, Anyiwo et al. (2018) surveyed Black adolescents aged 12 to18 about their television viewing patterns and their support of both mainstream gender roles (e.g., women prioritizing wife and mother roles) and the Strong Black Woman schema (i.e., a Black woman who is emotionally strong and willing to sacrifice her needs for the benefit of others). Findings revealed that viewing Black-oriented television programs was associated with more support of the Strong Black Woman schema, whereas viewing mainstream television programs was associated with less support of mainstream gender roles, among boys. Similarly, González-Velázquez et al. (2020) asked an ethnically/racially diverse sample of high school seniors (ages 15 to 20) questions about their well-being, empowerment, and identification with their ethnic group before and after watching the film *Black Panther*. They found that watching the film (and having a stronger ethnic/racial identity) was related to increased well-being and empowerment for Black youth. More research is needed to fully address how all Black youth, including those who hold multiple marginalized identities (e.g., Black queer youth), are engaging with the mediated messages they receive about their ethnic/racial group daily.

Latinx Youth. Limited research exists addressing how exposure to traditional media may be impacting the ethnic/racial beliefs and ethnic/racial identity of other youth of color. Like the research with Black youth, studies with Latinx youth have also examined how viewing mainstream media content versus content targeted to their ethnic/racial group (e.g., Spanish-language television) may impact Latinx youth differently. Rivadeneyra and colleagues (2007) examined potential links between types of media use and various self-esteem dimensions among Latinx high school students. They found that more frequent and more engaged television viewing (particularly with English-language soap operas) was related to lower social and appearance self-esteem. In other words, the more that Latinx youth viewed, for instance, messages about beauty standards (e.g., lighter skin being perceived as more beautiful), the more likely they were to be worried about others' perceptions of them and their perceptions of themselves.

Media images within Spanish-language television programs offer a more balanced view of Latinx communities than mainstream television programs (Rivadeneyra, 2006). When surveying Latinx adolescents, Rivadeneyra (2006) found that youth were more likely to feel that Spanish-language content has more characters that they can identify with, and these programs also focus on issues important to Latinx youth such as familial connections. More research is needed on how exposure to depictions of Latinx groups in both mainstream and Spanish-language media may be influencing Latinx youths' perceptions of their ethnic/racial group and their ethnic-racial identity.

Asian American/Pacific Islander (AAPI) Youth. Like Black and Latinx youth, scholars have also explored how AAPI youth may be impacted differently depending on whether they are watching mainstream media content or media targeted to AAPI populations. In a 2023 study, Mares examined whether viewing media content with ingroup celebrities (i.e., celebrities who share one's ethnic/racial group) may increase self-esteem and ingroup attitudes among two samples of Hispanic and Asian American adolescents ages 13 to 17. In Study 1, Asian American youth were randomly assigned to one of three conditions: no-exposure control (completing survey items before reading about and seeing pictures of celebrities); Hispanic-Celebrity condition (where they first read about and saw pictures of Hispanic celebrities and then responded to survey items); or Asian-Celebrity condition (where they read about and saw pictures of Asian and Asian American celebrities before responding to survey items). Mares (2023) found that among Asian American youth, those in the ingroup celebrity condition (i.e., the Asian-Celebrity condition) reported higher ratings of ingroup warmth and self-esteem compared to those in the control condition. In Study 2, another sample of Asian American adolescents was randomly assigned to either a no-exposure control, Hispanic-Celebrity, or

Asian-Celebrity condition. Exposure to ingroup celebrities among Asian American youth did not affect their ingroup warmth or identity pride as compared to those in the control condition. Perhaps one reason Study 1 findings differed from Study 2 findings is that Asian American adolescents may not always seek out Asian American celebrities as sources of identity affirmation. This is one of few studies that have centered AAPI youths' experiences with media content; further research is needed on how AAPI youth are affected by their groups' underrepresentation and misrepresentation in traditional media.

Native American/Indigenous Youth and Arab/MENA Youth. Like AAPI youth, literature on how exposure to traditional media may impact ethnic/racial beliefs and ethnic/racial identity among Native American/Indigenous youth is minimal. Fryberg et al. (2008) addressed the lack of research on these populations by exploring how viewing Native American/Indigenous mascots or advertisements impacts self-esteem and support of ingroup ethnic/racial stereotypes among American Indian high school students across multiple studies. American Indian high school students were assigned either to read text about American Indian mascots (e.g., Chief Wahoo), view media images of American Indians (e.g., *Pocahontas*), or read about stereotypically negative outcomes for American Indians (e.g., alcoholism). In one study, teens exposed to American Indian mascots reported lower levels of self-esteem than teens in a control condition; in a follow-up study, teens exposed to any of the media content about American Indians reported lower community worth than teens in a control condition. Further research is needed in these areas to gain a clearer picture of how viewing images of Native Americans/Indigenous Peoples affects Native American/Indigenous youths' perceptions of their ethnic/racial group. Since little research exists on how exposure to traditional media may impact Arab/MENA youths' self and ethnic/racial group perceptions, more work is needed centering these populations.

White Youth. Research on traditional media use among White youth has generally examined whether viewing pro-diversity content impacts their perceptions of people of color; less is known about how their overall media use impacts their perceptions of their own ethnic/racial group (Ward et al., 2024). Scholars who conduct work in this area report mixed results. Findings from some studies have suggested that viewing pro-diversity content leads White youth to have more favorable perceptions of people of color. For example, across two studies, White youth ages 3 to 6 who were exposed to videos featuring friendly nonverbal behavior between Black and White adults perceived the interactions more positively, viewed that Black adult more positively, and offered more positive perceptions of an unfamiliar Black adult than did White children who had viewed negative nonverbal behavior between Black and White adults (Castelli et al., 2008).

Additionally, listening to short positive stories involving African American characters led to less implicit bias toward African Americans for White youth (Gonzalez et al., 2017). However, other studies have found that viewing pro-diversity content had virtually no impact on White youths' perceptions of ethnic/racial minorities (e.g., Mares & McClain, 2020). More research is needed to understand how White youths' media use patterns may be impacting their self and ethnic/racial group perceptions.

Social Media and Ethnic/Racial Identity

Experiences with social media can also contribute greatly to how youth come to understand race and their own ethnic/racial identity. While overall rates of internet use are high, there are notable differences by race. African American adolescents report greater use of social media compared to White peers. Data suggest that Black youth spend the most daily social media time (2 hours 50 minutes) compared to Hispanic/Latinx (2 hours 19 minutes) and White adolescents (2 hours 5 minutes) (Rideout et al., 2022). Black adolescents may also use the internet more intensely, particularly being more likely to use social media platforms (Auxier & Anderson, 2022; Tynes & Mitchell, 2014). Similarly, Hispanic/Latinx youth are more likely than their White counterparts to report being online constantly (Vogels et al., 2022).

Identity Development

Research indicates that online spaces can play a significant role in youth development, particularly in areas such as identity formation, aspirations, and peer relationships, and may promote social capital, empowerment, and connectedness (Campos-Holland, 2017; Hernandez et al., 2023; Light & Falkenthal, 2013; Subrahmanyam & Šmahel, 2011). First, social media platforms provide a space for youth to explore various aspects of their identities that may not be available offline. The internet offers access to a wide range of content and exposure to content from different cultures and racial groups, which allows youth to challenge existing beliefs, stimulate curiosity, and encourage empathy across racial groups (Tynes et al., 2008; Tynes et al., 2015). These opportunities are especially important for youth of color who are looking to online spaces for support and affirmation. Online communities can validate their experiences with racism, allow them to access counter narratives, provide coping strategies, and reinforce positive racial identities (Tynes et al., 2018).

Second, social media platforms offer unique contexts where youth can internalize understandings of race and Whiteness, contributing to larger processes of racial socialization (Frey et al., 2022). The internet, which often reinforces Whiteness as the default experience (Bonilla-Silva, 2017; Brock, 2020), may significantly impact the racial socialization of White adolescents. Understanding how White adolescents reproduce and reinforce race-based norms and ideas within digital spaces is crucial for disrupting harmful socialization processes. For example, social platforms such as TikTok may recommend content based on racial characteristics, segregating White adolescents from others and limiting their exposure to diverse voices and perspectives. White adolescents might also use social media to find information that confirms existing biases rather than challenging them, fostering self-reinforcing echo chambers. Additionally, the use of likes, shares, and retweets of casually racist content constitutes a form of "weak-tie racism," and contributes to normalizing harmful race-based ideas within online spaces (Frey et al., 2022).

Online Racial Discrimination

Online interactions do not exist in a vacuum; they mirror and even amplify experiences happening offline (Reich et al., 2012). Online spaces create and recreate larger structural factors such as racism, which youth must negotiate in multiple ways. For example, unconscious biases are embedded within social media algorithms by the people who create these systems, which can happen even without overt racist intent and often reinforce existing racial stereotypes (Benjamin, 2019; Noble, 2018). Biased algorithms could perpetuate racism by recommending racially divisive content, could facilitate harassment and hate speech targeting specific racial or ethnic groups, and could enable advertisers to reinforce stereotypes or engage in discriminatory practices. Furthermore, the lack of diversity and representation online can exacerbate inequalities (Noble, 2018).

As a result, youth of color face a specific challenge in the form of online racial discrimination. This term refers to any form of online behavior that demeans, excludes, or attacks an individual or a group based on race. There are two primary types of online racial discrimination: Online-directed discrimination and online *vicarious* discrimination. Online-directed discrimination involves directly targeting individuals or groups with offensive content based on their race. This can include the race-related belittling or exclusion of individual users or groups of users through the use of videos, images, texts (e.g., using racial slurs), graphic representations (e.g., racist images), and symbols (Tynes et al., 2013). Online *vicarious* discrimination involves witnessing or being indirectly exposed to discriminatory content *targeted at others* based on their racial group membership. Unlike direct discrimination, where an individual is personally targeted, vicarious discrimination occurs when someone observes racist behavior directed toward others online. Online vicarious discrimination occurs more frequently than other types of experiences of racial discrimination, including online-directed discrimination and offline discrimination (English et al., 2020; Tynes et al., 2008), with more than 70% of both Black and White students reporting witnessing racist images, jokes, or language online targeting others (Tynes et al., 2008).

Online racial discrimination has been increasing. The Teen Life Online Survey, a longitudinal survey of internet usage among 340 African American, Latinx, Asian, and biracial adolescents, revealed an increase in both online directed and online vicarious discrimination experiences from 2010 to 2013 (Lozada et al., 2020). Here, 42% of youth reported having experienced at least one direct discriminatory incident in the first year of the study, 55% in the second year, and 58% in the third year. There was also a steady increase in vicarious discriminatory experiences, with 64% of youth reporting experiencing at least one vicarious discriminatory incident in the first year, 69% in the second year, and 68% in the third year. Online racial discrimination is also a global issue. Recent data reveal that a substantial percentage of children globally (8%–58%) were exposed to hate messages or violent images online in the past year, based on data from 31,790 children aged 12 to 16 years in 36 countries (Kardefelt-Winther et al., 2023). Unfortunately, both online racial discrimination and exposure to traumatic events online have been linked to poor mental health outcomes such as anxiety, depression, and trauma symptoms (i.e., Keum & Miller, 2017; Maxie-Moreman & Tynes, 2022; Tao & Fisher, 2022; Tynes et al., 2008; 2019; 2020), lower self-esteem (Thomas et al., 2023), decreases in academic motivation (Tynes et al., 2015), and conduct problems in school, such as rule-breaking (Tynes et al., 2014).

Youth's handling of online racial discrimination experiences is likely affected by other aspects of their identity, such as the strength of their ethnic/racial identity or their gender identity. Surveying 125 African American adolescents, Tynes et al. (2012) found that a strong ethnic identity lessened the link between online discrimination and anxiety, and also protected against the negative impact of vicarious online discrimination on depressive symptoms. However, it did not significantly reduce depressive symptoms in those directly targeted. Others have explored gender differences in online racial discrimination. Surveying a diverse sample of 10- to 17-year-olds, Tynes and Mitchell (2014) found that Black girls were more likely than Black boys to be harassed, threatened, or bothered online. Other researchers confirm these unique challenges faced by Black women and girls (Stewart et al., 2019).

Findings also indicate that social media use can be a positive source of support and activism concerning issues of racial identity and racial justice, and can increase consciousness of racial issues (e.g., Brock, 2012; Volpe et al., 2023). For example, interviews with Black African youth in

Australia found that social media use is an important source for reclaiming their racial dignity through recognizing and calling out anti-Blackness, through reversing the White gaze, and through expanding feelings of belonging and healing within the community (Gatwiri & Moran, 2022).

Taken together, social media have both positive and negative consequences for youths' racial identity and racial understanding. Future research should explore how technological advancements, such as artificial intelligence and augmented reality, shape racialized online experiences. Moreover, efforts should focus on developing effective strategies for promoting digital literacy, fostering inclusive online communities, and mitigating the harmful effects of online racism and discrimination. Although this chapter focused on gender and racial identities, we acknowledge that other identities, such as religious identity and sexual identity, are highly relevant during adolescence and could also be shaping and be shaped by media consumption. Further study is needed of these domains, as well.

References

Aladé, F., Lauricella, A. R., Kumar, Y., & Wartella, E. (2022). Impact of exposure to a counter-stereotypical STEM television program on children's gender-and race-based STEM occupational schema. *Sustainability*, *14*(9), 5631.

Anyiwo, N., Ward, L. M., Fletcher, K. D., & Rowley, S. (2018). Black adolescents' television usage and endorsement of mainstream gender roles and the strong Black woman schema. *Journal of Black Psychology*, *44*(4), 371–397. https://doi.org/10.1177/0095798418771818je

Archer, J., Rackley, K. R., Broyles Sookram, S., Nguyen, H., & Awad, G. H. (2022). Psychological predictors for watching television: The role of racial representation. *Psychological Reports*, *125*(5), 2571–2590. https://doi.org/10.1177/00332941211025266

Aubrey, J. S., & Roberts, L. (2020). Effects of media use on development of gender role beliefs. In J. Van den Bulck (Ed.), *The international encyclopedia of media psychology* (pp. 1–12). Wiley Blackwell ICA. https://doi.org/10.1002/9781119011071.iemp0081

Auxier, B., & Anderson, M. (2022). *Social media use in 2021*. Pew Research Center.

Bandura, A. (2001). Social cognitive theory: An agentic perspective. *Annual Review of Psychology*, *52*(1), 1–26. https://doi.org/10.1146/annurev.psych.52.1.1

Bates, A., Hobman, T., & Bell, B. T. (2020). "Let me do what I please with it ... don't decide my identity for me": LGBTQ+ youth experiences of social media in narrative identity development. *Journal of Adolescent Research*, *35*(1), 51–83. https://doi.org/10.1177/0743558419884700

Benjamin, R. (2019). *Race after technology: Abolitionist tools for the new Jim code*. John Wiley & Sons.

Berger, M. N., Taba, M., Marino, J. L., Lim, M. S. C., & Skinner, S. R. (2022). Social media use and health and well-being of lesbian, gay, bisexual, transgender, and queer youth: Systematic review. *Journal of Medical Internet Research*, *24*(9), e38449. https://doi.org/10.2196/38449

Bond, B. J. (2016). Fairy godmothers> robots: The influence of televised gender stereotypes and counter-stereotypes on girls' perceptions of STEM. *Bulletin of Science, Technology & Society, 36*(2), 91–97.

Bonilla-Silva, E. (2017). What we were, what we are, and what we should be: The racial problem of American sociology. *Social Problems, 64*(2), 179–187.

Brock, A. (2012). From the blackhand side: Twitter as a cultural conversation. *Journal of Broadcasting & Electronic Media, 56*(4), 529–549. https://doi.org/10.1080/08838151.2012.732147

Brock, J. (2020). *Distributed blackness: African American cybercultures*. New York University Press.

Campos-Holland, A. (2017). Sharpening theory and methodology to explore racialized youth peer cultures. In I. E. Castro, M. Swauger, & B. Harger (Eds.), *Researching children and youth: Methodological issues, strategies, and innovations* (pp. 223–247). Emerald Publishing Limited.

Capuzza, J. C., & Spencer, L. G. (2017). Regressing, progressing, or transgressing on the small screen? Transgender characters on US scripted television series. *Communication Quarterly, 65*(2), 214–230.

Castañeda, M. (2018). Television and its impact on Latinx communities. In I. Stavans (Ed.), *The Oxford handbook of Latino studies* (pp. 1–44). Oxford University Press. https://doi.org/10.1093/oxfordhb/9780190691202.013.28

Castelli, L., De Dea, C., & Nesdale, D. (2008). Learning social attitudes: Children's sensitivity to the nonverbal behaviors of adult models during interracial interactions. *Personality and Social Psychology Bulletin, 34*(11), 1504–1513. https://doi.org/10.1177/0146167208322769

Coyne, S. M., Linder, J. R., Rasmussen, E. E., Nelson, D. A., & Collier, K. M. (2014). It's a bird! It's a plane! It's a gender stereotype! Longitudinal associations between superhero viewing and gender-stereotyped play. *Sex Roles, 70*, 416–430.

Coyne, S., Lindner, J., Rasmussen, E., Nelson, D., & Birkbeck, V. (2016). Pretty as a princess: Longitudinal effects of engagement with Disney princesses on gender stereotypes, body esteem, and prosocial behavior in children. *Child Development, 87*(6), 1909–1925. https://doi.org/10.1111/cdev.12569

Coyne, S. M., Weinstein, E., Sheppard, J. A., James, S., Gale, M., Van Alfen, M., Ririe, N., Monson, C., Ashby, S., Weston, A., & Banks, K. (2023). Analysis of social media use, mental health, and gender identity among US youths. *JAMA Network Open, 6*(7), e2324389–e2324389. https://doi.org/10.1001/jamanetworkopen.2023.24389

Craig, S., Eaton, A., McInroy, L., Leung, V., & Krishnan, S. (2021). Can social media participation enhance LGBTQ+ youth well-being? Development of the social media benefits scale. *Social Media + Society, 7*(1), 1–13. https://doi.org/10.1177/2056305121988931

Craig, S. L., & McInroy, L. (2014). You can form a part of yourself online: The influence of new media on identity development and coming out for LGBTQ youth. *Journal of Gay & Lesbian Mental Health, 18*(1), 95–109. https://doi.org/10.1080/19359705.2013.777007

Dixon, T. L. (2019). Media stereotypes: Content, effects, and theory. In M. B. Oliver, A. A. Raney, & J. Bryant (Eds.), *Media effects: Advances in theory and research, fourth edition* (pp. 243–257). Routledge.

Dohnt, H., & Tiggemann, M. (2006). The contribution of peer and media influences to the development of body satisfaction and self-esteem in young girls: A prospective study. *Developmental Psychology, 42*(5), 929.

Döring, N., Reif, A., & Poeschl, S. (2016). How gender-stereotypical are selfies? A content analysis and comparison with magazine adverts. *Computers in Human Behavior, 55*, 955–962. https://doi.org/10.1016/j.chb.2015.10.001

England, D., Descartes, L., & Collier-Meek, M. (2011). Gender role portrayal and Disney princesses. *Sex Roles, 64*, 555–567. https://doi.org/10.1007/s11199-011-9930-7

English, D., Lambert, S., Tynes, B., Bowleg, L., Zea, M., & Howard, L. (2020). Daily multi-dimensional racial discrimination among black U.S. American adolescents. *Journal of Applied Developmental Psychology, 66*, 101068. https://doi.org/10.1016/j.appdev.2019.101068

Escobar-Viera, C. G., Whitfield, D. L., Wessel, C. B., Shensa, A., Sidani, J. E., Brown, A. L., Chandler, C. J., Hoffman, B. L., Marshal, M. P., & Primack, B. A. (2018). For better or for worse? A systematic review of the evidence on social media use and depression among lesbian, gay, and bisexual minorities. *JMIR Mental Health, 5*(3), e10496. https://doi.org/10.2196/10496

Fox, J., & Ralston, R. (2016). Queer identity online: Informal learning and teaching experiences of LGBTQ+ individuals on social media. *Computers in Human Behavior, 65*, 635–642. https://doi.org/10.1016/j.chb.2016.06.009

Frey, W. R., Ward, L. M., Weiss, A., & Cogburn, C. D. (2022). Digital white racial socialization: Social media and the case of whiteness. *Journal of Research on Adolescence, 32*(3), 919–937.

Fryberg, S. A., Markus, H. R., Oyserman, D., & Stone, J. M. (2008). Of warrior chiefs and Indian princesses: The psychological consequences of American Indian mascots. *Basic and Applied Social Psychology, 30*, 208–218. https://doi.org/10.1080/01973530802375003

Gatwiri, K., & Moran, C. (2022). Reclaiming racial dignity: An ethnographic study of how African youth in Australia use social media to visibilise anti-Black racism. *Australian Journal of Social Issues, 58*, 360–380. https://doi.org/10.1002/ajs4.224

Gehrau, V., Brüggemann, T., & Handrup, J. (2016). Media and occupational aspirations: The effect of television on career aspirations of adolescents. *Journal of Broadcasting & Electronic Media, 60*(3), 465–483.

Gerbner, G. (1998). Cultivation analysis: An overview. *Mass Communication and Society, 1*(3-4), 175–194.

Gerding, A., & Signorielli, N. (2014). Gender roles in tween television programming: A content analysis of two genres. *Sex Roles, 70*, 43–56.

Giaccardi, S., Heldman, C., Cooper, R., Cooper-Jones, N., Conroy, M., Esparza, P., Breckenridge-Jackson, I., Juliano, L., McTaggart, N., Phillips, H., & Seabrook, R. (2019). *See Jane 2019 report*. The Geena Davis Institute for Gender in Media. https://geenadavisinstitute.org/research/see-jane-2019/

Giaccardi, S., Ward, L. M., Seabrook, R. C., Manago, A., & Lippman, J. R. (2016). Media and modern manhood: Testing associations between media consumption and young men's acceptance of traditional gender ideologies. *Sex Roles, 75*, 151–163.

Giaccardi, S., Ward, L. M., Seabrook, R. C., Manago, A., & Lippman, J. R. (2017). Media use and men's risk behaviors: Examining the role of masculinity ideology. *Sex Roles, 77*, 581–592.

Gonzalez, A., Steele, J., & Baron, A. (2017). Reducing children's implicit racial bias through exposure to positive out-group exemplars. *Child Development, 88*(1), 123–130. https://doi.org/10.1111/cdev.12582

González-Velázquez, C. A., Shackleford, K. E., Keller, L. N., Vinney, C., & Drake, L. M. (2020). Watching *Black Panther* with racially diverse youth: Relationships between film viewing, ethnicity, ethnic identity, empowerment, and wellbeing.

Review of Communication, *20*(3), 250–259. https://doi.org/10.1080/15358593.2020.1778067

Hawkins, I., Coles, S. M., Saleem, M., Moorman, J. D., & Aqel, H. (2024). How reel middle Easterners' portrayals cultivate stereotypical beliefs and policy support. *Mass Communication and Society*, *27*(1), 1–25. https://doi.org/10.1080/15205436.2022.2062000

Hermann, E., Morgan, M., & Shanahan, J. (2022). Social change, cultural resistance: A meta-analysis of the influence of television viewing on gender role attitudes. *Communication Monographs*, *89*(3), 396–418. https://doi.org/10.1080/26895269.2023.2252410

Hernandez, J. M., Charmaraman, L., & Schaefer, H. S. (2023). Conceptualizing the role of racial–ethnic identity in US adolescent social technology use and well-being. *Translational Issues in Psychological Science*, *9*(3), 199–215. https://doi.org/10.1037/tps0000372

Herrmann, L., Bindt, C., Hohmann, S., & Becker-Hebly, I. (2024). Social media use and experiences among transgender and gender diverse adolescents. *International Journal of Transgender Health*, *25*(1), 36–49.

Hine, B., England, D., Lopreore, K., Skora Horgan, E., & Hartwell, L. (2018). The rise of the androgynous princess: Examining representations of gender in prince and princess characters of Disney movies released 2009–2016. *Social Sciences*, *7*(12), 245.

Hopper-Losenicky, K. (2017). *Inspiration and aspiration: Women in STEM careers reflect on role models, media portrayals, and influences on occupational goals* (Doctoral dissertation, Fielding Graduate University).

Humphries, K. D., Li, L., Smith, G. A., Bridge, J. A., & Zhu, M. (2021). Suicide attempts in association with traditional and electronic bullying among heterosexual and sexual minority U.S. high school students. *Journal of Adolescent Health*, *68*(6), 1211–1214. https://doi.org/10.1016/j.jadohealth.2020.12.133

Indremo, M., Jodensvi, A. C., Arinell, H., Isaksson, J., & Papadopoulos, F. C. (2022). Association of media coverage on transgender health with referrals to child and adolescent gender identity clinics in Sweden. *JAMA Network Open*, *5*(2), e2146531–e2146531. https://doi.org/10.1001/jamanetworkopen.2021.46531

Jordan, P., & Hernandez-Reif, M. (2009). Reexamination of young children's racial attitudes and skin tone preferences. *Journal of Black Psychology*, *35*(3), 388–403. https://doi.org/10.1177/0095798409333621

Kapidzic, S., & Herring, S. (2011). Gender, communication, and self-presentation in teen chatrooms revisited: Have patterns changed? *Journal of Computer-Mediated Communication*, *17*, 39–59. https://doi.org/10.1111/j.1083-6101.2011.01561.x

Kapidzic, S., & Herring, S. (2014). Race, gender, and self-presentation in teen profile photographs. *New Media + Society*, *17*(6), 958–976. https://doi.org/10.1177/1461444813520301

Kardefelt-Winther, D., Stoilova, M., Büchi, M., Twesigye, R., Smahel, D., Bedrosová, M., Kvardová, N., & Livingstone, S. (2023). *Children's exposure to hate messages and violent images online*. UNICEF Innocenti – Global Office of Research and Foresight.

Keum, B. T., & Miller, M. J. (2017). Racism in digital era: Development and initial validation of the perceived online racism scale (PORS v1. 0). *Journal of Counseling Psychology*, *64*(3), 310–321.

Korchmaros, J. D., Ybarra, M. L., & Mitchell, K. J. (2015). Adolescent online romantic relationship initiation: Differences by sexual and gender identification.

Journal of Adolescence, 40(1), 54–64. https://doi.org/10.1016/j.adolescence.2015.01.004

Lacroix, C. C. (2011). High stakes stereotypes: The emergence of the "Casino Indian" trope in television depictions of contemporary Native Americans. *The Howard Journal of Communications*, 22(1), 1–23. https://doi.org/10.1080/10646175.2011.546738

Light, M., & Falkenthal, J. (2013). Positive youth development in the 21st century: Exploring online environments. *Journal of Youth Development*, 8(1), 16–26.

Long, M., Steinke, J., Applegate, B., Knight Lapinski, M., Johnson, M. J., & Ghosh, S. (2010). Portrayals of male and female scientists in television programs popular among middle school-age children. *Science Communication*, 32(3), 356–382.

Lozada, F. T., Seaton, E. K., Williams, C. D., & Tynes, B. M. (2020). Exploration of bidirectionality in African American and Latinx adolescents' offline and online ethnic-racial discrimination. *Cultural Diversity and Ethnic Minority Psychology*, 27(3), 386–396. https://doi.org/10.1037/cdp0000355

Manago, A., Walsh, A., & Barsigian, L. (2023). The contributions of gender identification and gender ideologies to the purposes of social media use in adolescence. *Frontiers in Psychology*, 13, 1011951. https://doi.org/10.3389/fpsyg.2022.1011951

Mares, M.-L. (2023). Effects of ingroup and outgroup celebrities on Asian American and Hispanic teens' self-esteem and ingroup judgments. *Media Psychology*, 26(5), 579–611. https://doi.org/10.1080/15213269.2023.2169467

Mares, M.-L., & McClain, A. (2020). Using media to promote inclusive attitudes in childhood and (Eds.), *The international encyclopedia of media psychology*. John Wiley & Sons. https://onlinelibrary.wiley.com/doi/10.1002/9781119011071.iemp0082

Maxie-Moreman, A., & Tynes, B. (2022). Exposure to online racial discrimination and traumatic events online in Black adolescents and emerging adults. *Journal of Research on Adolescence*, 32(1), 254–269. https://doi.org/10.1111/jora.12732

McInroy, L. B., Beer, O. W. J., Scheadler, T. R., Craig, S. L., & Eaton, A. D. (2024). Exploring the psychological and physiological impacts of digital microaggressions and hostile online climates on LGBTQ + youth. *Current Psychology*, 43(3), 2586–2596. https://doi.org/10.1007/s12144-023-04435-1

McInroy, L. B., & Craig, S. L. (2015). Transgender representation in offline and online media: LGBTQ youth perspectives. *Journal of Human Behavior in the Social Environment*, 25(6), 606–617. https://doi.org/10.1080/10911359.2014.995392

McInroy, L. B., McCloskey, R. J., Craig, S. L., & Eaton, A. D. (2019). LGBTQ+ youths' community engagement and resource seeking online versus offline. *Journal of Technology in Human Services*, 37(4), 315–333. https://doi.org/10.1080/15228835.2019.1617823

McLaren, J. T., Bryant, S., & Brown, B. (2021). "See me! Recognize me!" An Analysis of transgender media representation. *Communication Quarterly*, 69(2), 172–191.

Mustafaj, M., & Dal Cin, S. (2023). Preexisting stereotypes and selection of counter-stereotypical genius representations in entertainment media. *Journal of Media Psychology: Theories, Methods, and Applications*, 36(1), 1–14. https://doi.org/10.1027/1864-1105/a000377

Noble, S. U. (2018). *Algorithms of oppression: How search engines reinforce racism*. New York University Press.

Pacilli, M., Tomasetto, C., & Cadinu, M. (2016). Exposure to sexualized advertisements disrupts children's math performance by reducing working memory, *Sex Roles*, *74*, 389–398. https://doi.org/10.1007/s11199-016-0581-6

Pang, K. C., Hoq, M., & Steensma, T. D. (2022). Negative media coverage as a barrier to accessing care for transgender children and adolescents. *JAMA Network Open*, *5*(2), e2138623. https://doi.org/10.1001/jamanetworkopen.2021.38623

Ramasubramanian, S., Doshi, M. J., & Saleem, M. (2017). Mainstream versus ethnic media: How they shape ethnic pride and self-esteem among ethnic minority audiences. *International Journal of Communication*, *11*, 1879–1899. https://ijoc.org/index.php/ijoc/article/view/6430

Ramón, A., Tran, M., & Hunt, D. (2023). *Hollywood diversity report 2023: Exclusivity in progress, part 2: television*. UCLA Entertainment & Media Research Initiative. https://socialsciences.ucla.edu/wp-content/uploads/2024/06/UCLA-Hollywood-Diversity-Report-2023-Television-11-9-2023.pdf

Reich, S. M., Subrahmanyam, K., & Espinoza, G. (2012). Friending, IMing, and hanging out face-to-face: Overlap in adolescents' online and offline social networks. *Developmental Psychology*, *48*(2), 356–368.

Rideout, V., Fox, S., Peebles, A., & Robb, M. B. (2021). Coping with COVID-19: How young people use digital media to manage their mental health. Common Sense Media. https://www.commonsensemedia.org/sites/default/files/research/report/2021-coping-with-covid19-full-report.pdf

Rideout, V., Peebles, A., Mann, S., & Robb, M. B. (2022). *Common Sense census: Media use by tweens and teens, 2021*. Common Sense.

Rideout, V. J., Peebles, A., Mann, S., & Robb, M. B. (2022). *The Common Sense Census: Media use by tweens and teens, 2022*. Common Sense Media. https://www.commonsensemedia.org/sites/default/files/research/report/8-18-census-integrated-report-final-web_0.pdf

Rivadeneyra, R. (2006). Do you see what I see? Latino adolescents' perceptions of the images on television. *Journal of Adolescent Research*, *21*(4), 393–414. https://doi.org/10.1177/0743558406288717

Rivadeneyra, R., Ward, L. M., & Gordon, M. (2007). Distorted reflections: Media exposure and Latino adolescents' conceptions of self. *Media Psychology*, *9*(2), 261–290. https://doi.org/10.1080/15213260701285926

Rogers, O., Mastro, D., Robb, M. B., & Peebles, A. (2021). *The inclusion imperative: Why media representation matters for kids' ethnic-racial development*. Common Sense.

Rose, J., Mackey-Kallis, S., Shyles, L., Barry, K., Biagini, D., Hart, C., & Jack, L. (2012). Face it: The impact of gender on social media images. *Communication Quarterly*, *60*(5), 588–607.

Roth-Cohen, O., Kanevska, H., & Eisend, M. (2022). Gender roles in online advertising. *Journal of Gender Studies*, *32*(2), 186–200. https://doi.org/10.1080/09589236.2022.2102970

Scharrer, E., Ramasubramanian, S., & Banjo, O. (2022). Media, diversity, and representation in the U.S.: A review of the quantitative research literature on media content and effects. *Journal of Broadcasting & Electronic Media*, *66*(4), 723–749. https://doi.org/10.1080/08838151.2022.2138890

Scharrer, E., & Warren, S. (2022). Adolescents' modern media use and beliefs about masculine gender roles and norms. *Journalism & Mass Communication Quarterly*, *99*(1), 289–315.

Selkie, E., Adkins, V., Masters, E., Bajpai, A., & Shumer, D. (2020). Transgender Adolescents' uses of social media for social support. *Journal of Adolescent Health*, *66*(3), 275–280. https://doi.org/10.1016/j.jadohealth.2019.08.011

Sink, A., & Mastro, D. (2017). Depictions of gender on primetime television: A quantitative content analysis. *Mass Communication and Society*, *20*(1), 3–22.
Slater, A., Halliwell, E., Jarman, H., & Gaskin, E. (2017). More than just child's play?: An experimental investigation of the impact of an appearance-focused internet game on body image and career aspirations of young girls. *Journal of Youth and Adolescence*, *46*, 2047–2059.
Smith, S. L., Choueiti, M., Prescott, A., & Pieper, K. (2012). *Gender roles & occupations: A look at character attributes and job-related aspirations in film and television*. Geena Davis Institute on Gender in Media.
Steele, J. R., & Brown, J. D. (1995). Adolescent room culture: Studying media in the context of everyday life. *Journal of Youth and Adolescence*, *24*(5), 551–576.
Steinke, J. (2017). Adolescent girls' STEM identity formation and media images of STEM professionals: Considering the influence of contextual cues. *Frontiers in Psychology*, *8*, 239856. https://doi.org/10.3389/fpsyg.2017.00716
Steinke, J., & Tavarez, P. M. P. (2017). Cultural representations of gender and STEM: Portrayals of female STEM characters in popular films 2002-2014. *International Journal of Gender, Science and Technology*, *9*(3), 244–277.
Stewart, A., Schuschke, J., & Tynes, B. (2019). Online racism: Adjustment and protective factors among adolescents of color. In H. Fitzgerald, D. Johnson, D. Qin, F. Villarruel, & J. Norder (Eds.), *Handbook of children and prejudice: Integrating research, practice, and policy* (pp. 501–513). Springer Nature.
Subrahmanyam, K., & Šmahel, D. (2011). *Digital youth: The role of media in development*. Springer.
Tao, X., & Fisher, C. (2022). Exposure to social media racial discrimination and mental health among adolescents of color. *Journal of Youth and Adolescence*, *51*, 30–44. https://doi.org/10.1007/s10964-021-01514-z
Terán, L., Shin, Y., & Jiao, J. (2023). Associations of adolescents' vocational anticipatory socialization: Exploring the roles of favorite television characters, gender, and parent-child communication. *Southern Communication Journal*, *88*(2), 148–159.
Thomas, A., Gale, A., & Golden, A. R. (2023). Online racial discrimination, critical consciousness, and psychosocial distress among Black and Latino adolescents: A moderated mediation model. *Journal of Youth and Adolescence*, *52*(5), 967–979.
Tompkins, T. L., Shields, C. N., Hillman, K. M., & White, K. (2015). Reducing stigma toward the transgender community: An evaluation of a humanizing and perspective-taking intervention. *Psychology of Sexual Orientation and Gender Diversity*, *2*(1), 34.
Tortajada, I., Araüna-Baró, N., & Martínez-Martínez, I.-J. (2013). Advertising stereotypes and gender representation in social networking sites. *Comunicar*, *21*(41), 177.
Tukachinsky, R., Mastro, D., & Yarchi, M. (2015). Documenting portrayals of race/ethnicity on primetime television over a 20-year span and their association with national-level racial/ethnic attitudes. *Journal of Social Issues*, *71*(1), 17–38. https://doi.org/10.1111/josi.12094
Turiel, O. (2022). Can hedonic technology use drive sexism in youth? Reconsidering the cultivation and objectification perspectives. *Behaviour & Information Technology*, *43*(2), 231–245. https://doi.org/10.1080/0144929x.2022.2159874
Tynes, B. M., Del Toro, J., & Lozada, F. T. (2015). An unwelcomed digital visitor in the classroom: The longitudinal impact of online racial discrimination on academic motivation. *School Psychology Review*, *44*(4), 407–424.

Tynes, B., English, D., Del Toro, J., Smith, N., Lozada, F., & Williams, D. (2020). Trajectories of online racial discrimination and psychological functioning among African American and Latino adolescents. *Child Development, 91*(5), 1577–1593. https://doi.org/10.1111/cdev.13350

Tynes, B. M., Giang, M. T., Williams, D. R., & Thompson, G. N. (2008). Online racial discrimination and psychological adjustment among adolescents. *Journal of Adolescent Health, 43*(6), 565–569.

Tynes, B. M., Lozada, F. T., Smith, N. A., & Stewart, A. M. (2018). From racial microaggressions to hate crimes: A model of online racism based on the lived experiences of adolescents of color. In G. Torino, D. Rivera, C. Capodilupo, K. Nadal, & D. Sue (Eds.), *Microaggression theory: Influence and implications* (pp. 194–212). John Wiley & Sons, Inc.

Tynes, B. M., & Mitchell, K. J. (2014). Black youth beyond the digital divide: Age and gender differences in internet use, communication patterns, and victimization experiences. *Journal of Black Psychology, 40*(3), 291–307.

Tynes, B., Rose, C., Hiss, S., Umaña-Taylor, A., Mitchell, K., & Williams, D. (2014). Virtual environments, online racial discrimination, and adjustment among a diverse, school-based sample of adolescents. *International Journal of Gaming and Computer-Mediated Simulations, 6*(3), 1–16. https://pmc.ncbi.nlm.nih.gov/articles/PMC4851344/

Tynes, B. M., Rose, C. A., & Markoe, S. L. (2013). Extending campus life to the internet: Social media, discrimination, and perceptions of racial climate. *Journal of Diversity in Higher Education, 6*(2), 102.

Tynes, B. M., Umana-Taylor, A. J., Rose, C. A., Lin, J., & Anderson, C. J. (2012). Online racial discrimination and the protective function of ethnic identity and self-esteem for African American adolescents. *Developmental Psychology, 48*(2), 343–355.

Tynes, B., Willis, H., Stewart, A., & Hamilton, M. (2019). Race-related traumatic events online and mental health among adolescents of color. *Journal of Adolescent Health, 65*(3), 371–377. https://doi.org/10.1016/j.jadohealth.2019.03.006

Uka, A. (2015). Students' educational and occupational aspirations are predicted by parents' and adolescents' characteristics. *European Journal of Social Science Education and Research, 2*(2), 56–67.

Valkenburg, P. M., & Peter, J. (2013). The differential susceptibility to media effects model. *Journal of Communication, 63*, 221–243.

Van Oosten, J., Vandenbosch, L., & Peter, J. (2017). Gender roles on social networking sites: Investigating reciprocal relationships between Dutch adolescents' hypermasculinity and hyperfemininity and sexy online self-presentations. *Journal of Children and Media, 11*(2), 147–166. https://doi.org/10.1080/17482798.2017.1304970

Vogels, E. A., Gelles-Watnick, R., & Massarat, N. (2022). *Teens, social media and technology 2022*. Pew Research Center.

Volpe, V., Benson, G., Ross, J., Briggs, A., Mejia-Bradford, S., Alexander, A., & Hope, E. (2023). Finding the bright side: Positive online racial experiences, racial identity, and activism for Black young adults. *Computers in Human Behavior, 144*, 107738.

Ward, L. M. (2004). Wading through the stereotypes: Positive and negative associations between media use and Black adolescents' conceptions of self. *Developmental Psychology, 40*(2), 284–294. https://doi.org/10.1037/0012-1649.40.2.284

Ward, L. M., Bridgewater, E., & Reynaga, M. (2024). Media influences. In W. Troop-Gordon and E. Neblett (Eds.), *Encyclopedia of adolescence* (Vol. 2,

2nd ed., pp. 246–256). Elsevier, Academic Press. https://doi.org/10.1016/B978-0-323-96023-6.00076-2

Ward, L. M., & Grower, P. (2020). Media and the development of gender stereotypes. *Annual Review of Developmental Psychology, 2*, 177–199. https://doi.org/10.1146/annurev-devpsych-051120-010630

Webb, L., Clary, L. K., Johnson, R. M., & Mendelson, T. (2021). Electronic and school bullying victimization by race/ethnicity and sexual minority status in a nationally representative adolescent sample. *Journal of Adolescent Health, 68*(2), 378–384. https://doi.org/10.1016/j.jadohealth.2020.05.042

Wiest, J. B. (2016). Entertaining genius: US media representations of exceptional intelligence. *MediaTropes, 6*(2), 148–170.

Ybarra, M. L., Mitchell, K. J., Palmer, N. A., & Reisner, S. L. (2015). Online social support as a buffer against online and offline peer and sexual victimization among U.S. LGBT and non-LGBT youth. *Child Abuse & Neglect, 39*, 123–136. https://doi.org/10.1016/j.chiabu.2014.08.006

Zhang, Q. (2010). Asian Americans beyond the model minority stereotype: The nerdy and the left out. *Journal of International and Intercultural Communication, 3*(1), 20–37. https://doi.org/10.1080/17513050903428109

Zheng, W., Yuan, C., Chang, W., & Wu, Y. (2016). Profile pictures on social media: Gender and regional differences. *Computers in Human Behavior, 63*, 891–898. https://doi.org/10.1016/j.chb.2016.06.041

Zhou, X. (2020). For better or for worse for females? A content analysis of gender-motivated comments on social media platforms. *Advances in Social Science, Education and Humanities Research, 466*, 1192–1199. https://www.atlantis-press.com/proceedings/isemss-20/125944167

8 Body Image

Jennifer Stevens Aubrey, Heather Gahler, and Kausumi Saha

In this chapter, we start from the radical position that all bodies are worthy and deserve respect, and further, children and adolescents deserve to live in a world that encourages this view. As such, we view body image as a social justice issue for several reasons. First, because adherence to dominant body ideals, such as thinness or athleticism, comes with privilege and power (Klebl et al., 2022), children likely learn that their goal is to be included in these preferred groups. Second, and related, such dynamics give rise to bias and prejudice based on weight. Not surprisingly, appearance-based bullying is the most common form of bullying that children and adolescents experience (Armitage, 2021), and other forms of bias and prejudice based on body size and appearance differences (including but not limited to ableism, fatphobia, and healthism) impact the health and well-being of all people, including children and adolescents (Harrison, 2021). Third, the cultural messages regarding attractiveness and beauty are quite exclusionary; there are many aspects of human difference that are systematically omitted from what is considered ideal, and these omissions can make children and adolescents feel that their bodies are invisible or less worthy than others (e.g., Sands & Wardle, 2003). In an ideal world, one that is not currently supported by Western media, children and adolescents would be exposed to cultural messages that encourage them to feel good about their own bodies, to celebrate their unique beauty regardless of what they look like, and to be accepting of others who may not look like themselves (Body Happy Org, n.d.). The media *could* be a powerful force for social justice in body image, but currently, we are far off from such a vision.

In this chapter, we will first examine the role of media in establishing cultural definitions of beauty, with a particular focus on differences in appearance and body ideals by race/ethnicity, gender/gender identity, and disability. Second, we will consider the role of developmental processes in relation to body image. Third, we will review the extensive research literature on media effects on body image, with a focus on the major theories that have been used to guide this research. Fourth, we will examine the existing research on media effects on the body image of children and adolescents who identify with marginalized social identities. Finally, we will consider the "body positivity" movement, at least how it is depicted in social media spaces, as a potential force in promoting social justice in body image.

Media, Body and Appearance Ideals, and Marginalized Identities

A major assumption of body image is that in addition to family and peers, the media largely define and reinforce what is considered attractive or ideal (Thompson et al., 1999). However, the media reinforce ideals that are quite homogenous, excluding all manner of human differences including both visible and invisible social categories. In the following, we will highlight research on body and appearance ideals by race/ethnicity, by gender/gender identity, and by ability.

Race and Ethnicity

Historically, mainstream appearance ideals have been Eurocentric, with a focus on slenderness (Holland & Tiggemann, 2016). In recent years, body ideals have shifted somewhat, with curvier body types (often referred to as "slim-thick") and fit-ideal body types (i.e., athletic and muscular) becoming prevalent and idealized (Belmonte et al., 2024; McComb & Mills, 2022). However, instead of ideals being more inclusive for all individuals, the research suggests that girls and women, especially, feel pressure to simultaneously adhere to multiple body ideals (curvy, fit-ideal, *and* thin; Betz et al., 2019; Gahler et al., 2023).

Because body image is grounded in one's broader identity, different cultural standards and appearance expectations account for systemic differences in body and appearance ideals by the racial and ethnic in-groups with which one identifies. Although there are systematic patterns in appearance ideals among racial and ethnic groups, we also acknowledge that not all individuals belonging to these groups hold these ideals. Like any cultural norm, there is variation within these overall patterns. With that in mind, White and Asian-American women generally idealize thinness. For White women, thinness has been a long-standing body ideal associated with purity, discipline, and Eurocentric beauty (Overstreet et al., 2010). For Asian and Asian-American women, thinness is often a component of stereotypical notions of beauty as well. In media representations, Asian women are often exoticized and depicted as hypersexual and submissive sexual objects; consequently, Asian-American women feel pressure to be small and petite (Brady et al., 2017).

A preference for slenderness is not universal across racial and ethnic groups. Black women's bodies have been historically marginalized and objectified (Lowy et al., 2021), but according to the "strong Black woman" stereotype, a heavier body weight symbolizes strength, independence, and resilience (Overstreet et al., 2010). Thus, an endorsement of the "strong Black woman" stereotype, might explain why Black women desire to have a small waist, but at the same time, a curvaceous upper and lower body shape (Poran, 2006; Romo et al., 2016). Similarly, Latinas also report greater preferences for curvaceous body types as opposed to thin ones (Bakhshi et al., 2014). Latina culture values a "buen cuerpo" ideal, consisting of a slender but curvy body, with a thin waist, big breasts, and ample hips (de Casanova, 2004; Romo et al., 2016).

Like body ideals, mainstream appearance ideals have been largely Eurocentric, with an underlying idealization of Eurocentric features such as blonde, straight hair and large, blue eyes (Awad et al., 2015; Jefferson & Stake, 2009). Eurocentric appearance standards put pressure on people to conform to beauty standards that are often phenotypically inappropriate for their racial and ethnic group. For example, in focus groups, some Black emerging-adult women identified hair as a constant source of concern (Awad et al., 2015). Many participants reported feeling pressure to forgo natural hairstyles in favor of treated, straightened hair as the latter is considered more closely aligned with White standards. Many also internalized the preference for a lighter skin tone, even among people of their own racial in-group (Awad et al., 2015). Some Asian-American emerging-adult women also preferred a phenotypically White face compared to a phenotypically East Asian face, and they perceived themselves as having a more phenotypically East Asian face than they objectively did (Thai et al., 2020).

Gender and Gender Identity

Although the media ideals that we have focused on so far have been largely defined for women and girls, the media also define body and appearance ideals for boys and men. While it is undesirable to be overweight for both girls and boys, for boys, it is also undesirable to be too thin or not sufficiently muscular (Labre, 2005). Thus, among men and boys, body dissatisfaction is typically tied to a desire for muscularity. The current ideal body for men is characterized by a mesomorphic body type, with well-defined abdominal and arm muscles, broad shoulders, and a thin waist (Kling et al., 2016). For example, 22% of young-adult men engage in some type of muscle-building behaviors, including eating more or differently to gain muscle, using weight-gain supplements, and even androgenic-anabolic steroid use (Nagata et al., 2019). Meanwhile, cultural pressures regarding men's bodies have increased dramatically in recent years. For example, advertisements for diet supplements, fitness programs, and grooming products all reinforce the idea that for men, just as it is for women, there is a need to improve one's body (Duggan & McCreary, 2004). Like girls, the need to conform to the muscular ideal emerges around the time that boys experience puberty. For example, in a study of preadolescent boys (average age = 11 years), those who consumed more sports magazines were more likely to report personal mesomorphic standards and perceived mesomorphic standards (i.e., muscular, lean, fit body shape) for men and boys in general (Rousseau et al., 2017).

In addition to cisgender adolescents, appearance and body ideals are relevant to gender-minority youth, including those who identify as non-binary, gender-queer, and transgender. Transgender folks, already prone to body dysmorphia, may face additional consequences of media-based assertions of the "ideal" transgender body (McGuire et al., 2016; Price, 2019), which is one that "passes" as their preferred gender identity and adheres to gendered appearance norms (Heiden-Rootes et al., 2023). Mainstream discourses advance the "wrong body" narrative of the subjective transgender identity, one that needs to be fixed by various bodily modifications (Barker-Plummer, 2013). Media representations of transgender characters are shown to either be in various stages of change or transformation, or having already achieved the cisgender ideal that they "should" be (Lovelock, 2017; Price, 2019).

Disability

An oft-ignored marginalized group in the media is persons with visible and invisible disabilities. Individuals with visible physical disabilities are more prone to negative body image due to the societal devaluation of their bodies, and this is directly related to the severity of impairment (Argyrides et al., 2023; Shpigelman & HaGani, 2019). In general, the media define appearance and body ideals that assume an abled body, leaving those with disabilities invisible. Media scholars often call this "symbolic annihilation," when representations of certain groups, in this case disabled folks, are simply absent from mainstream discourse (Gerbner & Gross, 1976). Rendering a group invisible essentially maintains its lower status in society.

Taken together, children are attuned to the differing body and appearance ideals that are illustrated in the media. Indeed, by preadolescence (usually considered 9–12 years old), children use the media to gather appearance norms and information so that they can cope with their body concerns (Rousseau et al., 2018). Further, by this age, girls have internalized body ideals from the media, and this is further linked to their body dissatisfaction (Sands & Wardle, 2003). For children and adolescents who do not conform to the Eurocentric, cisgender, and abled-bodied standards that they see in the media, they are likely to feel left out. Some will challenge the ideals, and in the spirit of social justice, resistance should be encouraged (Body Happy Org, n.d.). However, many children and adolescents just want to fit in, and the dominant media system is not serving their best interests. In the next section, we will discuss the development of body image in childhood and adolescence.

Development of Body and Appearance Concerns

During early childhood, children typically process their environment perceptually, which means that they attend to what people, places, and things look like more so than what they conceptually mean (Elkind, 1975). Thus, children are attuned to how people look. People whose appearance deviates from the norms that they have internalized will likely draw their attention. By the age of five, children often develop a weight bias, believing that thinner people are more intelligent, friendly, successful, and strong-willed than fat people (Damiano et al., 2015). Weight bias may be eventually internalized and applied to the self. For example, Davison et al. (2003) found that children who exhibited a weight bias at 5 and 7 years were more likely to have higher dietary restraint, more maladaptive eating attitudes, and a greater likelihood of dieting at 9 years.

During middle childhood (approximately 6–9 years), children start to compare themselves to others, usually their peers, on aspects such as physical/athletic abilities and appearance (Neves et al., 2021). Such early comparisons are the basis of body image development. By preadolescence (approximately 9–12), children begin to experience body (dis)satisfaction as they make subjective evaluations of their own bodies in relation to others (Smolak, 2004). Thus, if they have unease about how their bodies and appearance compares to others, they will start to become preoccupied with their physical appearance, and they might start to take actions (e.g., diet, exercise, cosmetics) to live up to the idealized standards that they have internalized.

By adolescence, body and appearance concerns are normative. Over 70% of adolescent girls want to be thinner (compared to preadolescent age-groups in which the percentage generally ranges from 40% to 60%), and over 60% of adolescent girls have attempted to lose weight (Wertheim & Paxton, 2012). Likewise, for boys, the preference for a large and muscular ideal body peaks in adolescence (Ricciardelli, 2012). During and after puberty, adolescents experience changes to their bodies and appearance, which can bring them further in line or out of line with sociocultural standards of attractiveness. Boys' bodies tend to cooperate with the body standards that they internalize; "filling out" brings them closer to masculine appearance ideals (Ricciardelli, 2012). For girls, puberty generally brings their bodies out of alignment with feminine body standards (Wertheim & Paxton, 2012). Thus, because their bodies are rapidly changing, adolescents are sensitive to understanding the sociocultural appearance ideals for bodies, particularly for the members of their social group (e.g., age, gender, race/ethnicity).

Likewise, peers are an essential sources of appearance information, and their feedback on adolescents' appearance can be quite potent. During adolescence, acceptance from peers is a primary reason why adolescents are drawn to social media (Webb & Zimmer-Gembeck, 2014), and social media, in turn, provide them with a plethora of information about how they should look (Choukas-Bradley et al., 2022).

Taken together, even young children learn what people should look like from the media, and from that early exposure, many develop weight stigma. As early as middle childhood, and certainly by adolescence, youth have internalized mediated ideals related to appearance and bodies and apply the ideals to themselves. In Table 8.1, we summarize the relevant developmental milestones and associated changes in different facets of body image that can describe children from non-marginalized identity groups.

Table 8.1 Developmental changes related to body image.

	Early Childhood (0–5 years)	Middle Childhood (6–9 years)	Preadolescence (9–12 years)	Adolescence (13–18 years)
Developmental Changes	Young children are perceptual thinkers, making them sensitive to other people's appearances, especially if they appear out of the ordinary.	Social comparison to peers starts to occur.	Social comparison to peers continues and increases in frequency.	The major developmental task is the construction of a coherent identity, and body image is an important aspect of that identity. Feedback from peers is an important source of information about appearance. Concerns with reputation and status among one's peer group are heightened, and for many adolescents, appearance will be relevant to these concerns.

(Continued)

Table 8.1 (Continued)

	Early Childhood (0–5 years)	Middle Childhood (6–9 years)	Preadolescence (9–12 years)	Adolescence (13–18 years)
Weight Concerns	Development of weight bias (i.e., internalized a cultural bias against fat people) occurs by age 5.	Girls learn to strive for a slim body type; boys learn to strive for a lean, muscular body type (i.e., mesomorphic).	On average, girls want to be thinner than they are, whereas boys are fairly split on wanting to lose weight or gain weight.	Pubertal increases in weight typically cause boys to come more aligned with dominant body ideals for men (i.e., "filled out"). Pubertal changes typically cause girls to feel more misaligned with the dominant thinness body ideal for many women.
Body Satisfaction/ Image	Although difficult to measure body satisfaction in young children, by 1.5–2 years, they are aware of their own appearance and how other people respond to it.	Children's conceptions of their ideal appearance become relatively stable. Subjective evaluations of one's own bodies leads to body satisfaction or dissatisfaction. Girls typically experience more body dissatisfaction than boys.	Body (dis)satisfaction will likely affect self-esteem. Body image schemas (e.g., "thinness" schema, "muscular" schema) are in place. Actions (e.g., diet, exercise, cosmetics) to "fix" appearance will typically start.	Body and appearance concerns are normative and stable. For girls, body satisfaction is more likely to be related to appearance; for boys, it is more likely to be related to functional aspects of the body (i.e., "what the body can do").

Source: Authors

Note: These are generalizations that would not necessarily describe all children, nor will they describe many children from marginalized social groups. The generalizations provided in this table were informed by five review articles on the development of body image (see McCabe, 2012; Ricciardelli, 2012; Smolak, 2004; 2012; Wertheim & Paxton, 2012).

Effects of Media on Body Image

The role that media (both traditional and social) plays in one's body image, both in terms of impacting the concept of, as well as the ongoing negotiation with, one's own body image, has been studied extensively for the past several decades. In the following, we provide a brief overview of the existing literature, focusing on research with youth younger than 18 years where possible and drawing on studies from young adults (i.e., roughly ages 18–29) to fill in gaps when necessary. We review this literature through three theoretical lenses: the *tripartite model* (Thompson et al., 1999), *social comparison theory* (Festinger, 1954), and *objectification theory* (Fredrickson & Roberts, 1997).

The Tripartite Model

The Tripartite Model is an integrative theoretical framework that describes three major sources of cultural and societal beauty standards on individuals' body image: peers, family, and media (Thompson et al., 1999). Each of the three sources lead to both internalization of appearance ideals and social comparison, and these two constructs, in turn, predict individuals' body image.

The internalization of media ideals occurs when individuals buy into, or apply to themselves, the ideals of attractiveness that they have learned through the media (Thompson & Stice, 2001). These ideals may relate to both one's body shape and size, and, more broadly, their appearance, which might include their facial features, hair, and skin. Decades of research has shown that media exposure is predictive of the internalization of media ideals (see Grabe et al., 2008; Mingoia et al., 2017 for meta-analyses). By early adolescence, children's internalization of these ideals from the media is predictive of their body dissatisfaction and disordered eating (e.g., Keery et al., 2004; Zimmer-Gembeck et al., 2023).

Recently, the conceptualization of the internalization of media ideals has widened to include the sociocultural ideals that one might learn from social media (Roberts et al., 2022). Adolescents use highly visual forms of social media, such as Instagram and Snapchat, that focus on physical appearance. Additionally, body ideals, as defined by social media, include not only the thin ideal, but also an athletic/fit ideal (with defined musculature; Roberts et al., 2022) as well as a slim-thick ideal (McComb & Mills, 2022), and instead of social media broadening ideals, they instead appear to reinforce pressure to adhere to multiple ideals at the same time (e.g., Donovan et al., 2020; Roberts et al., 2022). As such, social media use and exposure are also associated with the internalization of body ideals (Mingoia et al., 2017), with downstream consequences for body dissatisfaction, self-objectification, and appearance comparison (Prichard et al., 2023).

The quantifiable metrics of social media in terms of followers, likes, and comments make it particularly salient for adolescents, who are typically interested in popularity and social status (Choukas-Bradley et al., 2022). Such quantifiable feedback also encourages youth to compare themselves not only to their own peers, but also to influencers (i.e., prominent individuals who have a high number of followers) and celebrities. Indeed, social comparison is another mediating pathway linking media use and exposure and body image outcomes, a process that can be further explicated by social comparison theory.

Social Comparison Theory

Social comparison theory assumes that people are driven by a need to evaluate themselves, and they satisfy this need by engaging in comparisons to others (Festinger, 1954). Even when there are objective standards that people could use to evaluate their bodies (e.g., BMI, objective health criteria), people consistently choose to compare themselves to others to know where they stand (Fardouly et al., 2017). **Upwards comparisons** occur when individuals compare themselves to those viewed as superior on appearance standards, and these types of comparisons will typically have a negative effect on their body image and self-esteem (see Myers & Crowther, 2009, for a meta-analysis). **Downward comparisons** occur when individuals compare themselves to those who are inferior to their internalized appearance standards, and these comparisons generally have positive effects on individuals' body image (Myers & Crowther, 2009).

Although interpersonal social comparisons are most common (i.e., comparing oneself to those encountered face to face), the second most common comparison is to models who are featured in the media (Fardouly et al., 2017). The media provide ample opportunities for upward-mediated comparisons. Although adolescents typically recognize the unattainability of media models, they are still affected by their images. Social media influencers, in particular, foster the social comparison process because users see them as more realistic and natural than traditional celebrities (Fardouly et al., 2017; Prichard et al., 2023).

Research suggests that social comparison with media models, both from traditional media and social media comparison targets, is associated with negative body-image outcomes among adolescents (Keery et al., 2004; Rodgers et al., 2015). Further, in early adolescence (10–13 years old), both boys and girls engage in appearance comparison conversations about online media models with peers, which directly impact online appearance comparison in later adolescence (15–17 years old; Zimmer-Gembeck et al., 2023).

Objectification Theory

Objectification theory was developed to understand the experiences and consequences of sexual objectification, which occurs when one is treated as a body or a collection of body parts valued for its use to or consumption by others (Fredrickson & Roberts, 1997). Although men can be objectified, objectification functions within a historical system of male power that allows for the pervasiveness of objectification of women. Mediated depictions of sexual objectification are quite common in both traditional and social media. In general, media portrayals are considered sexually objectifying when the visual media highlights bodies and body parts, especially when depicting them as the target of a sexualized gaze (Calogero, 2012).

Self-objectification, defined as a third-person perspective on the self, such that people see themselves as objects to be consumed by others, is the primary consequence of sexual objectification (Calogero, 2012; Fredrickson & Roberts, 1997). Media consumption has been linked to chronic levels of self-objectification in adolescents (see Karsay et al., 2018, for meta-analysis). Once activated, self-objectification is linked to a variety of negative outcomes, including proximal consequences such as body shame, appearance anxiety, reduced interoceptive awareness, and distal consequences such as depression, disordered eating, and sexual dysfunction (Moradi & Huang, 2008).

Fredrickson and Roberts (1997) argued that self-objectification co-occurs with puberty, especially among girls from minoritized groups, as this is when their maturing bodies start to become subjected to a sexualized gaze. Although self-objectification has been measured in children as young as 5 to 7 years old (Perez et al., 2018), the evidence suggests that self-objectification increases with age (Daniels et al., 2020). Moreover, media use and exposure are linked to self-objectification in adolescent samples, but the limited research on the links between self-objectification and media exposure among preadolescent children has yielded inconsistent findings (e.g., Rousseau et al., 2017). Taken together, the research supports Fredrickson and Roberts (1997) theorizing that puberty is a turning point in self-objectification.

Media Effects on Body Image Among Children and Adolescents Who Identify with Marginalized Social Groups

The theoretical frameworks that were described above have been mostly used to examine media effects on body image among White, cisgender, able-bodied people. It is not well-understood whether these theories apply to children and adolescents who identify with marginalized social groups, and in our view of body image as a social justice issue, this is an imperative next step in the research. In the following, we will summarize what we know about research on media effects on body image among the marginalized identities that we discussed earlier in this chapter that were based on race/ethnicity, gender, and disability.

Racial and Ethnic Minority Youth

Research that focuses specifically on racial-minority or ethnic-minority children and adolescents is scarce, but among the existing studies, the findings typically illustrate either an acculturation effect (i.e., adopting the values, perceptions, and behaviors of the majority group) or a resistance effect (i.e., rejecting the values, perceptions, and behaviors of the majority group) on body image. Reflective of the first camp, one focus group study of non-Western minority children (ages 8–12) who were living in the Netherlands showed that children's body preferences were reflective of Western body ideals (Veldhuis et al., 2017). That is, their preferences for thin and "normal" bodies were reinforced by the media that they viewed, suggesting that the children had acculturated to the body ideals of the Western media environment to which they were exposed. The media have an acculturating effect on the body image of racial minority adolescents as well. For example, Gentles and Harrison (2006) reported that Black adolescent girls felt pressured by media to achieve a thin body ideal, and they felt frustrated that their attempts to resist this pressure were undermined by peers who had embraced the media-reinforced thin ideal.

At the same time, it is encouraging that youth can and do resist these mediated ideals. For example, among a racially diverse sample of children (ages 7–12), the internalization of media ideals (i.e., wanting the media ideal to be one's own personal ideal) was correlated with body dissatisfaction among the White children in the sample but not among the Black children or the children who identified with other racial groups (Harrison, 2009). As an explanation for this difference, Harrison suggested that the youth of color were likely consuming media with ideals that are more relevant to their own racial/ethnic identities and thus more likely to accept a wider range of body ideals beyond the thin ideal. Indeed, adolescents have expressed the idea of resisting "White" body ideals in qualitative studies. In an interview study, Black emerging-adult and teen women challenged White cultural norms of beauty about hair texture/thickness, nose, lips, and skin color, because they saw them as discriminating toward them and their racial in-group (Ringrose et al., 2019). Similarly, although Latina women reported as much body dissatisfaction as White women, ethnic identity protects against the negative impacts of media-based ideals (Umaña-Taylor et al., 2002). For instance, in an investigation of the effects of mainstream media on Latina adolescents' body image, Schooler and Daniels (2014) found that ethnic identity had a larger effect on body image than media exposure, and a stronger ethnic identity was correlated with higher body satisfaction overall.

Gender Minority Youth

Extensions of the above theories to gender-minority youth would need to carefully examine how subculture ideals may vary depending on one's gender self-presentation (Rodgers & Rousseau, 2022). The patterns of relationships between media use and body image may be less clear among gender-minority groups due to the heterogeneity of these identities combined with the paucity of existing research. Although we are not aware of any research that has examined the effects of mediated ideals on gender-minority youths' body image, research does suggest that they have worse body image than their cisgender peers (The Trevor Project, 2023). Thus, it is critical that future research examines how the mediated appearance and body ideals of gender minorities translate to their body image and mental health.

Physically Disabled Youth

Not surprisingly, research on the effects of media portrayals of disabled bodies is practically non-existent. One study by Tamari (2017) showed that a portrayal of the use of modern prosthetics among Paralympic athletes had some positive consequences for disabled audiences. The "prosthetic-aesthetic" had the effect of shifting the image of the disabled body from being hidden and camouflaged to one that is more exhibited and empowered (p. 25). Thus, such research provides a hopeful vision for normalizing disabled bodies in the media.

Social Media and Body Positivity

Although social media are often criticized for promoting unrealistic and unattainable appearance ideals, some, such as Instagram and TikTok, have simultaneously popularized body positivity (Cohen et al., 2019). The "body positivity" movement seemingly rejects narrowly defined and inaccessible body ideals in favor of a more inclusive and positive conceptualization of body image. The primary goals of body positivity are to increase visibility of otherwise underrepresented bodies in media (Cohen et al., 2019; Lazuka et al., 2020), as well as to normalize body attributes (e.g., cellulite, stretch marks) that do not conform to societal beauty ideals (Cohen et al., 2019). In a content analysis of 342 videos tagged #bodypositivity, Harriger et al. (2023) found that about one-third of the videos featured a theme that they considered encouraging of a positive body image (i.e., body appreciation, body acceptance and love, broad conceptualizing of beauty, self-adaptive investment, inner positivity, and filtering information in a body-protective manner). Indeed, the majority of videos highlighted body acceptance and love.

At the same time, body positivity has been criticized for keeping the focus on appearance (Webb et al., 2017) and for creating pressure to love one's body (Hallward et al., 2023). As a response to these criticisms, body neutrality has more recently been popularized on social media. Body positivity, body neutrality shifts the perspective from loving one's body to a focus on body functionality (Pellizzer & Wade, 2023). On TikTok, body neutrality is communicated by four main themes: Size Inclusivity (i.e., people's activities/preferences should not be based on body size), Adaptive Self-Investment (i.e., self-care focused on health), Body Appreciation (i.e., respect for what one's body can do), and No Judgment (i.e., a person's worth should not be based on appearance; Aubrey et al., 2024). Despite its emerging popularity, examinations of the effects of messages related to body neutrality are a needed step in future research (Pellizzer & Wade, 2023).

Research on the effects of body positivity messages so far has been mixed. Cohen et al. (2019) found that viewing body-positive posts on Instagram led participants to make more positive statements about their appearance compared to viewing thin-ideal or body-neutral posts; however, they also showed that body-focused messaging, even if positive, produced more self-objectification than neutral non-body messaging. Using a sample of undergraduate women, Westenberg and Oberle (2023) failed to find a significant effect of body-positivity TikTok videos on participants' body dissatisfaction. In a series of experiments with emerging adult women, Legault and Sago (2022) tested several body positivity messages to see what framing was the most effective in boosting body positivity. Participants viewed messages that either pressured women to feel good about their bodies (i.e., "You MUST accept your body or you will never be happy"), that highlighted the basic need of body acceptance from others (i.e., "There are lots of people out there who appreciate you just the way you are"), or that focused on body autonomy (i.e., "You are the author of your own happiness"). The pressuring messages produced less agency and lower acceptance of one's body compared to the other messages. Thus, this research suggests that not all body positivity messages will result in felt body positivity.

Conclusion

Despite the criticisms of body positivity, there is potential in this movement insofar as it challenges the homogenous and restrictive appearance ideals that dominate the media (Harriger et al., 2023). Media content that counters exclusionary ideals and provides more inclusive representations are key for children and adolescents, particularly those who identify with marginalized groups. In the spirit of social justice, "social media platforms provide opportunities for harnessing advocacy efforts to address and combat weight stigma, unrealistic appearance ideals, and content that promotes disordered eating behaviors" (Harriger et al., 2023, p. 225).

The existing research on body positivity, albeit nascent, implies an important role for researchers. Given that body positivity requires careful messaging strategies to be effective (Legault & Sago, 2022), researchers must test message strategies and then promote effective guidelines to social media content creators. Social media campaigns to raise awareness regarding the damaging effects of exposure to exclusionary media ideals should also be informed by research. Although there is still a long way to go before social justice in body image for children and adolescents is achieved, such research provides a hopeful way forward.

References

Argyrides, M., Koundourou, C., Angelidou, A., & Anastasiades, E. (2023). Body image, media influences, and situational dysphoria in individuals with visible physical disabilities. *International Journal of Psychological Research*, 16(1), 78–88. https://doi.org/10.21500/20112084.6014

Armitage, R. (2021). Bullying in children: Impact on child health. *BMJ Pediatrics Open*, 5(1), e000939–e000939. https://doi.org/10.1136/bmjpo-2020-000939

Aubrey, J. S., Zeng, J., Saha, K., Gahler, H., & Dajches, L. (2024). The body positive... or the body neutral?: A content analysis of body positivity and body neutrality hashtagged videos on TikTok. *Body Image*, 50, 101737. https://doi.org/10.1016/j.bodyim.2024.101737

Awad, G. H., Norwood, C., Taylor, D. S., Martinez, M., McClain, S., Jones, B., Holman, A., & Chapman-Hilliard, C. (2015). Beauty and body image concerns among African American college women. *Journal of Black Psychology*, 41(6), 540–564. https://doi.org/10.1177/0095798414550864

Bakhshi, S., Shamma, D., & Gilbert, E. (2014). Faces engage us. *Conference on Human Factors in Computing Systems - Proceedings*, 965–974. https://doi.org/10.1145/2556288.2557403

Barker-Plummer, B. (2013). Fixing Gwen: News and the mediation of (trans)gender challenges. *Feminist Media Studies*, 13(4), 710–724. https://doi.org/10.1080/14680777.2012.679289

Belmonte, A., Hopper, K. M., & Aubrey, J. S. (2024). Instagram use and endorsement of a voluptuous body ideal: A serial mediation model. *Sex Roles: A Journal of Research*. https://doi.org/10.1007/s11199-024-01442-9

Betz, D., Sabik, N. J., & Ramsey, L. R. (2019). Ideal comparisons: Body ideals harm women's body image through social comparison. *Body Image*, 29, 100–109.

Body Happy Org (n.d.) Why does body image matter? https://www.bodyhappy-org.com/why-does-body-image-matter

Brady, J. L., Kaya, A., Iwamoto, D., Park, A., Fox, L., & Moorhead, M. (2017). Asian American women's body image experiences: A qualitative intersectionality study. *Psychology of Women Quarterly*, 41(4), 479–496. https://doi.org/10.1177/0361684317725311

Calogero, R. M. (2012). Objectification theory, self-objectification, and body image. In Cash, T. (Ed.), *Encyclopedia of body image and human appearance* (pp. 574–580). Academic Press. https://doi.org/10.1016/B978-0-12-384925-0.00091-2

Choukas-Bradley, S., Roberts, S. R., Maheux, A. J., & Nesi, J. (2022). The perfect storm: A developmental–sociocultural framework for the role of social media in adolescent girls' body image concerns and mental health. *Clinical Child and Family Psychology Review*, 25, 681–701. https://doi.org/10.1007/s10567-022-00404-5

Cohen, R., Irwin, L., Newton-John, T., & Slater, A. (2019). #bodypositivity: A content analysis of body positive accounts on Instagram. *Body Image*, 29, 47–57. https://doi.org/10.1016/j.bodyim.2019.02.007

Damiano, S. R., Paxton, S. J., Wertheim, E. H., McLean, S. A., & Gregg, K. J. (2015). Dietary restraint of 5-year-old girls: Associations with internalization of the thin ideal and maternal, media, and peer influences. *The International Journal of Eating Disorders*, 48(8), 1166–1169. https://doi.org/10.1002/eat.22432

Daniels, E. A., Zurbriggen, E. L., & Ward, L. M. (2020). Becoming an object: A review of self-objectification in girls. *Body Image*, 33, 278–299. https://doi.org/10.1016/j.bodyim.2020.02.016

Davison, K. K., Markey, C. N., & Birch, L. L. (2003). A longitudinal examination of patterns in girls' weight concerns and body dissatisfaction from ages 5 to 9 years. *The International Journal of Eating Disorders*, 33(3), 320–332. https://doi.org/10.1002/eat.10142

de Casanova, E. M. (2004). "No ugly women": Concepts of race and beauty among adolescent women in Ecuador. *Gender & Society*, 18(3), 287–308. https://doi.org/10.1177/0891243204263351

Donovan, C. L., Uhlmann, L. R., & Loxton, N. J. (2020). Strong is the new skinny, but is it ideal?: A test of the tripartite influence model using a new measure of fit-ideal internalisation, *Body Image*, 35, 171–180. https://doi.org/10.1016/j.bodyim.2020.09.002

Duggan, S. J., & McCreary, D. R. (2004). Body image, eating disorders, and the drive for muscularity in gay and heterosexual men: The influence of media images. *Journal of Homosexuality*, 47, 45–58.

Elkind, D. (1975). Perceptual development in children: The work of Jean Piaget provides psychologists with important tools for analyzing perceptual skills and performances. *American Scientist*, 63(5), 533–541.

Fardouly, J., Pinkus, R. T., & Vartanian, L. R. (2017). The impact of appearance comparisons made through social media, traditional media, and in person in women's everyday lives. *Body Image*, 20, 31–39. https://doi.org/10.1016/j.bodyim.2016.11.002

Festinger, L. (1954). A theory of social comparison processes. *Human Relations*, 7(2), 117–140. https://doi.org/10.1177/001872675400700202

Fredrickson, B. L., & Roberts, T.-A. (1997). Objectification theory: Toward an understanding women's lived experiences and mental health risks. *Psychology of Women Quarterly*, 21, 173–206.

Gahler, H., Dajches, L., Terán, L., Yan, K., & Aubrey, J. S. (2023). Instagram influences: An examination of the tripartite influence model of body image among a racially diverse sample of young-adult women. *Computers in Human Behavior*, 145, 107785. https://doi.org/10.1016/j.chb.2023.107785

Gentles, K. A., & Harrison, K. (2006). Television and perceived peer expectations of body size among African American adolescent girls. *The Howard Journal of Communications*, 17(1), 39–55. https://doi.org/10.1080/10646170500487939

Gerbner, G., & Gross, L. (1976). Living with television: The violence profile. *Journal of Communication*, 26(2), 172–194. https://doi.org/10.1111/j.1460-2466.1976.tb01397.x

Grabe, S., Ward, L. M., & Hyde, J. S. (2008). The role of the media in body image concerns among women: A meta-analysis of experimental and correlational studies. *Psychological Bulletin*, 134(3), 460–476. https://doi.org/10.1037/0033-2909.134.3.460

Hallward, H., Feng, O., & Duncan, L. R. (2023). An exploration and comparison of #BodyPositivity and #BodyNeutrality content on TikTok. *Eating Behaviors*, *50*, 1–7. https://doi.org/10.1016/j.eatbeh.2023.101760.

Harriger, J. A., Wick, M. R., Sherline, C. M., & Kunz, A. L. (2023). The body positivity movement is not all that positive on TikTok: A content analysis of body positive TikTok videos. *Body Image*, *46*, 256–264. https://doi.org/10.1016/j.bodyim.2023.06.003

Harrison, D. (2021). *Belly of the beast: The politics of anti-fatness as anti-blackness*. Penguin.

Harrison, K. (2009). The multidimensional media influence scale: Confirmatory factor structure and relationship with body dissatisfaction among African American and Anglo American children. *Body Image*, *6*(3), 207–215. http://doi.org/10.1016/j.bodyim.2009.04.001

Heiden-Rootes, K., Linsenmeyer, W., Levine, S., Oliveras, M., & Joseph, M. (2023). A scoping review of the research literature on eating and body image for transgender and nonbinary adults. *Journal of Eating Disorders*, *11*(1), 111–140. https://doi.org/10.1186/s40337-023-00828-6

Holland, G., & Tiggemann, M. (2016). A systematic review of the impact of the use of social networking sites on body image and disordered eating outcomes. *Body Image*, *17*, 100–110. https://doi.org/10.1016/j.bodyim.2016.02.008

Jefferson, D., & Stake, J. E. (2009). Appearance self-attitudes of African-American and European American women: Media comparisons and internalization of beauty ideals. *Psychology of Women Quarterly*, *33*(4), 396–409. https://doi.org/10.1111/j.1471-6402.2009.01517.x

Karsay, K., Knoll, J., & Matthes, J. (2018). Sexualizing media use and self-objectification: A meta-analysis. *Psychology of Women Quarterly*, *42*(1), 9–28.

Keery, H., van den Berg, P., & Thompson, J. K. (2004). An evaluation of the tripartite influence model of body dissatisfaction and eating disturbance with adolescent girls. *Body Image*, *1*(3), 237–251. https://doi.org/10.1016/j.bodyim.2004.03.001

Klebl, C., Rhee, J. J., Greenaway, K. H., Luo, Y., & Bastian, B. (2022). Beauty goes down to the core: Attractiveness biases moral character attributions. *Journal of Nonverbal Behavior*, *46*(1), 83–97. https://doi.org/10.1007/s10919-021-00388-w

Kling, J., Rodgers, R. F., & Frisén, A. (2016). Young men's endorsement and pursuit of appearance ideals: The prospective role of appearance investment. *Body Image*, *16*, 10–16.

Labre, M. P. (2005). The male body ideal: Perspectives of readers and non-readers of fitness magazines. *The Journal of Men's Health & Gender*, *2*, 223–229.

Lazuka, R. F., Wick, M. R., Keel, P. K., & Harriger, J. A. (2020). Are we there yet? Progress in depicting diverse images of beauty in Instagram's body positivity movement. *Body Image*, *34*(1), 85–93. https://doi.org/10.1016/j.bodyim.2020.05.001

Legault, L., & Sago, A. (2022). When body positivity falls flat: Divergent effects of body acceptance messages that support vs. undermine basic psychological needs. *Body Image*, *41*, 225–238. https://doi.org/10.1016/j.bodyim.2022.02.013

Lovelock, M. (2017). Call me Caitlyn: Making and making over the 'authentic' transgender body in Anglo-American popular culture. *Journal of Gender Studies*, *26*(6), 675–687. https://doi.org/10.1080/09589236.2016.1155978

Lowy, A. S., Rodgers, R. F., Franko, D. L., Pluhar, E., & Webb, J. B. (2021). Body image and internalization of appearance ideals in black women: An update and call for culturally-sensitive research. *Body Image*, *39*, 313–327. https://doi.org/10.1016/j.bodyim.2021.10.005

McCabe, M. P. (2012). Body image development –boy children. In T. F. Cash (Ed.), *Encyclopedia of body image and human appearance* (pp. 207–211). Elsevier.

McComb, S. E., & Mills, J. S. (2022). The effect of physical appearance perfectionism and social comparison to thin-, slim-thick-, and fit-ideal Instagram imagery on young women's body image. *Body Image*, *40*, 165–175. https://doi.org/10.1016/j.bodyim.2021.12.003

McGuire, J. K., Doty, J. L., Catalpa, J. M., & Ola, C. (2016). Body image in transgender young people: Findings from a qualitative, community-based study. *Body Image*, *18*, 96–107. https://doi.org/10.1016/j.bodyim.2016.06.004

Mingoia, J., Hutchinson, A. D., Wilson, C., & Gleaves, D. H. (2017). The relationship between social networking site use and the internalization of a thin ideal in females: A meta-analytic review. *Frontiers in Psychology*, *8*, 1351.

Moradi, B., & Huang, Y.-P. (2008). Objectification theory and psychology of women: A decade of advances and future directions. *Psychology of Women Quarterly*, *32*(4), 377–398. https://doi.org/10.1111/j.1471-6402.2008.00452.x

Myers, T. A., & Crowther, J. H. (2009). Social comparison as a predictor of body dissatisfaction: A meta-analytic review. *Journal of Abnormal Psychology*, *118*(4), 683–698. https://doi.org/10.1037/a0016763

Nagata, J. M., Murray, S. B., Bibbins-Domingo, K., Garber, A. K., Mitchison, D., & Griffiths, S. (2019). Predictors of muscularity-oriented disordered eating behaviors in U.S. Young adults: A prospective cohort study. *The International Journal of Eating Disorders*, *52*(12), 1380–1388. https://doi.org/10.1002/eat.23094

Neves, C. M., Filgueiras Meireles, J. F., Morgado, F. F. R., Campos, P. F., & Ferreira, M. E. C. (2021). Child body concerns and behavior scale: Development and psychometric properties of a body image scale for children. *Perceptual and Motor Skills*, *128*(1), 220–242. https://doi.org/10.1177/0031512520948285

Overstreet, N. M., Quinn, D. M., & Agocha, V. B. (2010). Beyond thinness: The influence of a curvaceous body ideal on body dissatisfaction in black and white women. *Sex Roles*, *63*(1-2), 91–103. https://doi.org/10.1007/s11199-010-9792-4

Pellizzer, M. L., & Wade, T. D. (2023). Developing a definition of body neutrality and strategies for an intervention. *Body Image*, *46*, 434–442. https://doi.org/10.1016/j.bodyim.2023.07.006

Perez, M., Kroon Van Diest, A. M., Smith, H., & Sladek, M. R. (2018). Body dissatisfaction and its correlates in 5- to 7-year-old girls: A social learning experiment. *Journal of Clinical Child and Adolescent Psychology*, *47*, 757–769. http://dx.doi.org/10.1080/15374416.2016.1157758

Poran, M. A. (2006). The politics of protection: Body image, social pressures, and the misrepresentation of young black women. *Sex Roles*, *55*(11-12), 739–755. https://doi.org/10.1007/s11199-006-9129-5

Prichard, I., Taylor, B., & Tiggemann, M. (2023). Comparing and self-objectifying: The effect of sexualized imagery posted by Instagram Influencers on women's body image. *Body Image*, *46*, 347–355. https://doi.org/10.1016/j.bodyim.2023.07.002

Price, S. (2019). Nia Nal the super girl: Transgender representation and body image. *Popular Culture Studies Journal*, *7*(2), 85–106.

Ricciardelli, L. A. (2012). Body image development – Adolescent boys. In T. F. Cash (Ed.), *Encyclopedia of body image and human appearance* (pp. 180–186). Elsevier.

Ringrose, J., Tolman, D., & Ragonese, M. (2019). Hot right now: Diverse girls navigating technologies of racialized sexy femininity. *Feminism & Psychology*, *29*(1), 76–95. https://doi.org/10.1177/0959353518806324

Roberts, S. A., Maheux, A. J., Hunt, R. A., Ladd, B. A., & Choukas-Bradley, S. (2022). Incorporating social media and muscular ideal internalization into the tripartite influence model of body image: Towards a modern understanding of adolescent girls' body dissatisfaction. *Body Image*, *44*, 239–244. https://doi.org/10.1016/j.bodyim.2022.03.002

Rodgers, R. F., McLean, S. A., & Paxton, S. J. (2015). Longitudinal relationships among internalization of the media ideal, peer social comparison, and body dissatisfaction: Implications for the tripartite influence model. *Developmental Psychology*, *51*(5), 706–713. https://doi.org/10.1037/dev0000013

Rodgers, R. F., & Rousseau, A. (2022). Social media and body image: Modulating effects of social identities and user characteristics. *Body Image*, *41*, 284–291. https://doi.org/10.1016/j.bodyim.2022.02.009

Romo, L. F., Mireles-Rios, R., & Hurtado, A. (2016). Cultural, media, and peer influences on body beauty perceptions of Mexican American adolescent girls. *Journal of Adolescent Research*, *31*(4), 474–501. https://doi.org/10.1177/0743558415594424.

Rousseau, A., Gamble, H., & Eggermont, S. (2017). The role of appearance schematicity in the internalization of media appearance ideals: A panel study of preadolescents. *Journal of Adolescence*, *60*, 27–38. http://dx.doi.org/10.1016/j.adolescence.2017.07.011

Rousseau, A., Trekels, J., & Eggermont, S. (2018). Preadolescents' reliance on and internalization of media appearance ideals: Triggers and consequences. *The Journal of Early Adolescence*, *38*(8), 1074–1099. https://doi.org/10.1177/0272431617714330

Sands, E. R., & Wardle, J. (2003). Internalization of ideal body shapes in 9-12-year-old girls. *The International Journal of Eating Disorders*, *33*(2), 193–204. https://doi.org/10.1002/eat.10121

Schooler, D., & Daniels, E. A. (2014). "I am not a skinny toothpick and proud of it": Latina adolescents' ethnic identity and responses to mainstream media images. *Body Image*, *11*(1), 11–18. https://doi.org/10.1016/j.bodyim.2013.09.001

Shpigelman, C., & HaGani, N. (2019). The impact of disability type and visibility on self concept and body image: Implications for mental health nursing. *Journal of Psychiatric and Mental Health Nursing*, *26*(3–4), 77–86. https://doi.org/10.1111/jpm.12513

Smolak, L. (2004). Body image in children and adolescents: Where do we go from here? *Body Image*, *1*(1), 15–28. https://doi.org/10.1016/S1740-1445(03)00008-1

Smolak, L. (2012). Body image development – Girl children. In T. F. Cash (Ed.), *Encyclopedia of body image and human appearance* (pp. 180–186). Elsevier.

Tamari, T. (2017). Body image and prosthetic aesthetics: Disability, technology and paralympic culture. *Body & Society*, *23*(2), 25–56. https://doi.org/10.1177/1357034X17697364

Thai, M., Lee, A. J., Axt, J. R., Hornsey, M. J., & Barlow, F. K. (2020). Discrepancies in East Asians' perceived actual and ideal phenotypic facial features. *Asian American Journal of Psychology*, *11*(3), 117–125. https://doi.org/10.1037/aap0000181

The Trevor Project. (2023). *2023 U.S. national survey on the mental health of LGBTQ young people*. https://www.thetrevorproject.org/survey-2023/

Thompson, J. K., Heinberg, L. J., Altabe, M., & Tantleff-Dunn, S. (1999). *Exacting beauty: Theory, assessment, and treatment of body image disturbance.* American Psychological Association. https://doi.org/10.1037/10312-000

Thompson, J. K., & Stice, E. (2001). Thin-ideal internalization: Mounting evidence for a new risk factor for body-image disturbance and eating pathology. *Current Directions in Psychological Science, 10,* 181–183.

Umaña-Taylor, A. J., Diversi, M., & Fine, M. A. (2002). Ethnic identity and self-esteem of Latino adolescents: Distinctions among the Latino populations. *Journal of Adolescent Research, 17*(3), 303–327. https://doi.org/10.1177/0743558402173005

Veldhuis, J., te Poel, F., Pepping, R., Konijn, E. A., & Spekman, M. L. C. (2017). "Skinny is prettier and normal: I want to be normal"—Perceived body image of non-Western ethnic minority children in the Netherlands. *Body Image, 20,* 74–86. https://doi.org/10.1016/j.bodyim.2016.11.006

Webb, J. B., Vinoski, E. R., Bonar, A. S., Davies, A. E., & Etzel, L. (2017). Fat is fashionable and fit: A comparative content analysis of fatspiration and health at every size® Instagram images. *Body Image, 22,* 53–64. https://doi.org/10.1016/j.bodyim.2017.05.003

Webb, J. B., & Zimmer-Gembeck, M. J. (2014). The role of friends and peers in adolescent body dissatisfaction: A review and critique of 15 years of research. *Journal of Research on Adolescence, 24*(4), 564–590. https://doi.org/10.1111/jora.12084

Wertheim, E. H., & Paxton, S. J. (2012). Body image development – Adolescent girls. In T. F. Cash (Ed.), *Encyclopedia of body image and human appearance* (pp. 187–193). Elsevier.

Westenberg, J. M., & Oberle, C. D. (2023). The impact of body-positivity and body-checking TikTok videos on body image. *The Journal of Social Media in Society, 12*(1), 49–60.

Zimmer-Gembeck, M. J., Hawes, T., Scott, R. A., Campbell, T., & Webb, H. J. (2023). Adolescents' online appearance preoccupation: A 5-year longitudinal study of the influence of peers, parents, beliefs, and disordered eating. *Computers in Human Behavior, 140.* https://doi.org/10.1016/j.chb.2022.107569

9 Aggression

Marina Krcmar, Toni Lane Hines, and Olivia Buckley

Research on the effects of media violence on children and youth spans more than a century, with one of the earliest examinations emerging in the 1920s from what came to be known as the Payne Fund studies. The 1933 Payne Fund studies—twelve volumes of research conducted by psychologists, sociologists, and educators—linked exposure to media violence (at the time, film and comic books) to aggression in children. Little if any attention was paid to individual differences in whether media effects differed by age, gender, or other aspects of diversity. Early research also tended to ignore how perpetrators and victims were represented.

More recent research has attended to these important questions given the need to consider issues such as underrepresentation (see Chapter 3) and differential effects on various racial, ethnic, and other underrepresented groups (see Chapter 7). Clearly, neither a single chapter nor indeed a full book can adequately cover that breadth of research on media violence and youth. Nevertheless, to provide an overview appropriate for students of and scholars in media effects, the current chapter seeks to use a framework of focus on underrepresentation in media violence, both in the content that is shown and who is affected.

With that in mind, we start by reviewing research that examines how violence and aggression are represented in media that targets children and adolescents. Next, we review older forms of media and move more-or-less chronologically through emerging forms. We briefly consider some of the more classic research that examines media such as television and film. Although this earliest research tended not to consider the importance of marginalized groups' representation and effects, the arrival of video games onto the media scene exposed children to a more diverse representation in both positive and negative ways. In a related vein, the last two decades have also seen a rise in attention among researchers to not only media aggression, but to moral reasoning in children and how moral judgment and development can be influenced by media exposure. Violent content in the media—in the stories told in film, TV, or games or in the comments, videos, or other content shared on the internet—brings up key questions about morality. Finally, we consider our most recent form of media—one that has captured more attention from adolescents than other more traditional media formats, social media, specifically, cyberbullying. For the section on cyberbullying and beyond, we caution readers of the book that there may be potentially triggering discussions related to self-harm.

Representations of Violence in Media

Media violence includes any depictions of behaviors intended to harm another by way of physical aggression or relational aggression (e.g., Archer & Coyne, 2005). Whereas *physical aggression* refers to a fairly obvious set of bodily harms inflicted on others, *relational aggression* is a subtle indirect form of social aggression mostly given through manipulation, bullying, or social exclusion; it is not physical (Coyne & Stockdale, 2014). Physical aggression is therefore somewhat self-explanatory, as it is aggression that is clear and tangible in nature such as hitting or biting, but relational aggression is more difficult to define, and to identify. Both relational and physical aggression have been prominently depicted in children's television. For example, 92% of programs for children between the ages of two and 12 have been found to contain relational aggression (Coyne & Stockdale, 2014).

This prevalent form of relational aggression is often depicted in ways that are related to gender with females shown exhibiting more relational aggression than males (Coyne & Stockdale, 2014), suggesting a bias in depictions. In real life, relational aggression is more often committed by females, as well; whereas men are more likely to use physical aggression (Crick, 1996; Crick & Grotpeter, 1995, 1996; Crick et al., 2006; Werner & Crick, 2004). Although a meta-analysis by Casper and colleagues (2020) did not find significant gender differences in experiences of relational aggression or victimization in a narrow age range of adolescents, with a mean age of 13.03 and little variance, this does not account for children or adolescents of all ages and may only speak to those in that age range. For instance, a study by O'Dell and colleagues (2024) focusing on at-risk youth of various races/ethnicities with a mean age of 16.75 found girls engaged in more relational aggression than boys and boys engaged in more overt aggression than girls.

Viewing relational aggression on television has been correlated with higher levels of relational aggression utilization, for at least one year after exposure, in females but not males (Coyne et al., 2019). *Social Cognitive Theory* (Bandura, 2009) suggests that not only can behaviors be emulated from media but identification with similar others might be one factor increasing the likelihood of a behavior being emulated. Also consistent with Social Cognitive Theory, learning violent behaviors is more likely when the behaviors go unpunished and relational aggression in children's television is often portrayed without consequence (Martins & Wilson, 2012). Additional factors also make learning aggression through media more likely: Relational aggression is committed by attractive (Martins & Wilson, 2012) female characters (Linder & Lyle, 2011) in media targeting young children, a pattern mirrored in teen television programs as well (Coyne & Stockdale, 2014). Thus, in both child and adolescent media, relational aggression is extensive, and portrayed as an effective and normative tool to increase social power by popular, attractive females, resulting in few consequences (Coyne & Stockdale, 2014). For example, in the popular teen drama *Georgia and Ginny*, the main character was exiled from her friend group resulting in her relapse of self-harm. While her friends never directly harmed her, the social isolation was a form of relational regression.

Although the overall frequency of physical aggression in the media may be cause for concern (i.e., how many acts of violence occur per hour?), recent critics of violence in the media are more concerned with specific factors relating to representation, such as the graphicness of the violence. Netflix's popular teen show *13 Reasons Why*, for instance, was so graphic and controversial that it had to be edited after release (Martins & Riddle, 2022). A recent content analysis focusing on children's media examined 765 shows across 21 channels pertaining to the amount and nature of violence in children's programs and found when looking at only children's programs (i.e., all programs originally produced and marketed to children and adolescents under 18), 80% of shows contained at least one act of violence, with 16% of those containing "blood and gore" (Martins & Riddle, 2022). Alternatively, a 2019 study by Taggart and colleagues focusing on 88 popular children's television programs for ages two to five years old found that 64% of children's television shows in the sample contained no violence at all, suggesting that violence in programs targeting children likely increases as the target audience gets older.

In addition to television violence, video games are another important point of focus as 85% of U.S teens report playing and four out of every ten identify as gamers (Gottfried & Sidoti, 2024). Importantly, research has shown games influence players in many ways including evoking stereotypes (Burgess et al., 2011) and reinforcing negative attitudes regarding minoritized social groups (Yang et al., 2014). Therefore, video games may well be a source of increased stigmatization, stereotyping, and racism. A 2011 content analysis by Burgess and colleagues of top-selling video game magazines and 149 video game covers found overt gender- and race-based stereotyping. Specifically, females from minoritized racial and ethnic groups were found to be virtually absent in game representation, and males from minoritized racial and ethnic groups were more often portrayed as aggressive or as athletes as opposed to their White counterparts who were often shown using technology or in military combat (Burgess et al., 2011). Males from underrepresented racial and ethnic groups were found to be underrepresented overall and when depicted were more often shown using guns as compared to their White counterparts (Burgess et al., 2011). More specifically, depictions of Black males are particularly problematic, being disproportionately shown as aggressive (Yang et al., 2014).

Effects of Violence in TV and Film on Aggressive Outcomes

Whereas it is important to consider the representation of violence in media, especially as it relates to issues of race, gender, equity, vulnerability, risk, and empowerment, these issues are crucial specifically because of the research on the *effects* of these depictions. In fact, although recent research has looked at newer forms of technology such as video games and social media, early research and children's own lived experiences suggest that the lives of children and adolescents are also shaped by their exposure to more traditional screen media, including television and film. Indeed, very young children spend more time watching traditional screen media than any other media form with children two and under in the United States averaging three hours of screen time daily and 3- to 5-year-olds 2.5 hours daily (Chen & Adler, 2019). However, there are considerable differences in exposure that are related to race, education, and other factors. For example, in the United States, African American individuals compared to their White counterparts on average spend more time watching television on any day of the week whereas Hispanic/Latinx and Asian individuals on average spend less time watching television on any day of the week (Bureau of Labor Statistics, 2024). Additionally, individuals with a high school diploma or less spend more time watching television than individuals with higher degrees (some college degree or above; Bureau of Labor Statistics, 2024). Combined with research earlier in the chapter on problematic race representations, this finding is particularly concerning suggesting that all children are at risk of experiencing outcomes associated with these depictions, but some outcomes are more likely among heavy viewers.

As early as 1982, the National Institute of Mental Health conducted a review of the empirical research on the effects of television and film violence on children and found that exposure to screen violence caused children to be more *fearful*; to learn *aggression* (developing aggressive thoughts, attitudes, or behavior) and to be less sensitive to the pain and suffering of others, a process referred to as *desensitization* (Huesmann & Eron, 1986). Each of these effects have been supported in the ensuing decades and has been shown to occur in both the short- and long-term, suggesting that some effects of violent media occur right after exposure whereas others are cumulative in nature (Anderson, 2016). To the latter point, then, about long-term risks, consistent exposure to screen media in childhood could influence aggression in adolescence (Bushman & Huesmann, 2006). In fact, a classic study from the 1980s demonstrated that children who watched a lot of TV violence when they were eight years old were more likely to be arrested and prosecuted for criminal acts as adults (Huesmann & Eron, 1986). Furthermore, longitudinal research found that early exposure to screen violence was a better predictor of later aggression than the reverse–that is, early aggression did not as strongly predict later interest in screen violence (Huesmann & Eron, 1986; Huesmann et al., 2003).

Of course, exposure to screen violence is just one of the many predictors of aggression but it is one statistically significant predictor. In a large-scale study of 1,990 adolescents, media violence exposure was one of the strongest predictors of aggression, after the personality trait of impulsivity and exposure to family conflict (Khurana et al., 2019). The large-scale scoping review of the effects of exposure to community and media violence in children and adolescents from minoritized racial and ethnic groups by Jipguep and Sanders-Phillips (2003) suggested that exposure to higher levels of both community and screen violence is likely to contribute to childhood and adolescent aggression among low-income and minoritized groups when both violent screen media and community violence are present, rather than when only one of those is present. It is important to note, however, that more recent research finds little to no relationship between the effects of media violence and race. In addition to exposure to screen and community violence, another risk factor is the problematic depictions of characters of color in video games and television discussed above. If youth identify with these characters (Ellithorpe & Bleakley, 2016; see Chapter 7) the confluence of all of these risk factors becomes increasingly problematic. Overall, then, risk factors including negative representation, the potential for identification with such representations (given a dearth of other options), and exposure to media can all increase the potential for vulnerability in youth.

Effects of Video Game Violence

Video games have become omnipresent in the lives of adolescents, making them an intrinsic part of modern youth culture. The societal view of video games has often been ambivalent, with the medium being celebrated for its potential educational benefits and simultaneously criticized for purported links to aggressive behavior. Media portrayals of video games within the news frequently oscillate between these poles, shaping public opinion and, at times, affecting legislative responses. The advent of video games dates back to the 1970s; however, the emergence of notably violent video games did not occur until the 1990s. Scholarly inquiry into the potential detrimental effects commenced in the 1980s. Nonetheless, it was the succession of school shootings that unfolded in the late 1990s, and the finding that many of the school shooters engaged in violent video game play, that heightened public scrutiny and concern (Anderson et al., 2007).

Another notable comparison of the effects of video game violence lies between males and females in terms of their video game play. While males have traditionally played more games and more violent games, this gap is narrowing. In 2023, a poll conducted by a gaming industry group found that 46% of all video gamers were female, while in 2006 only 38% of gamers were female (Entertainment Software Association, 2023). While it's difficult to celebrate greater use of violent games among females, this trend does signify a possible decrease in gender disparity in the gaming industry itself, perhaps exemplified by what was known as Gamer-gate, reflecting a movement towards empowerment and diversity in gaming culture. Gamer-gate was a campaign and controversy that emerged in 2014 in which video game critics who focused attention toward sexism and misogyny in games and gaming were severely harassed (Ferguson & Glasgow, 2021). Still, in 2023, men spent more hours on average per week playing video games than women (Statista, 2024).

Despite increases in equity of opportunities and representation, gender differences suggest a historical—and to some extent ongoing, pattern. Male gamers exhibit a higher likelihood of engaging with violent video games, implying a form of greater male agency in choosing and interacting with media that reflects cultural power and control dynamics. A study by Yang et al. (2014) found that playing violent video games as a male avatar increased aggression in both female and male players more than playing as a female avatar. This effect, attributed to the priming of aggressive stereotypes associated with male characters, was stronger among male players, possibly due to greater identification with the male avatar. ***Priming theory*** suggests that exposure to certain stimuli, like the gender of an avatar, can call to mind existing schema such as stereotypes that can influence how individuals respond to subsequent related stimuli. Thus, problematic imbalances in representation may support a power imbalance in the broader society.

In addition to considering the amount and consequences of gaming engaged in by various groups, Anderson et al. (2010) have argued for a causal connection between violent video game play and increased aggression. Their argument is supported by a thorough meta-analysis across a wide range of literature examining various aggressive outcomes including thoughts, emotions, physiological arousal, desensitization towards violence, and both aggressive and prosocial (or positive) behaviors. This extensive review included data from more than 130 studies with over 130,000 participants, concluding that a positive correlation exists between exposure to video game violence and heightened aggressive responses, while also finding a negative correlation with exposure and empathy and prosocial actions (Anderson et al., 2010). Greitemeyer and Mügge's (2014) subsequent meta-analysis corroborates these assertions with 98 independent studies and 36,965 participants. They found that time spent with violent video games increases aggression and aggression-related variables and decreases prosocial outcomes.

A study conducted by Coyne et al. (2023) examined the relationship between time spent playing video games and physical aggression in the context of additional factors through a longitudinal analysis of adolescents. They found that 28% of the sample were classified as "multi-risk," characterized by initially high levels of physical aggression that persisted into emerging adulthood despite a slight decline over time. Multi-risk individuals faced numerous risk factors linked to aggression, such as male gender, lower income, maternal hostility, bullying victimization, and stressful home environments. Interestingly, although moderately high use of violent video games among this group initially correlated with higher physical aggression, the majority (75%) of those in the multi-risk group either abstained from gaming or played minimally. Those who did engage in moderate gaming showed a decline in aggression levels over time, suggesting a potential ceiling effect. Overall, while time spent playing violent video games was initially associated with aggression in this high-risk group, other risk factors like family environment and victimization likely exerted a more substantial influence.

Taken together, therefore, we can conclude that (1) most studies find a statistical link between media violence exposure and aggression; (2) the size of that relationship is usually rather small, although it is "significant," meaning there is a very low likelihood that the relationship is found in research and not in real life; (3) media violence is only one contributor to aggression, and, in fact, the size of its influence is likely to be smaller than family and community factors. Thus, interventions focusing solely on reducing video game use may not effectively mitigate aggression in these adolescents.

Moral Reasoning

Whereas decades of research have focused on the effects of exposure to media depictions on specific aggressive behaviors and cognitions, as described above, less research has focused on how media influence our judgment of and reasoning about right and wrong, that is, on moral judgment. Moral reasoning covers a breadth of topics from cheating and fairness to loyalty and respect for authority (Haidt & Joseph, 2004), and one area that receives a lot of research attention is the moral category of harm/care.

This category is integrally linked to research on the effects of media violence due to the implication of violent depictions for the potential for harm. Yet, research on this topic often focuses on adults (c.f., Tamborini et al., 2010; Tamborini et al., 2012), and thus combing through the literature to assess only those studies that focus on children and adolescents (i.e., youth), and even further focusing on violence, can prove challenging.

In this section, we will begin first with a general conceptualization of moral judgment and reasoning. Second, using this conceptualization, we will discuss some of the theories concerning and adjacent to moral reasoning that have focused on youth. Third, we will shift our focus specifically to violence, which is a subset of moral reasoning and judgment. Then finally, we will present research that while not framed as about moral reasoning, per se, can be broadly classified as being so through the lens of violence as a subset of morality.

Media scholars Weber et al. (2012) adopt a rather straightforward conception of *morality* as a set of norms utilized as an overriding guide to behaviors enacted by those in a given social group. Others assume that a given behavior is or is not moral (e.g., causing unprovoked physical harm to another is immoral) and then have simply applied moral theory to a given problem. For example, researchers have explored media content depicting justified and unjustified violence in the context of moral reasoning (e.g., Hartmann et al., 2010; Krcmar & Valkenburg, 1999), studying such depictions as protagonists engaging in violence for an ostensibly defensible reason like defending others or fighting against evil. While labeling behaviors as good or bad ignores the role of culture and circumstance in those determinations (Mares & Woodard, 2001), in the interest of space, in this chapter we will discuss two key theories—Moral Foundations Theory and the Model of Intuitive Morality and Exemplars (MIME)—that have been applied to research on the effects of media violence on moral reasoning because those theories are most often used in research in this area.

Morality in children has often been studied using **Moral Foundations Theory** (MFT) (Haidt & Joseph, 2004) because the theory attempts to avoid the pitfall of cultural relativism by focusing on moral intuitions (i.e., moral "gut feelings" that something is wrong) rather than cultural standards (although see critiques, e.g., Harper & Rhodes, 2021). MFT argues that our immediate and reflexive and automatic moral *judgments* may be innate but also are influenced over time by our proximal environment such as interpersonal exchanges (Haidt & Joseph, 2004) and exposure to mediated content (Tamborini, 2011). Although the theory argues for six moral foundations, we focus here only on the harm/care foundation due to its connection with media violence. Haidt and Joseph (2004, 2008) note the need to care for others and protect them from harm as a primary moral foundation across cultures. Research on the effects of film violence dating back to the Payne studies of the 1930s (Lowery & DeFleur, 1995) has focused on the effects of exposure to violations of the harm/care foundation of morality, long before MFT was developed. Nevertheless, interpreting even this older media violence research through the lens of MFT is beneficial because MFT implies a potential media effect due to the environmental influences on one's reflexive moral intuitions. In other words, even our quick, reflexive moral judgments and reasoning can be influenced over time by environmental inputs.

The Model of Intuitive Media Exemplars (MIME; Tamborini, 2011) relies on MFT (Haidt & Joseph, 2004) but extends it to argue that media content, as a key part of many individuals' proximal environment around the world, is processed morally, and can influence the short- and long-term salience of these moral intuitions (Eden et al., 2021; Tamborini et al., 2011). That is, exposure to violence primes intuitive harm/care judgments in the direction of the depiction (i.e., supportive of harm norms vs. care norms). Applications of MIME suggest that children of different ages and in different developmental stages do respond differently to moral media (Cingel & Krcmar, 2019; Cingel et al., 2020; Krcmar & Cooke, 2001; Vieira & Krcmar, 2011). Furthermore, moral foundations themselves have been found to have a developmental trajectory (Cingel & Krcmar, 2020, 2023; Haidt & Bjorklund, 2008), with harm/care being one of the earlier foundations to be engaged by children.

Because this foundation arrives early in children, early exposure to violent media has been found to have a negative effect on children's moral judgment and reasoning from the preschool years. For example, Krcmar and Valkenburg (1999) found that children exposed to violent media were more likely to judge provoked violence (i.e., when another character acted aggressively first) as more correct, compared to children who did not view much violent media content. Furthermore, using moral developmental theory, Krcmar and Cooke (2001) found that children judged both provoked or unprovoked violence as wrong, although the age of the child combined with whether or not that violence was shown as punished was key in influencing *how* wrong children judged it to be. Specifically, older children were more swayed by whether or not the violence had a fair motive; whereas younger children were influenced by whether or not an authority figure punished the violence.

In addition, Krcmar and Curtis (2003) found that children were more likely to view violence as a correct solution to problems after exposure to a cartoon with a physically violent ending, compared to children who watched the exact same cartoon without the violent ending, making them more vulnerable to and at risk for solving problems through aggressive means. Krcmar and Vieira (2005) reported a similar finding, specifically that overall violent video game exposure was related to less developmentally advanced moral judgments and reasoning among children. More recently, Cingel and Krcmar (2019) found that effects of a prosocial television narrative on 4- to 6-year-olds' moral reasoning about violence were not mediated by comprehension of events, motives, and emotions. In other words, in this study, children were influenced by prosocial narratives even when they could not show a clear understanding of the message. This suggests that children may be learning at an intuitive level even if they can't articulate it.

Thus, overall, it appears that exposure to media violence can have a negative effect on both the moral judgments and reasoning of children. If we apply the theories of MFT and MIME we would argue that media depictions that show or imply that violence or aggression is acceptable under certain circumstances seem to influence children's conceptions of right and wrong. In other words, portrayals in which violence seems to have a justifiable motive, seems to solve a problem, or that involves a trusted adult can shape beliefs about whether and which forms of violence are seen as morally acceptable.

Cyberbullying

While traditional screen media and interactive media such as video games remain an important source of entertainment and information for children and adolescents, the rise of social media over the last decade has encouraged a generation of children and adolescents to be online—in some cases continuously—throughout the day (Anderson & Jiang, 2018). The effects of that online behavior have been explored in hundreds of studies; however, in a chapter on aggression, it seems appropriate to explore one area in particular: cyberbullying. Scholars have defined *online aggression* as any behavior or act of aggression with the intent to harm someone who does not wish to be harmed by way of electronic media (DeWall et al., 2013; Grigg, 2010). *Cyberbullying* is a form of online aggression (Olson & Bellmore, 2021), also referred to as online or electronic bullying, in which bullying takes place by method of technology (e.g., texting, social sites, instant messages, sexting, etc.) (Notar et al., 2013). Sending hurtful messages via text or social networking sites, posting mean content, and exclusion from online groups are examples of cyberbullying enacted via computers or cellular devices (Olson & Bellmore, 2021).

Kowalski et al. (2014) argued that like bullying itself, cyberbullying has three key qualities: intention, repetition, and an imbalance of power between the victim and aggressor (Olweus, 1993). These imbalances in power are often caused or exacerbated by race, gender, and other factors that themselves can create bias, a point we will return to in this chapter and that connects to Chapters 3 and 7, as well. While these three characteristics are present in cyberbullying, Olweus and Limber (2018) note differences between electronic and face-to-face environments and propose that repetition and imbalance of power can differ from face-to-face to electronic aggression. For example, affordances of social media platforms allow for easy and intense repetition through reposting, and social status and anonymity provide additional strategies for imbalance of power not defined in traditional bullying (Olson & Bellmore, 2021). Despite these differences, a majority of research finds a relationship between cyberbullying and traditional bullying (e.g., Brown & Demaray, 2014; Cho et al., 2019; Waasdorp & Bradshaw, 2015). For example, Waasdorp and Bradshaw (2015) found online bullying most likely occurs in correlation with verbal and relational bullying.

Inconsistencies in scales, platforms, and measurements of adolescent cyberbullying make it hard to definitively estimate the frequency of cyberbullying (Olson & Bellmore, 2021). However, in a review of 58 unique U.S studies, estimates of adolescent cyberbullying victimization can range between 9% to 40% (e.g., Aboujaoude et al., 2015; Kowalski et al., 2014) and 3% to 72% (Selkie et al., 2016), while perpetration can range between 1% and 41% (Selkie et al., 2016). Other countries also present wide ranges in cyberbullying involvement, for instance, cybervictimization rates in Spain range between 2% and 30% and cyber aggression rates range between 1% and 44% (Zych et al., 2016). Despite these wide variations in frequency estimates, research examining the effects has been more consistent.

General Effects of Cyberbullying on Adolescent Victims

When considering the effects of cyberbullying, research has examined effects on victims, characteristics of perpetrators, and even effects on bystanders. The negative effects of cyberbullying on adolescent victims are clear in the literature (Olson & Bellmore, 2021): Adolescent victims of cyberbullying experience depressive symptoms (Bonanno & Hymel, 2013; Kowalski et al., 2014; Wright, 2015), anxiety (Rose & Tynes, 2015; Wright, 2015), and low self-esteem (Özdemir, 2014). Longitudinal studies also find an association between cyberbullying victimization and depression (Gámez-Guadix et al., 2013). Other effects of cyberbullying victimization include academic difficulties (Kowalski & Limber, 2013), suicidal ideation and behaviors (Messias et al., 2014), and physical issues such as headaches and fatigue (Kowalski & Limber, 2013). The strongest links with cyberbullying victimization have been found to be suicidal ideation and stress (Kowalski et al., 2014); with a review of 26 studies finding youth cyberbullying victims are 2.5 times more likely to attempt suicide or 2.3 times as likely to self-harm in comparison to nonvictims (John et al., 2018).

In almost every study in which gender is reported, adolescent females are at greater risk for effects, suggesting a particular susceptibility among girls. For example, Wang et al. (2018) found a stronger link between experiencing cyberbullying and suicidal thoughts and behaviors among Asian American girls than boys. Espinoza (2015) found Latina girls had higher levels of distress and anger from daily cybervictimization than their Latino high schooler counterparts, which aligns with findings of daily cyberbullying outcomes of predominantly White youth (e.g., Bauman et al., 2013). In addition, Romero and colleges (2018) found for both Latino and Latina adolescents cybervictimization increased the likelihood of suicide attempts but Latina girls were more likely to be cybervictimized than Latino males. A meta-analysis of 57 studies from 17 countries found the link between cyberbullying victimization and depression to be stronger among girls compared to boys (Hu et al., 2021).

Female adolescents also receive more pressure to engage in sexting than males (Englander & McCoy, 2017), which opens the door to revenge porn as a way of cyberbullying. Although there is limited research on adolescent outcomes of revenge porn, among adults, revenge porn has been associated with depression, posttraumatic stress disorder, anxiety, and suicidal ideation (Olson & Bellmore, 2021), suggesting that similar results are likely among those under 18, whose vulnerability may be even greater.

The experience of *online harassment* also varies by gender; for example, 15% of teenage girls have been a target of four of the six online harassment behaviors (such as being more likely to receive unwanted explicit images) while only 6% of teen boys have (Anderson, 2018). Once again, this would suggest a power imbalance, one that replicates power imbalances offline as well. Thus, simply being female online can pose a threat to well-being.

While gender is clearly one risk factor, racial and ethnic identity has also been examined in terms of cyberbullying and the results have been largely mixed (Espinoza & Ismail, 2021). While some studies have found no difference in rates of cyberbullying involvement by race or ethnicity (e.g., Bauman et al., 2013; Duarte et al., 2018; Stoll & Block, 2015), some have found significant differences. In their summary review on the topic, Espinoza and Ismail (2021) identified multiple inconsistencies within the findings regarding ethnic differences and cyberbullying involvement, pointing out contradictions between two national studies, one finding that those who did not identify with one of the racial groups provided on a survey (i.e., chose "other") were more likely to be cybervictimized and the other finding the opposite. For example, Messias et al. (2014), in their nationally representative study of US 9th to 12th grade students, found cyberbullying victims who identified as "other" (including ethnicities such as Asian, American Indian, and Pacific Islander), were more likely to experience victimization versus those who were Caucasian, Hispanic, or African American. Black youth who report cyberbullying involvement have been found more likely than White and Latino adolescents to be cyberbullied via sharing of private information, while cyberbullying is more likely to occur for Latino adolescents through online gaming context (U.S. Department of Education, 2015). Thus, although the research evidence is less consistent in this area, being a person of color also may pose a risk in terms of cyberbullying victimization, either in terms of whether one is bullied or how.

Still other studies look at cyberbullying and its correlates within rather than across racial and ethnic groups. Wang et al. (2018), for instance, found that school climate (such as perception of school community) had an effect on the relationship between cybervictimization and suicidal thoughts for Asian youth. In regard to Arab American adolescent males, links between cyberbullying and physical and psychological health were found such as cyberbullying perpetration predicted physical complaints (Albdour et al., 2019). Among Black or African American adolescents, Cho et al. (2019) found that those who talked more with their friends about problems they were experiencing were less likely to be cyberbullied than those who did so less (Figure 9.1).

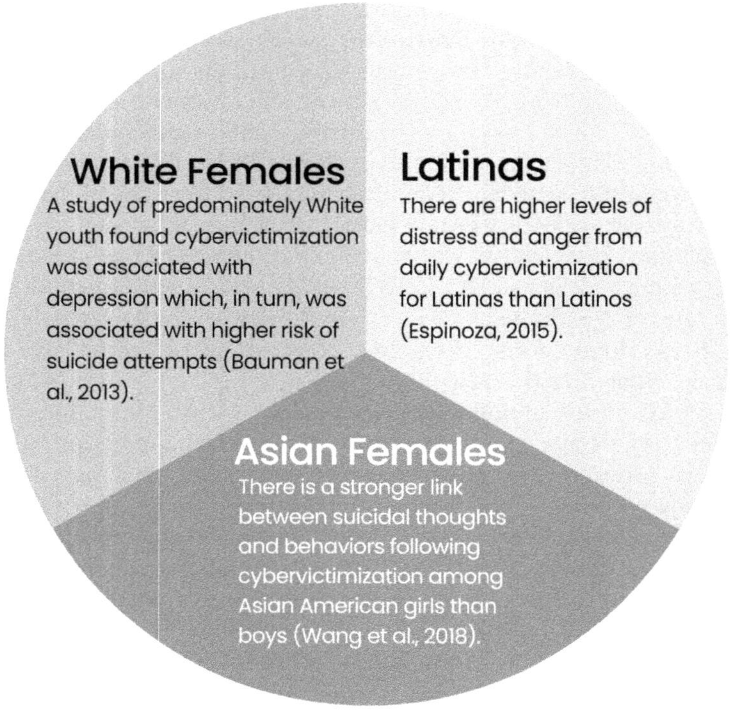

White Females
A study of predominately White youth found cybervictimization was associated with depression which, in turn, was associated with higher risk of suicide attempts (Bauman et al., 2013).

Latinas
There are higher levels of distress and anger from daily cybervictimization for Latinas than Latinos (Espinoza, 2015).

Asian Females
There is a stronger link between suicidal thoughts and behaviors following cybervictimization among Asian American girls than boys (Wang et al., 2018).

Figure 9.1 Ethnicity and cyberbullying among girls and young women.
Source: Authors

Despite the clearly negative effects of cyberbullying on a number of racial groups, at least one finding offers hope: Ethnic identification can buffer the negative impact of online discrimination on mental health for adolescents, especially among African American youth (Tynes et al., 2012), as also discussed in Chapter 7. Alternatively, low ethnic identity exploration can be related to increased externalization problems, such as aggression and impulsivity, as shown in Latino adolescents (Umaña-Taylor et al., 2015). Therefore, stronger identification with one's racial group may serve as a protective factor, empowering youth against cyberbullying.

Adolescents with learning disabilities are more at risk to engage in and be victims of cyberbullying than those who do not have learning disabilities (Mishna, 2003). In addition, the presence of one or more particular disabilities may intensify the negative outcome already associated with cyberbullying for disabled youth (Eldridge et al., 2021), specifically illustrated by more emotional loneliness and less self-efficacy reported by disabled cyber victims than non-disabled (Heiman et al., 2015). Research indicates that among disabled youth, cyberbullying participation in any form may be associated with emotional issues and psychological distress (Eldridge et al., 2021), such as depression (Didden et al., 2009; Wright, 2017).

Cyberbullying: Perpetrators and Bystanders

Some research attempts to identify which youth are more likely to perpetrate cyberbullying. For instance, low overall levels of life satisfaction and loneliness are also associated with youth cyberbullying perpetration in many studies (e.g., Kowalski et al., 2014). Other research suggests that perpetration is associated with substance use among adolescents (Kumar & Goldstein, 2020). Perpetrators of cyberbullying usually have normative beliefs about aggression, that is, they believe aggression to be a justified way to solve problems, and they show high levels of moral disengagement (Kowalski et al., 2014). Therefore, although there is no research on the connection between cyberbullying and moral judgment and reasoning, it seems likely that high moral disengagement would be associated with more permissive moral judgment and lower levels of moral reasoning.

Perhaps somewhat surprisingly, those who are perpetrators of cyberbullying are also more likely than their peers to be victims, suggesting a cyclical pattern (e.g., Brown & Demaray, 2014; Cho et al., 2019; Waasdorp & Bradshaw, 2015). In addition, Waasdorp and Bradshaw (2015) found cyberbullying online occurred more frequently when adolescents were also experiencing verbal and relational bullying offline. Lastly, cyberbullying has been consistently associated with physical symptoms and negative academic outcomes regarding attendance and low school climate perceptions (Espinoza & Ismail, 2021).

Social networking sites provide a space where adolescents view cyberbullying even if they are not the victim or perpetrator (Bastiaensens et al., 2013). The publicness and scale or reach afforded by social media put adolescents in a bystander of cyberbullying role just by seeing a post and committing no further action (Olson & Bellmore, 2021). In a study of adolescents between the ages of 12 and 17 years, 90% admitted to being bystanders of cyberbullying by viewing and ignoring incidents, 80% reported defending the cyberbullying victim, and 21% admitted reinforcing cyberbullying by way of joining in (Lenhart et al., 2011). Despite gender, race/ethnicity, and disability-based differences noted above, cyberbullying may be so widespread that few adolescents, regardless of identity group, are immune from exposure and many may become desensitized.

Conclusion

Research on media violence has a long history, dating back almost 100 years (Lowery & DeFleur, 1995). Whereas the oldest studies did not focus much on diversity, inclusion, agency, victimization, and/or power, as these are all concepts that have become more prominent in research in only the last few decades, more recent research has tapped into important findings. In the media violence literature, research on the representation of violence in the media finds evidence for overt racial stereotyping, especially in video games (Burgess et al., 2011), and finds gender differences with male characters depicted as more physically violent than female characters while the reverse is true for relational violence. Since children from minoritized racial and ethnic groups identify with characters of color more than with White characters (Ellithorpe & Bleakley, 2016), this suggests they have few good options in video games. The effects of media violence have also been found to be compounded by community-level violence (Jipguep and Sanders-Phillips, 2003), although media violence was a weaker predictor of aggression than family- and community-based factors subsequent research (Coyne et al., 2023). Finally, more recent research on cyberbullying suggests differences in both vulnerability and agency. For example, adolescent females, compared to males, are at greater risk for both victimization and negative effects (Wang et al., 2018). These findings would suggest that victimization occurs more for marginalized or minoritized teens.

Overall, then, media violence continues to be a cause for concern for children and adolescents. But hope exists through several mechanisms. First, a meta-analysis of 51 studies (Jeong et al., 2012) found that media literacy interventions had positive effects on outcomes including media knowledge, criticism, perceived realism, influence, behavioral beliefs, attitudes, self-efficacy, and behavior. Although this large-scale meta-analysis did not focus on violent media, per se, we might extrapolate that despite the sheer amount of media violence that children are exposed to, education from parents, schools, and other trusted adults can mitigate effects (see Chapters 4 and 5). Second, while lack of positive and diverse representations remains a problem, at least some evidence exists that strong racial identification can act as a buffer (Tynes et al., 2012). Finally, recent research on social media broadly and cyberbullying more specifically finds that perpetration, victimization, and bystanding are prevalent, but that being socially connected offline can be a protective factor against cyberbullying and provide support to cyberbullying victims (McLoughlin & Hermens, 2018). These final findings point towards the need for continued positive representations in media across gender and racial/ethnic groups as well as the need for education, social connection, and support for all adolescents as they navigate the current landscape of media that contains violence and aggression in multiple forms.

References

Aboujaoude, E., Savage, M. W., Starcevic, V., & Salame, W. O. (2015). Cyberbullying: Review of an old problem gone viral. *The Journal of Adolescent Health: Official Publication of the Society for Adolescent Medicine, 57*(1), 10–18. https://doi.org/10.1016/j.jadohealth.2015.04.011

Albdour, M., Hong, J. S., Lewin, L., & Yarandi, H. (2019). The impact of cyberbullying on physical and psychological health of Arab American adolescents. *Journal of Immigrant and Minority Health, 21*, 706–715. https://doi.org/10.1007/s10903-018-00850-w.

Anderson, C. A. (2016). Media violence effects on children, adolescents and young adults. *Health Progress (Saint Louis, Mo.), 97*(4), 59–62.

Anderson, M. (2018, Sept. 27). *A majority of teens have experienced some form of cyberbullying.* Pew Research Center. https://www.pewresearch.org/internet/2018/09/27/a-majority-of-teens-have-experienced-some-form-of-cyberbullying/

Anderson, C. A., Gentile, D. A., & Buckley, K. E. (2007). *Violent video game effects on children and adolescents: Theory, research, and public policy.* Oxford University Press.

Anderson, M., & Jiang, J. (2018, May 31). *Teens, social media & technology 2018.* Pew Research Center. https://www.pewresearch.org/internet/2018/05/31/teens-social-media-technology-2018/

Anderson, C. A., Shibuya, A., Ihori, N., Swing, E. L., Bushman, B. J., Sakamoto, A., Rothstein, H. R., & Saleem, M. (2010). Violent video game effects on aggression, empathy, and prosocial behavior in eastern and western countries: A meta-analytic review. *Psychological Bulletin, 136*(2), 151–173. https://doi.org/10.1037/a0018251

Archer, J., & Coyne, S. M. (2005). An integrated review of indirect, relational, and social aggression. *Personality and Social Psychology Review, 9*(3), 212–230. https://doi.org/10.1207/s15327957pspr0903_2

Bandura, A. (2009). Social cognitive theory of mass communication. In J. Bryant, & M. B. Oliver (Eds.), *Media effects: Advances in theory and research* (3rd ed., pp. 94–124). Routledge.

Bastiaensens, S., Vandebosch, H., Poels, K., Van Cleemput, K., DeSmet, A., & De Bourdeaudhuij, I. (2013). Cyberbullying on social network sites. An experimental study into bystanders' behavioural intentions to help the victim or reinforce the bully. *Computers in Human Behavior*, 31, 259–271. https://doi.org/10.1016/j.chb.2013.10.036.

Bauman, S., Toomey, R. B., & Walker, J. L. (2013). Associations among bullying, cyberbullying and suicide in high school students. *Journal of Adolescence*, 36(2), 341–350. https://doi.org/10.1016/j.adolescence.2012.12.001

Bonanno, R. A., & Hymel, S. (2013). Cyber bullying and internalizing difficulties: Above and beyond the impact of traditional forms of bullying. *Journal of Youth and Adolescence*, 42, 685–697. https://doi.org/10.1007/s10964-013-9937-1

Brown, C. F., & Demaray, M. K. (2014). Cyber victimization in middle school and relations to social emotional outcomes. *Computers in Human Behavior*, 35, 12–21. https://doi.org/10.1016/j.chb.2014.02.014

Bureau of Labor Statistics. (2024). *American time use survey.* https://www.bls.gov/tus/

Burgess, M. C. R., Dill, K. E., Stermer, S. P., Burgess, S. R., & Brown, B. P. (2011). Playing with prejudice: The prevalence and consequences of racial stereotypes in video games. *Media Psychology*, 14(3), 289–311. https://doi.org/10.1080/15213269.2011.596467

Bushman, B. J., & Huesmann, L. R. (2006). Short-term and long-term effects of violent media on aggression in children and adults. *Archives of Pediatrics & Adolescent Medicine*, 160(4), 348–352. https://doi.org/10.1001/archpedi.160.4.348

Casper, D. M., Card, N. A., & Barlow, C. (2020). Relational aggression and victimization during adolescence: A meta-analytic review of unique associations with popularity, peer acceptance, rejection, and friendship characteristics. *Journal of Adolescence*, 80(1), 41–52. https://doi.org/10.1016/j.adolescence.2019.12.012

Chen, W., & Adler, J. L. (2019). Assessment of screen exposure in young children, 1997 to 2014. *JAMA Pediatrics*, 173(4), 391–393. https://doi.org/10.1001/jamapediatrics.2018.5546

Cho, S., Lee, H., Peguero, A. A., & Park, S. (2019). Social-ecological correlates of cyberbullying victimization and perpetration among African American youth: Negative binomial and zero inflated negative binomial analyses. *Children and Youth Services Review*, 101(7), 50–60. https://doi.org/10.1016/j.childyouth.2019.03.044

Cingel, D., & Krcmar, M. (2023). Developing a scale of moral intuition development in children. *Journal of Communication*, 73(2). https://doi.org/10.1080/15213269.2019.1601570

Cingel, D. P., & Krcmar, M. (2019). Prosocial television, preschool children's moral judgments, and moral reasoning: The role of social moral intuitions and perspective-taking. *Communication Research*, 46(3), 355–374. https://doi.org/10.1177/0093650217733846

Cingel, D. P., & Krcmar, M. (2020). Considering moral foundations theory and the model of intuitive morality and exemplars in the context of child and adolescent development. *Annals of the International Communication Association*, 44(2), 120–138. https://doi.org/10.1080/23808985.2020.1755337

Cingel, D. P., Sumter, S. R., Stoeten, E., & Mann, S. (2020). Can television help to decrease stigmatization among young children? The role of theory of mind and general and explicit inserts. *Media Psychology*, 23(3), 342–364.

Coyne, S. M., Ehrenreich, S. E., Holmgren, H. G., & Underwood, M. K. (2019). "We're not gonna be friends anymore": Associations between viewing relational aggression on television and relational aggression in text messaging during adolescence. *Aggressive Behavior*, 45(3), 319–326. https://doi.org/10.1002/ab.21821

Coyne, S. M., & Stockdale, L. (2014). Meanness and manipulation in the media: Portrayals and effects of viewing relational aggression in the media. In D. A. Gentile (Ed.), *Media violence and children: A complete guide for parents and professionals* (2nd ed., pp. 209–228). Praeger/ABC-CLIO.

Coyne, S. M., Warburton, W., Swit, C., Stockdale, L., & Dyer, W. J. (2023). Who is most at risk for developing physical aggression after playing violent video games? An individual differences perspective from early adolescence to emerging adulthood. *Journal of Youth and Adolescence*, 52(4), 719–733.

Crick, N. R. (1996). The role of overt aggression, relational aggression, and prosocial behavior in the prediction of children's future social adjustment. *Child Development*, 67, 2317–2327. https://doi.org/10.1111/j.1467-8624.1996.tb01859.x

Crick, N. R., & Grotpeter, J. K. (1995). Relational aggression, gender, and social-psychological adjustment. *Child Development*, 66(3), 710–722. https://doi.org/10.2307/1131945

Crick, N. R., & Grotpeter, J. K. (1996). Children's treatment by peers: Victims of relational and overt aggression. *Development and Psychopathology*, 8(2), 367–380. https://doi.org/10.1017/S0954579400007148

Crick, N. R., Ostrov, J. M., & Werner, N. E. (2006). A longitudinal study of relational aggression, physical aggression, and children's social-psychological adjustment. *Journal of Abnormal Child Psychology*, 34(2), 131–142. https://doi.org/10.1007/s10802-005-9009-4

DeWall, C. N., Anderson, C. A., & Bushman, B. J. (2013). Aggression. In H. Tennen, J. Suls, & I. B. Weiner (Eds.), *Handbook of psychology: Personality and social psychology* (pp. 449–466). John Wiley & Sons Inc.

Didden, R., Scholte, R. H., Korzilius, H., Moor, J. M., Vermeulen, A., O'Reilly, M., & Lancioni, G. E. (2009). Cyber bullying among students with intellectual and developmental disability in special education settings. *Developmental Neurorehabilitation*, 12(3), 146–151. https://doi.org/10.1080/17518420902971356

Duarte, C., Pittman, S. K., Thorsen, M. M., Cunningham, M. R., & Ranney, M. L. (2018). Correlation of minority status, cyberbullying, and mental health: A cross-sectional study of 1031 adolescents. *Journal of Child and Adolescent Trauma*, 11(1), 39–48. https://doi.org/10.1007/s40653-018-0201-4

Eden, A., Tamborini, R., Aley, M., & Goble, H. (2021). Advances in research on the model of intuitive morality and exemplars (MIME). In P. Vorderer & C. Klimmt (Eds.), *The Oxford handbook of entertainment theory* (pp. 231–249). Oxford University Press.

Eldridge, M. A., Demaray, M. L. K., Emmons, J. D., & Riffle, L. N. (2021). Cyberbullying and cybervictimization among youth with disabilities. In M.F. Wright, & L.B. Schiamberg, (Eds.) *Child and adolescent online risk exposure* (pp. 255–281). Elsevier Academic Press.

Ellithorpe, M. E., & Bleakley, A. (2016). Wanting to see people like me? Racial and gender diversity in popular adolescent television. *Journal of Youth and Adolescence*, 45(7), 1426–1437. https://doi.org/10.1007/s10964-016-0415-4

Englander, E. K., & McCoy, M. (2017). Pressured sexting and revenge porn in a sample of Massachusetts adolescents. *International Journal of Technoethics*, 8(2), 1625. https://doi.org/10.4018/IJT.2017070102

Entertainment Software Association. (July, 2023). Distribution of video gamers in the United States from 2006 to 2023, by gender [Graph]. In *Statista*. Retrieved July 30, 2024, from https://www-statista-com.wake.idm.oclc.org/statistics/232383/gender-split-of-us-computer-and-video-gamers/

Espinoza, G. (2015). Daily cybervictimization among Latino adolescents: Links with emotional, physical and school adjustment. *Journal of Applied Developmental Psychology*, 38, 39–48. https://doi.org/10.1016/j.appdev.2015.04.003

Espinoza, G., & Ismail, F. R. (2021). Cyberbullying perpetration and victimization among ethnic minority youth in the United States: Similarities or differences across groups? In M. F. Wright & L. B. Schiamberg (Eds.), *Child and adolescent online risk exposure: An ecological perspective* (pp. 209–231). Elsevier Academic Press. https://doi.org/10.1016/B978-0-12-817499-9.00011-9

Ferguson, C. J., & Glasgow, B. (2021). Who are GamerGate? A descriptive study of individuals involved in the GamerGate controversy. *Psychology of Popular Media*, 10(2), 243–247. https://doi.org/10.1037/ppm0000280

Gámez-Guadix, M., Orue, I., Smith, P. K., & Calvete, E. (2013). Longitudinal and reciprocal relations of cyberbullying with depression, substance use, and problematic internet use among adolescents. *The Journal of Adolescent Health: Official Publication of the Society for Adolescent Medicine*, 53(4), 446–452. https://doi.org/10.1016/j.jadohealth.2013.03.030

Gottfried, J., & Sidoti, O. (2024, May 9). *Teens and video games today*. Pew Research Center. https://www.pewresearch.org/internet/2024/05/09/teens-and-video-games-today/

Greitemeyer, T., & Mügge, D. O. (2014). Video games do affect social outcomes: A meta-analytic review of the effects of violent and prosocial video game play. *Personality & Social Psychology Bulletin*, 40(5), 578–589. https://doi.org/10.1177/0146167213520459

Grigg, D. W. (2010). Cyber-aggression: Definition and concept of cyberbullying. *Journal of Psychologists and Counselors in Schools*, 20(2), 143–156. https://doi.org/10.1375/ajgc.20.2.143

Haidt, J., & Bjorklund, F. (2008). Social intuitionists answer six questions about moral psychology. In W. Sinnott-Armstrong (Ed.), *Moral psychology, vol. 2. The cognitive science of morality: Intuition and diversity* (pp. 181–217). Boston Review.

Haidt, J., & Joseph, C. (2004). Intuitive ethics: How innately prepared intuitions generate culturally variable virtues. *Daedalus*, 133(4), 55–66. http://www.jstor.org/stable/20027945

Haidt, J., & Joseph, C. (2008). The moral mind: How five sets of innate intuitions guide the development of many culture-specific virtues, and perhaps even modules. In P. Carruthers, S. Laurence, & S. Stich (Eds.), *The innate mind vol. 3. Foundations and the future* (pp. 367–391). Oxford University Press. https://doi.org/10.1093/acprof:oso/9780195332834.003.0019

Harper, C. A., & Rhodes, D. (2021). Reanalysing the factor structure of the moral foundations questionnaire. *British Journal of Social Psychology*, 60(4), 1303–1329.

Hartmann, T., Toz, E., & Brandon, M. (2010). Just a game? Unjustified virtual violence produces guilt in empathetic players. *Media Psychology*, 13(4), 339–363. https://doi.org/10.1080/15213269.2010.524912

Heiman, T., Olenik-Shemesh, D., & Eden, S. (2015). Cyber bullying involvement among students with ADHD: Relation to loneliness, self-efficacy and social support. *European Journal of Special Needs Education*, *30*(1), 15–29. https://doi.org/10.1080/08856257.2014.943562

Hu, Y., Bai, Y., Pan, Y., & Li, S. (2021). Cyberbullying victimization and depression among adolescents: A meta-analysis. *Psychiatry Research*, *305*, 114198.

Huesmann, L. R., & Eron, L. D. (1986). *Television and the aggressive child: A cross-national comparison*. Erlbaum.

Huesmann, L. R., Moise-Titus, J., Podolski, C. L., & Eron, L. D. (2003). Longitudinal relations between children's exposure to TV violence and their aggressive and violent behavior in young adulthood: 1977–1992. *Developmental Psychology*, *39*(2), 201–221.

Jeong, S. H., Cho, H., & Hwang, Y. (2012). Media literacy interventions: A meta-analytic review. *Journal of Communication*, *62*(3), 454–472. https://doi.org/10.1111/j.1460-2466.2012.01643.x

Jipguep, M.-C., & Sanders-Phillips, K. (2003). The context of violence for children of color: Violence in the community and in the media. *The Journal of Negro Education*, *72*(4), 379–395. https://doi.org/10.2307/3211190

John, A., Glendenning, A. C., Marchant, A., Montgomery, P., Stewart, A., Wood, S., ... & Hawton, K. (2018). Self-harm, suicidal behaviours, and cyberbullying in children and young people: Systematic review. *Journal of Medical Internet Research*, *20*(4), e9044.

Khurana, A., Bleakley, A., Ellithorpe, M. E., Hennessy, M., Jamieson, P. E., & Weitz, I. (2019). Media violence exposure and aggression in adolescents: A risk and resilience perspective. *Aggressive Behavior*, *45*(1), 70–81.

Kowalski, R. M., Giumetti, G. W., Schroeder, A. N., & Lattanner, M. R. (2014). Bullying in the digital age: A critical review and meta-analysis of cyberbullying research among youth. *Psychological Bulletin*, *140*(4), 1073–1137. https://doi.org/10.1037/a0035618

Kowalski, R. M., & Limber, S. P. (2013). Psychological, physical, and academic correlates of cyberbullying and traditional bullying. *The Journal of Adolescent Health: Official Publication of the Society for Adolescent Medicine*, *53*(1 Suppl), S13–S20. https://doi.org/10.1016/j.jadohealth.2012.09.018

Krcmar, M., & Cooke, M. C. (2001). Children's moral reasoning and their perceptions of television violence. *Journal of Communication*, *51*(2), 300–316. https://doi.org/10.1111/j.1460-2466.2001.tb02882.x

Krcmar, M., & Curtis, S. (2003). Mental models: Understanding the impact of fantasy violence on children's moral reasoning. *Journal of Communication*, *53*(3), 460–478.

Krcmar, M., & Valkenburg, P. M. (1999). A scale to assess children's moral interpretations of justified and unjustified violence and its relationship to television viewing. *Communication Research*, *26*, 608–634.

Krcmar, M., & Vieira, E. T. Jr (2005). Imitating life, imitating television: The effects of family and television models on children's moral reasoning. *Communication Research*, *32*, 1–28.

Kumar, V. L., & Goldstein, M. A. (2020). Cyberbullying and adolescents. *Current Pediatrics Reports*, *8*(3), 86–92. https://doi.org/10.1007/s40124-020-00217-6

Lenhart, A., Madden, M., Smith, A., Purcell, K., & Zickuhr, K. (2011). *Teens, kindness and cruelty on social network sites*. Pew Research Center. http://www.pewinternet.org/2011/11/09/teens-kindness-and-cruelty-on-social-network-sites/

Linder, J. R., & Lyle, K. A. (2011). A content analysis of indirect, verbal, and physical aggression in television programs popular among school-aged girls. *American Journal of Media Psychology*, *4*, 24–42.

Lowery, S., & DeFleur, M. (1995). *Milestones in mass communication research: Media effects*. 3rd ed. Longman.

Mares, M. L., & Woodard, E. H. (2001). Prosocial effects on children's social interactions. In D.G Singer & J.L. Singer (Eds.), *Handbook of Children and the Media* (pp.183–206). Sage.

Martins, N., & Riddle, K. (2022). Reassessing the risks: An updated content analysis of violence on U.S. children's primetime television. *Journal of Children and Media*, *16*(3), 368–386. https://doi.org/10.1080/17482798.2021.1985548

Martins, N., & Wilson, B. J. (2012). Mean on the screen: Social aggression in programs popular with children. *Journal of Communication*, *62*(6), 991–1009. https://doi.org/10.1111/j.1460-2466.2011.01599.x

McLoughlin, L. T., & Hermens, D. F. (2018). Cyberbullying and social connectedness. *Frontiers for Young Minds*, *6*(54), 1–6. https://doi.org/10.3389/frym.2018.00054.

Messias, E., Kindrick, K., & Castro, J. (2014). School bullying, cyberbullying, or both: Correlates of teen suicidality in the 2011 CDC youth risk behavior survey. *Comprehensive Psychiatry*, *55*(5), 1063–1068. https://doi.org/10.1016/j.Comppsych.2014.02.005

Mishna, F. (2003). Learning disabilities and bullying: Double jeopardy. *Journal of Learning Disabilities*, *36*(4), 336–347. https://doi.org/10.1177/00222194030360040501

Notar, C. E., Padgett, S., & Roden, J. (2013). Cyber bullying: A review of the literature. *Universal Journal of Educational Research*, *1*(1), 1–9. https://doi.org/10.13189/ujer.2013.010101

O'Dell, C., Charles, N. E., & Barry, C. T. (2024). Gender differences in links between antisocial features and forms and functions of aggression among at-risk youth. *Journal of Psychopathology and Behavioral Assessment*, *46*(2), 357–372. https://doi.org/10.1007/s10862-024-10134-3

Olson, C., & Bellmore, A. (2021). Online aggression and romantic relationships in adolescence. In M. F. Wright & L. B. Schiamberg (Eds.), *Child and adolescent online risk exposure: An ecological perspective* (pp. 97–127). Elsevier Academic Press.

Olweus, D. (1993). *Bullying at school*. Blackwell.

Olweus, D., & Limber, S. P. (2018). Some problems with cyberbullying research. *Current Opinion in Psychology*, *19*, 139–143. https://doi.org/10.1016/j.Copsyc.2017.04.012

Özdemir, Y. (2014). Cyber victimization and adolescent self-esteem: The role of communication with parents. *Asian Journal of Social Psychology*, *17*(4), 255–263. https://doi.org/10.1111/ajsp.12070

Romero, A. J., Bauman, S., Borgstrom, M., & Kim, S. E. (2018). Examining suicidality, bullying, and gun carrying among Latina/o youth over 10 years. *American Journal of Orthopsychiatry*, *88*(4), 450–461. https://doi.org/10.1037/ort0000323.

Rose, C. A., & Tynes, B. M. (2015). Longitudinal associations between cyber-victimization and mental health among US adolescents. *Journal of Adolescent Health*, *57*(3), 305–312. https://doi.org/10.1016/j.jadohealth.2015.05.002

Selkie, E. M., Fales, J. L., & Moreno, M. A. (2016). Cyberbullying prevalence among US middle and high school-aged adolescents: A systematic review and quality assessment. *The Journal of Adolescent Health: Official Publication of the Society for Adolescent Medicine*, 58(2), 125–133. https://doi.org/10.1016/j.jadohealth.2015.09.026

Statista. (February 16, 2024). Weekly time spent playing video games according to adults in the United States as of December 2023, by gender (in hours) [Graph]. In *Statista*. Retrieved July 30, 2024, from https://www-statista.com.wake.idm.oclc.org/statistics/202847/gaming-time-average-week-adults-usa-gender/

Stoll, L. C., & Block, R. Jr (2015). Intersectionality and cyberbullying: A study of cybervictimization in a midwestern high school. *Computers in Human Behavior*, 52, 387–397. https://doi.org/10.1016/j.chb.2015.06.010

Tamborini, R. (2011). Moral intuition and media entertainment. *Journal of Media Psychology: Theories, Methods, and Applications*, 23(1), 39–45. https://doi.org/10.1027/1864-1105/a000031

Tamborini, R., Bowman, N. D., Eden, A., Grizzard, M., & Organ, A. (2010). Defining media enjoyment as the satisfaction of intrinsic needs. *Journal of Communication*, 60(4), 758–777. https://doi.org/10.1111/j.1460-2466.2010.01513.x

Tamborini, R., Eden, A., Bowman, N. D., Grizzard, M., & Lachlan, K. A. (2012). The influence of morality subcultures on the acceptance and appeal of violence. *Journal of Communication*, 62(1), 136–157. https://doi.org/10.1111/j.1460-2466.2011.01620.x

Tynes, B. M., Umaña-Taylor, A. J., Rose, C. A., Lin, J., & Anderson, C. J. (2012). Online racial discrimination and the protective function of ethnic identity and self-esteem for African American adolescents. *Developmental Psychology*, 48(2), 343–355. https://doi.org/10.1037/a0027032

U.S. Department of Education. (2015). *Student reports of bullying and cyberbullying: Results from the 2013 School Crime Supplement to the National Crime Victimization Survey.* (NCES 2015056). https://nces.ed.gov/pubs2015/2015056.pdf

Umaña-Taylor, A. J., Tynes, B. M., Toomey, R. B., Williams, D. R., & Mitchell, K. J. (2015). Latino adolescents' perceived discrimination in online and offline settings: An examination of cultural risk and protective factors. *Developmental Psychology*, 51(1), 87–100. https://doi.org/10.1037/a0038432

Vieira, E. T., & Krcmar, M. (2011). The influences of video gaming on US children's moral reasoning about violence. *Journal of Children and Media*, 5(02), 113–131.

Waasdorp, T. E., & Bradshaw, C. P. (2015). The overlap between cyberbullying and traditional bullying. *The Journal of Adolescent Health: Official Publication of the Society for Adolescent Medicine*, 56(5), 483–488. https://doi.org/10.1016/j.jadohealth.2014.12.002

Wang, C., La Salle, T., Wu, C., Anh Do, K., & Sullivan, K. E. (2018). School climate and parental involvement buffer the risk of peer victimization on suicidal thoughts and behaviors among Asian American middle school students. *Asian American Psychological Association*, 9(4), 296–307. https://doi.org/10.1037/aap0000138

Weber, R., Popova, L., & Mangus, J. M. (2012). Universal morality, mediated narratives, and neural synchrony. In R. Tamborini (Ed.), *Media and the moral mind* (pp. 26–42). Taylor and Francis. https://doi.org/10.4324/9780203127070-10

Werner, N. E., & Crick, N. R. (2004). Maladaptive peer relationships and the development of relational and physical aggression during middle childhood. *Social Development*, 13(4), 495–514. https://doi.org/10.1111/j.1467-9507.2004.00280.x

Wright, M. F. (2015). Cyber victimization and perceived stress: Linkages to late adolescents' cyber aggression and psychological functioning. *Youth & Society*, *47*(6), 789–810. https://doi.org/10.1177/0044118X14537088

Wright, M. F. (2017). Cyber victimization and depression among adolescents with intellectual disabilities and developmental disorders: The moderation of perceived social support. *Journal of Mental Health Research in Intellectual Disabilities*, *10*(2), 126–143. https://doi.org/10.1080/19315864.2016.1271486

Yang, G. S., Gibson, B., Lueke, A. K., Huesmann, L. R., & Bushman, B. J. (2014). Effects of avatar race in violent video games on racial attitudes and aggression. *Social Psychological and Personality Science*, *5*(6), 698–704. https://doi.org/10.1177/1948550614528008

Zych, I., Ortega-Ruiz, R., & Marín-López, I. (2016). Cyberbullying: A systematic review of research, its prevalence and assessment issues in Spanish studies. *Psicología Educativa*, *22*(1), 5–18. https://doi.org/10.1016/j.pse.2016.03.002

10 News/Politics

Lynn Schofield Clark

In August 2023, a US judge in the state of Montana sided with young environmental activists who argued that the state has a legal obligation to address climate change and protect natural resources for future generations. The judge ruled that the state had violated young people's rights when preventing analysis of climate effects in environmental reviews of fossil fuel projects. The Montana case, filed by 16 young people ranging in age from 5 to 22, was the first youth-led climate trial in the United States and is viewed as a model for how young people can engage with the US legal system (Hanson & Brown, 2023). Sariel Sandoval, a plaintiff who is an enrolled member of the Confederated Salish and Kootenai tribes and was 17 at the time of the trial, wanted "to hold the state accountable" (Twumasi, 2024). Claire Vlases, another plaintiff who was 17 when *Held vs. Montana* went to trial, explained that although she was too young to vote, "There are three branches of government for a reason … If I'm not able to use the other two, this is my way, and it's a way for kids, to have their voices heard" (Clark, 2023).

Around the world, young people may or may not have been familiar with this case, as many young people do not follow news regularly at all (Newman et al., 2023). But research suggests that given strong levels of climate concern among youth, many young people, and perhaps especially those from the global South, would be enthusiastic to learn of it (Bowman, 2019; Unigwe, 2019).

Given that by 2020 some 1.4 million protesters had joined youth strikes for climate change worldwide, those young people who had previously sought out news about climate activism may have heard about the case (Boulianne et al., 2020). This is both because youth involvement in the climate change movement has become a topic of regular media coverage (Boykoff, 2006; von Zabern & Tulloch, 2021), and because, thanks to algorithmic norms, the feeds of those interested in climate change activism are structured to "attract" news of the Montana case to their feed (Thorson, 2020). But in the feeds of other young people, there might be

DOI: 10.4324/9781003453123-12

misinformation or no information at all. Young people, like those of all ages, live in specific news and information ecosystems that are comprised of sources that include face-to-face, online, and school-based conversations among peers, friends, and family members as well as via social media feeds and legacy media sources (Lee et al., 2013; Shah et al., 2017). News most often comes to young people second hand or via hearsay from their peers or family members. And platforms such as Instagram, TikTok, and YouTube allow for the acceleration of news sharing as well as the sharing of other kinds of information, as well as news avoidance and the spread of disinformation, in ways that scholars are continuously seeking to better understand, as this chapter will discuss.

This chapter focuses on young people, news, and politics: an area that has seen an increased level of scholarly interest over the past decade (Fillol & Pereira, 2020). Although the chapter includes references to children and to the ways that people continue to change and grow throughout their lives, much of the existing research has focused on middle adolescence to young adulthood (approximately ages 15–25), and thus the chapter will give particular emphasis to this time in life. And although the chapter uses the term politics, we focus more broadly on youth civic engagement, which, following the definition offered by the Center for Information and Research on Civic Learning and Engagement, encompasses the ways that young people engage in "a wide range of actions and behaviors that improve communities and help solve problems"(CIRCLE, 2024). Although civic engagement can include political participation that happens through the formal electoral processes of voting, it can also include volunteering, serving in community organizations, participating in social movements, and participating in commodity activism such as boycotting (refusing to buy certain goods) or buycotting (deliberately shopping at ethical companies instead) (Vromen et al., 2016). And although much of the existing research on youth and politics has focused on the late democratic societies of the West, an increasing body of scholarship is considering youth, media, and politics in contexts of the East and the global South (Cheruiyot et al., 2021).

Because minoritized and low-income young people are among the least likely to feel that their voices are heard in political and civic spaces (Marchi, 2012; Rubin et al., 2009), in this chapter we are also interested in politics in a sense that is somewhat apart from societal institutions. This is because some young people of color and LGBT young people view their daily lived experiences as political. Youth advocates, educators, and some scholars who study youth and politics note that recognizing and thriving within systems of social inequity requires addressing both internalized and structural experiences of racism through critical consciousness development (Yosso & Solorzano, 2006). Engaging in activities that foster a heightened awareness of inequalities and injustices, then, is viewed as an important aspect of what Watts et al. (1999), in their studies of young Black men, have termed sociopolitical development (see also Watts & Hipolito-Delgado, 2015). Sociopolitical development can strengthen critical consciousness and can lead to *youth activism*, which is a phrase that refers to efforts by young people between the ages of 12 and 25 who seek to change the institutions, policies, and cultural norms that affect their lives by expressing dissent from prevailing norms and advocating for different policies, often through actions that are disruptive and that seek to mobilize members of the public to their cause (O'Brien et al., 2018). Young people of color and other young people experiencing marginalization due to gender identity, neurodiversity, or physical disability can and do develop political efficacy in ways that differ from the mainstream and thus challenge existing notions of the relationships between youth, news, and politics. The role that media play in these processes is an important emergent area for research, particularly as today's young people are the most racially and ethnically diverse generation in US history (Parker et al., 2019).

This chapter therefore begins with a discussion of the ways that social media have changed youth experiences with news, both through the restructuring of traditional news organizations (such as the US's *CNN, The New York Times, Fox News,* and others) and through the rise of alternative formats and practices through which young people encounter and share news, like via TikToks, Instagram Stories, or texting news to a friend. The chapter discusses how the topics of youth and news and youth and politics have been studied in the past. We then turn to three areas of research that have been of particular interest to those studying youth, politics, and news in recent years: (1) youth involvement in social movements and youth uses of social media for political expression, (2) youth engagement in political institutions as traditionally conceived and their efforts to leverage media outlets in this work, and (3) growing concerns about the spread of disinformation and endeavors to respond to this challenge. Each of these topics have been central in areas of youth digital media and civic literacy, as was discussed in Chapter 5. But because it is also important to recognize the limitations of literacy efforts alone within a rapidly changing media landscape, this chapter also aligns with the interventions that ask: who is responsible for shaping the media environment for young people, and how can that environment best support both youthful thriving and youthful participation in the decisions that affect their lives, both now and in the future? We begin by exploring how news itself has been undergoing change.

News and Young People

The platforms of social media have dramatically changed the ways that people of all ages encounter and engage with news. The Reuters Digital News Report of 2024 found that social media are the main gateway for news for both older and younger news consumers, following trends reported over the past several years (Madden et al., 2017; Newman et al., 2023). This trend is particularly marked in the global South, where the proportion reporting that they use TikTok for news has grown rapidly in Africa, Latin America, and parts of Asia (see Figure 10.1).

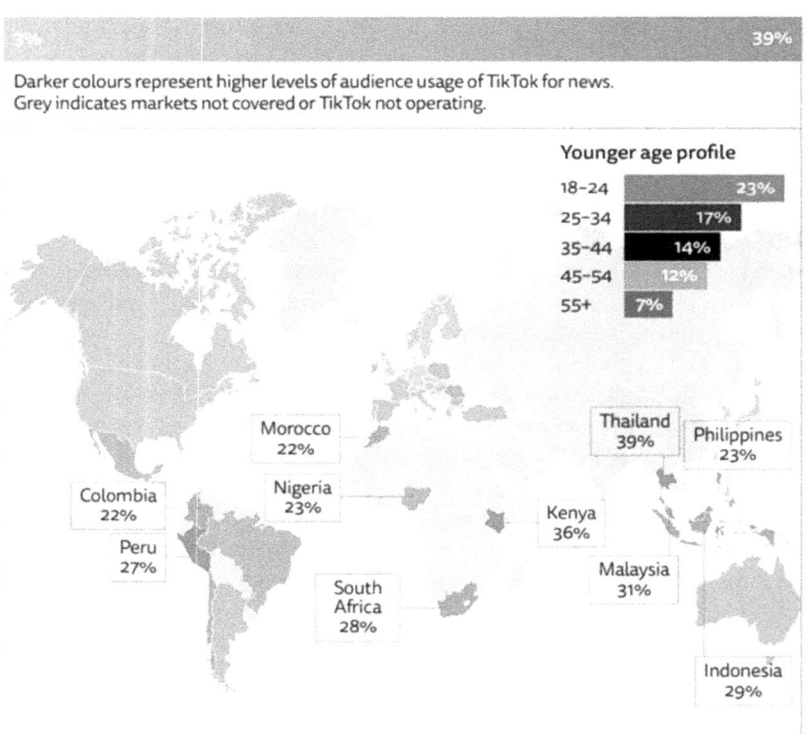

Figure 10.1 Using TikTok for news by age.
Source: *Reuters Digital News Report 2024* (reproduced with permission)

It used to be that people would seek out the news from reputable news sources, reading the daily newspaper that was delivered to their door or tuning in to a news broadcast on a local radio or television station. Today, more people say that they have a "news-finds-me" attitude, and some people cannot identify where the news they encounter may have actually originated (Boczkowski et al., 2017; Gil de Zúñiga et al., 2017; Kalogeropoulos et al., 2019; Kligler-Vilenchik et al., 2022). Additionally, rather than setting aside a particular time in the day for news, people now read, watch, or listen to news in short bursts, checking for news when they're on the go in the car or on a train, clicking on stories that are of interest to them or scrolling through quick news "snacks" when they have just a brief moment to digest what they're seeing or hearing. Few people report taking the time to share, like, comment on, or recommend news stories to others in their social circles (Costera Meijer & Groot Kormelink, 2015). Today's traditional news organizations—those of print, broadcast, and cablecast news—have thus come to be viewed by audiences as one of many sources of input within their personalized news repertoires (Peters et al., 2022). Many news organizations are shuttering, including some such as *BuzzFeed* that attempted to harness social media logics (Darcy, 2023). News avoidance is on the rise, as documented in a five-nation comparative study tracing the cognitive and emotional reasons for the practice (Edgerly, 2017; Villi et al., 2022). In response, scholars have turned their attention to shoring up traditional news sources and to studying the news making and sharing that takes place outside traditional news media structures (Bengtsson & Johansson, 2020; Cheruiyot et al., 2021).

The shift to social media platforms as a primary source for news is largely driven by the youngest generations, but numerous studies have been documenting a declining interest in news among all populations for more than a decade, noting that this trend is happening more rapidly among young people when compared with adults. As they have become more platform-dependent, news organizations have sought to balance the delivery of factual information and positive emotions as they adapt to the logic of platforms like TikTok and Instagram, experimenting with story length, format, and with youthful reporters (Hendrickx, 2023; Røsok-Dahl & Kristine Olsen, 2024).

Social media platforms are both responding to and further contributing to the declining interest in news. When Instagram announced that the platform would no longer recommend "political content" unless users opted in to seeing it in 2024, for example, news accounts on those sites experienced a decline in shares, comments, likes, reach, and video views, with shares from major news accounts falling 26% week over week, on average, according to analyses (Maheshwari & Isaac, 2024).

Another way that social media contribute to the decline in news is less direct. News organizations increasingly rely on metrics and data to shape their news delivery strategies (Hermida, 2020). Social media users whose behaviors suggest that they are less likely to engage with and pay for news become less likely to be targeted with news content by news organizations (Thorson, 2020). As a result, the news preferences of young people are of less interest to news organizations. In this way, as Thorson (2020) has argued, the insights that news organizations glean from user data indirectly limit the possibilities for incidental news exposure among young people.

But this lack of interest in young audiences among legacy news organizations is hardly new. News organizations only rarely have been wholeheartedly focused on the young audience for news in the past, as Buckingham (2002) pointed out several decades ago in his review of youth encounters with industry-produced youth news. There have been several prominent exceptions in the past, however, of news programs produced with young people in mind or with substantial numbers of young people in the audience. Carter (2004), for example, recounted the story of *Children's Express*, an endeavor launched by former Wall Street lawyer and business entrepreneur Bob Clampitt in 1975. *Children's Express* partnered professional news organizations with trained young people who wrote and delivered news, but the organization ended its run in 2001. In the UK, the BBC's *Newsround* was regularly viewed by 55% of all 5- to 7-year-olds in 1972, according to *Radio Times* article (Carter, 2004). Also in the UK, Channel 4 offered *First Edition*, a news program for primary school students with Jon Snow, from 1997 to 2002, and from 1995 to 2000 it offered the Emmy, Peabody, Children's BAFTA, and Prix Europa award-winning program *Wise Up!* (Buckingham, 2002). Christensen (2013) and Jensen (2013) have detailed the long history of the Danish Broadcasting Service's *News for Children* and related efforts to center children's voices and concerns, and Hendershot (2004) traced the history of *Nick News with Linda Ellerbee*, the longest-running US news program serving 8- to 13-year-olds, which aired from 1992 to 2015 on the Nickelodeon channel. In 1990, Channel One News offered a controversial new model in which schools were offered satellite receivers and televisions in exchange for the promise that schools would record and then play daily advertising-sponsored news content in classrooms (Greenberg & Brand, 1993). But overall, funds for television news programs for children started to fall by the wayside in the early 2000s, as commercial news media systems saw their profit margins wane years before the social media transformation (Clark & Marchi, 2017). Fortunately, some scholarship is finding that news media today are taking young people more seriously than they once did (Boulianne et al., 2020; Poot & Bauwens, 2023), although there is also evidence that many news stories continue to trivialize young people and are dismissive of their concerns, which provides further disincentive for young people to seek out and share news from traditional news organizations (Mampaey et al., 2021).

With the rise of social media, boundaries between news and entertainment have been blurring (Lee-Wright et al., 2012). Young people, particularly those in their teen and young adult years, often encounter news via comedy, with the stars of late-night television and satirical news programs holding special influence. *The Daily Show*, *Last Week Tonight with John Oliver*, and the Weekend Update with Colin Jost and Michael Che on *Saturday Night Live* each introduce young people to news stories (Baym, 2005; Jones, 2010; Penney, 2019), as do original political memes and short videos that quote or link to these commercial productions. The 2023 Reuters Institute for the Study of Journalism found that 55% of TikTok users and 52% of Instagram users get their news from these social media outlets and other influencers on these platforms, with YouTube and Snapchat also playing an important role (Newman et al., 2023). The most successful youth-based news influencers around the world are overwhelmingly White and cisgender males who talk with mostly male guests. While young independent journalists Hugo Travers, Jack Kelly, and Vitus Spehar get attention, topping the list as most mentioned news-related accounts in the United States are many leaders who espouse conservative or libertarian perspectives, including Tucker Carlson, Joe Rogan, Tim Pool, and Alex Jones, among others (Newman et al., 2023) (see Figure 10.2).

Despite a current interest in young people's news consumption practices, youth and news was generally considered a marginalized topic in the field until the rise of social media (Buckingham, 2017). Changes in news distribution and consumption patterns, coupled with the documented

YOUTH-BASED NEWS INFLUENCERS AROUND THE WORLD

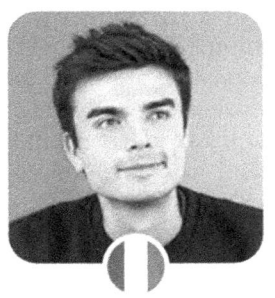
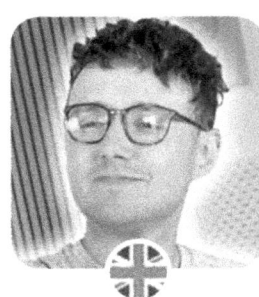
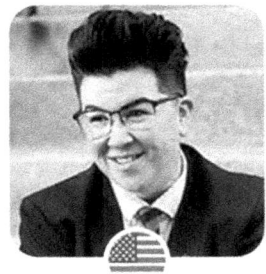

Hugo Travers　　　　　Jack Kelly　　　　　Vitus Spehar

Figure 10.2 Youth-based news influencers around the world.

Source: Reuters Digital News Report 2024 (reproduced with permission)

large declines in trust in news (Brosius et al., 2022; Matsa, 2022), are giving rise to urgent concerns regarding the future of news and its role in relation to thriving democratic societies. Thus scholars continue to argue that concerns about youth encounters with news are as much about the present as they are about an imagined future (Darcy, 2023).

With social media, young people can speak back to news organizations and reporters, they can repackage traditional news in the creation of their own commentary, and they can use their own creativity to produce and share user-generated content that highlights their own views on what they think is important for others to know. YouTube, Instagram, and TikTok have thus become important venues for the production and sharing of youth perspectives, with political expression being just one of many areas of creativity (Raby et al., 2018). We will return to the topic of youth creativity and political expression, but first, we turn to a review of how youth and news, and youth and politics, have been approached within distinct scholarly traditions.

Frameworks for Researching Young People, News, and Politics

The reason that youth and news is a relatively recent area of interest may be rooted in the fact that two schools of thought have tended to govern the studies of young people, news, and politics. The first body of research has viewed young people as vulnerable and in need of protection. Scholars have explored the purported traumatizing effects for children who are not developmentally ready to encounter information about war, death, natural disasters, school shootings, and health threats such as those related to epidemics and pandemics like COVID-19 (Strasser et al., 2022). Other scholars in this approach have considered youthful vulnerability to propaganda, noting that bad actors can leverage youthful enthusiasm for political ends (Appleby, 2013; Yani, 2021). Young people are often viewed in this approach as "citizens-in-waiting," to use Gordon and Taft's (2011) term: in need of protection until they enter adulthood and are developmentally ready to engage in the age-bound acts of citizenship that include voting, serving in the military, serving on a jury, and living independently of one's guardians. But researcher Cindy Carter, who has studied news among children, has argued that this approach has led parents to believe that viewing and discussing news with children can be problematic. Rather than inculcating a sense of civic awareness, parents are more concerned about monitoring a child's emotional responses to the news, watching for psychological or physiological symptoms that the child may be suffering, and parents feel that they are to then "provide reassurance that the child is personally safe" (Carter, 2004, p. 78). She argues that given the dominance of this concern, parents may not see their role as needing "to explain, analyse or critique the reporting of a traumatic event in the news," which in turn, she argues, underestimates children's ability to understand, critique, and cope with traumatic news (Carter, 2004, p. 78).

Following the critiques of Carter and others, a second and more recent body of research has centered the voices and experiences of young people themselves in relation to news. Consistent with the United Nations' Convention on the Rights of the Child, scholars in this approach have considered the ways that young people seek out opportunities to express their views and participate in other forms of civic action such as volunteering in one's community or participating in acts of protest (Middaugh et al., 2017). In addition to viewing information as a right, scholars in this approach have explored the settings and structures that help students to learn through civic engagement endeavors, youth participatory action research, and other methods that best equip young people for participation (Mihailidis, 2018). While this chapter reviews literature from both approaches, it is ultimately rooted in the assumption that young people's views, practices, and experiences matter, and that young people have insights to share on how best to engage both them and their peers in the present day and in the future.

Similar to the scholarship on youth and news, there are differing frameworks that have guided the study of youth and politics. In general, research in this area has tended to embrace either a human development, lineage/socialization, a generational/cohort, or a life course approach. **Human development research** has demonstrated that experiences with politics in the formative years of childhood, adolescence, and young adulthood can shape life-long political behaviors (Gerber et al., 2003). One way that this area has connected with news is in studies that have found that US young people may first come into an awareness of political issues through direct experience with or news coverage of school shootings. In one study of 18- to 24-year-olds, for example, almost two-thirds (64%) said that they had paid some or a lot of attention to news about the 2018 shooting in Parkland, Florida at Stoneman Douglas high school (CIRCLE, 2019). In addition to heightened awareness of issues directly related to youth well-being, there is increasing evidence that involving young people in activities of political participation has a positive effect on the development of both political efficacy and civic knowledge (Jimenez et al., 2023; Padilla et al., 2022).

Lineage or socialization approaches look at how political values, attitudes, and behaviors are propagated from one generation to the next, usually by caregivers and educators (Braungart & Braungart, 1986; Hooghe, 2004). These scholars have observed that parents often do not embrace direct or intensive efforts to influence the political orientations of their children, but role modeling and the ways that parents subtly reward preferred political behaviors do have a significant influence on young people (Bengtson et al., 1985). Schools also can play a role in political socialization, particularly via programs that encourage children to bring assignments home for work with parents, thus initiating a "trickle up" phenomenon in which the school facilitates both the child's and the parent's socialization into politics (McDevitt & Chaffee, 2002).

A third group of scholars have considered **generational or cohort approaches**. This approach explores the experiences of groups who were born around the same time and thus experienced significant world events at similar points in their lives. A classic cohort study of the 20th century was Lowenberg's (1983) psychoanalytic explanation for the rise of Nazism among the large cohort of young men who had experienced wartime hunger and deprivation and then witnessed the humiliation and disappointment of their fathers who returned from the first world war to high unemployment and a depressed economy. Scholars in the cohort or generational approach have explored how youth experiences cohered to give shape to the Arab Spring (Hoffmann & Jamal, 2014) and how common experiences of poverty and exclusion from policymaking processes led to political violence in Nigeria (Onimisi, 2024; Urdal, 2006).

Life course scholars bring together human development and sociological approaches, exploring the ways that awareness and comprehension of political issues and current events might increase both as cognitive development occurs through childhood and adolescence and as young people encounter differing life trajectories or pathways to differing outcomes (Mayer, 2009). Looking at the adolescent years in the life course, scholars have noted that the quality of political understanding is related to various factors such as intelligence, family background, gender, race, and class, while political orientation is influenced by socializing factors including family, friends, teachers, and media (Amnå, 2012). This approach tends to take a view that development of political interest and awareness is more plastic than is sometimes assumed, as sociohistorical contexts and political upheavals can play an important role in focusing and cultivating political interests at any age (Flanagan & Sherrod, 1998).

In the next sections, we explore three areas of research that have been of particular interest to those studying youth, politics, and news in recent years: youth involvement in social movements and in political expression online, growing concerns about the spread of disinformation with various explorations regarding how best to combat this problem, and youth engagement in political institutions as traditionally conceived and the communication infrastructures that have emerged to support these endeavors. Each of these areas have been treated with greater or less attention within youth digital media and civic literacy endeavors, as is discussed further in Chapter 5 of this volume.

Youth and Social Movements

A great deal of scholarship has acknowledged that young people have provided leadership in social and political revolutions, markedly so since the 1830s (Braungart & Braungart, 1986). In a 2021 poll conducted at the Harvard Kennedy School, 36% of young Americans reported that they consider themselves to be politically active, representing a 150% increase from 2009 (Harvard Youth Poll, 2021). Beyond the United States, researchers are also finding that youth are increasingly politically engaged both offline and online (UNICEF, 2020). In addition to youth involvement in the climate change movements, scholars have explored young adult participation in the Arab Spring, in protests supporting young undocumented immigrant "Dreamers," in the 2011 in Occupy Wall Street, and in the #MeToo and trans rights and the Black Lives Matter movements (Bennett & Segerberg, 2013; Howard et al., 2016; Milkman, 2017; Papacharissi, 2015; Tufekci, 2017).

Today, scholars observe that the rise of youth movements must be understood as an interaction between life course development, shared cohort experiences, and sociopolitical trends. This approach suggests that political consciousness largely emerges in relation to both personal and historical experiences with politics and society. And although a few decades ago scholars bemoaned a purported lack of political engagement and interest among young people, in recent years scholars have pointed out that we may be witnessing a change rather than a decline in citizenship norms, with heightened youth interest in social movements, protests, volunteering, and other forms of civic engagement (Loader, 2007; Youniss et al., 2002; Zukin et al., 2006). Loader et al. (2014) argued further that with social media we have seen the rise of "networked young citizens," who participate in personalized political actions as well as lifestyle politics: for example, choosing to eat vegetarian as a protest against eating animal products or biking to work instead of driving to protest the fossil fuel industry while reinforcing the need for alternative modes of transportation. Today's young adults leverage digital media for participatory politics, or "peer-based acts through which individuals and groups seek to exert both voice and influence on issues of public concern" (Cohen & Kahne, 2011 p. vi). They also leverage contacts with reporters, seeking to garner attention for youth civic engagement to engage in connective journalism: sharing news stories about youth civic and political action with their peers, often as a precursor to their own actions (Clark & Marchi, 2017). Additionally, the number of 18 to 24 year olds participating in a march or demonstration increased dramatically from 2016 to 2018 and again to 2020, with Black and Latinx youth having a higher rate of political media creation and engagement than White and Asian youth (CIRCLE, 2020).

Social media spaces have been of particular interest to those studying the emergence of new forms of youthful political expression, or in how young people create and share political messages with their peers on social media sites like Instagram, YouTube, or TikTok. Sreekumar and Vadrevu (2013) argued that memes hold the potential for enhancing political engagement among a citizenry that is often seen as depoliticized and apathetic, and that humor has become a key feature of young peoples' political expression online (Vraga et al., 2015; Vromen et al., 2016). Although Penney (2019) acknowledged that some young people who are concerned with politics avoid humor because they fear political meme-sharing will make their own concerns seem less important, other scholars such as Kligler-Vilenchik and Literat (2018) have pointed out that young people can experience a taste of political agency as they experiment with online political expression and can participate in reimagining politics (see also Bowyer et al., 2017; Kahne & Middaugh, 2012). Researchers have found a strong connection between online and offline political participation among young people (Boulianne & Theocharis, 2020).

For a time, scholars were particularly interested in positive outcomes associated with political expression online, but in more recent years there has been a renewed focus on far-right activism. Marwick and Lewis (2017) reported on memes produced and shared on 4Chan and Reddit that featured racist and antisemitic jokes targeting racial and gendered minority groups while spreading conspiracy theories and misinformation. Miller-Idriss (2020) pointed out that young people stumble across extremist ideas in many places in their everyday lives, including through humorous memes, "trad" or traditionally minded and ideologically conservative YouTube cooking programs, and through music festivals, gaming tournaments, music lyrics, and symbols on t-shirts. The mainstreaming of far-right ideologies has meant that young people move in and out of extremist movement actions more fluidly than in the past. As Miller-Idriss argues, this suggests that there is an urgent need for teaching about radicalization and for helping young people to recognize radical codes and symbols at an early age. This focus has also aligned with the issue that has garnered perhaps the greatest amount of attention in relation to questions of youth, news, and politics in recent years: disinformation.

Disinformation: The Dark Side of Youth, News, and Politics

Given that young people learn of major world events like the Russian invasion of Ukraine and the Israeli-Hamas war via TikTok, some scholars of youth and politics are particularly concerned about the vulnerability of young people to sources of disinformation. Disinformation has been defined as including "all forms of false, inaccurate, or misleading information designed, presented and promoted to intentionally cause public harm or for profit" (European Commission, 2018, p. 3). Freelon and Wells (2020) point out that this definition excludes messages that can cause unintentional harm (misinformation) and messages intended to harm without deception (such as those of racism, xenophobia, or gender-related discrimination), and they go on to argue that any discussion of heightened concerns about youth and disinformation needs to be understood in the context of increased polarization; rising distrust in societal institutions of governance, science, and of the press; and the expansion of conservative voice through radio, cable television, and the internet with the repeal of the Fairness Doctrine: the US law that used to require television channels to devote equal time to contrasting viewpoints on issues of public importance. Each of these factors has provided fertile ground for disinformation's spread.

One 2020 study found that 76% of 14- to 24-year-olds had encountered disinformation online at least once a week, which represented a rise of 50% over the previous two years (Vodafone Foundation Germany, 2020). Younger children report concern regarding their ability to judge truthfulness online, but one study across ten countries found that relatively large proportions of older children reported high critical evaluation skills (Howard et al., 2021).

Young people encounter disinformation on social media sites because disinformation spreads faster and further than truthful information, at least in part because emotionally charged content spreads more rapidly than regular content. One instance that circulated widely on Instagram, for example, involved the manipulation of a photo of gun control activist Emma Gonzales, a survivor of the 2017 Parkland school shooting. Gonzalez had been photographed ripping up a shooting range target, but a manipulated photo showed her ripping up the US constitution (Howard et al., 2021). Greta Thunberg has been similarly targeted, as she has been falsely accused of alleged associations with antifa and has been depicted as mentally unsound (Aashka et al., 2020).

Howard et al. (2021) have argued that disinformation among parents, caregivers, and educators can have a negative effect on children even when young people themselves are not directly exposed to it. They note that harmful consequences include violence against ethnic minority children as well as victimization of children, both of which rise in concert with the spread of manipulated images that stereotype and discredit them. They also note that the circulation of anti-vaccine conspiracy theories had the effect of reducing parental plans to vaccinate their children, thus putting children at risk. They argue that there is a great need for more research into the questions of how susceptible children are to disinformation, and how such disinformation affects their development, well-being, and rights.

Research has found that those adults who identify as conservative are disproportionately more likely to be targeted by those purveying disinformation (Faris et al., 2017; Freelon & Lokot, 2020; Howard, 2018) and that they are more likely to believe and share disinformation (Alcott & Gentzkos, 2017; Grinberg, et al., 2019; Guess et al., 2019). There is also evidence that Black US social media users were disproportionately targeted with disinformation (DiResta et al., 2018; Howard, 2018).

Responding to Disinformation

Disinformation is one of the most pressing issues in the realm of news and politics, and not just for young people. While there are signs that international bodies and local groups are taking the problems of disinformation seriously, there is still much more to be done. After many tech companies strengthened their efforts to combat myths about the Coronavirus, in 2023 platforms such as YouTube and Twitter cut their safety, policy, content moderation, and disinformation teams, with little accountability to the public for such actions (Myers & Grant, 2023; Timberg et al., 2020). Scholars tend to agree on important interventions, but recognize the challenges in expecting that stakeholders will cooperate. For example, technology companies could be required to offer transparency and accountability on their content policies, grant more access to researchers, and invest more heavily in content moderation and media literacy. Policymakers could be pressed to regulate those companies so that children's rights to safe spaces, to freedom of expression, and to reliable information are guaranteed, and so that disinformation is addressed quickly and with accountability. Trusted news organizations can be funded to deepen their historic role as fact-checkers and verifiers of news. Educators could be expected to incorporate digital media literacy into the curriculum as part of the expectation of full participation in society, including ensuring that young people have the right not only to information but to pathways that enable their voices on issues to be heard. Scholars as well as youth advocates, educators, and policymakers struggle to surface these and other options for public consideration in a polarized environment that has politicized news and evidence. But there are also areas of research that may help in these endeavors.

Youth, the Vote, and the Courts: The Role of Organizations in Social Change

While research in political expression and extremist political communication has adopted cohort and life course approaches to news and politics, socialization and human development scholarship has been the starting point for research focused on the intentions of parents and of schools. But to return to one of the quotations that began this chapter, it is also important to think about the access that young people have to the various branches of government while they are still young. Several community, not-for-profit, and nongovernmental organizations provide spaces for the cultivation of youth voice and for an expanded focus on youth involvement in adult social movements, in some cases seeking a lowering of the voting age or inclusion of youth voices and experiences in the courts (Painter et al., 2024; Russell, 2016). In many cases, these efforts have involved young people in media production. In her study of the grassroots citizen media project Ciudad Comuna, for example, Brough (2020) explores the ways that hip hop, graffiti, and digital media were leveraged to enhance participation in participatory budgeting in the city of Medellin, Colombia. Jimenez et al. (2023) similarly trace efforts to leverage social media to garner the attention of local lawmakers and advocate for community resources. There are also activist groups on the far right that provide media and structural support for social movements. Turning Point USA, for example, has spent thousands aiming to get young conservatives elected onto university student government ballots. That organization also courts controversy to garner media attention and thus raise awareness of its work. At the same time, though, the organization eschews transparency in their work, encouraging the students it supports to downplay their connection to the organization and to under-report Turning Point's contributions to youth efforts to avoid scrutiny (Mayer, 2017; Vasquez, 2017).

Returning to the example of the Held vs. Montana case that was introduced at the beginning of this chapter, then, it is worth noting that the first youth-led climate court case was the result of more than a decade's worth of work on behalf of the organization known as Our Children's Trust. Our Children's Trust was started in 2010 by Julia Olson, an environmental attorney in Eugene, Oregon. Olson had been inspired by the work of Mary Cristina Wood, a law professor at the University of Oregon who had argued that lawsuits to address climate change could build on the public trust doctrine: a legal principle that establishes that certain natural and cultural resources are preserved for public use (Wood, 2007, 2009). The public trust doctrine, with roots in ancient Roman law, was subsequently strengthened in England and became part of US common law (Langbein et al., 2009). The organization, which has pending litigation in Alaska, Florida, Utah, and Virginia as well as one against the U.S. Environmental Protection Agency, has created social media and arts toolkits as well as short animation and news releases. They promote and hold online educational events and coordinate fundraising efforts. The organization's documentary, YouthVGov, is a complement to #youthvgov high school curriculum resources, and has been available at schools throughout the United States and is now available on Netflix. The not-for-profit also offers tips on how to write letters to the editor for school and other news publications, and maintains an Instagram with more than 15,000 followers, a Facebook page with 29,000 followers, a Twitter/X feed with more than 12,000 followers, and a small presence on TikTok via the hashtag #youthvgov. The organization also shares common efforts with several related not-for-profits and NGOs that place youth voice at the forefront, including EarthJustice and Earth Guardians as well as the international civil disobedience movement Extinction Rebellion which is based in the U.K. Extinction Rebellion offers a blog featuring a monthly newsletter that provides updates on the organization's climate action as well as "must reads:" reports filed by journalists as well as academics that detail fallout from the latest climate-related disasters and predictions for the future. Our Children's Trust has supported or represented young people in legal actions, many of which involve climate lawsuits, in all fifty US states as well as in seven other countries. Tracing the role of organizations supportive of youth voice is a relatively recent area of interest for those interested in youth, news, and politics, and is a promising one.

Conclusions: Signs of Hope

As this chapter has discussed, the scholarship focused on youth, news, and politics has been expanding rapidly as media systems undergo transformations and as concepts related to politics, youth civic engagement, and democracy also are undergoing change. People of all ages are more reliant than ever on social media platforms for their encounters with news, raising many questions about the viability of legacy news organizations and the role of social media and video platforms like TikTok, Instagram, and YouTube in news delivery. And in contrast to the broadcast and print legacy news experiments of the past that engaged young people in the creation and distribution of news for youth, there is, as of now, no commitment on the part of the most prominent platforms to supporting news creation or distribution for young people - or for those of any age, in fact. Experiments are occurring, and the breadth and depth of youthful political expression is encouraging. But the most successful young news influencers to date in many Western contexts are those that combine video and podcasting, have a libertarian or conservative orientation, and are White and male: hardly reflective of the burgeoning diverse youth population or of its political needs and desires (CIRCLE, 2022; Kruikemeier & Shehata, 2017).

Some studies of youth and news, like those of youth and politics, focus on young people as vulnerable populations in need of adult guidance regarding information about violence and wars as well as guidance on propaganda and political systems, approaching young people as "citizens in waiting," as this chapter has discussed. A growing body of research, particularly studies focused on older teens and young adults, are considering the rights of children to information and to participation in the decisions that affect their lives, working within the life course framework of research that brings together human development and sociological approaches. Much of the scholarship on youth and social movements falls into this latter framework. In addition to the example of climate change activism that opened this chapter, for example, there are researchers who are analyzing youth involvement in social movements that address LGBTQ rights, immigration, racism, and gun control, and analyses are increasingly focused on efforts to recruit young people into conservative movements as well, as this chapter has discussed.

Youth presence in social movements and their interest in related issues has also fueled research into the ways that new forms of political expression are emerging through political memes, video shorts, and commentary, all of which continue to be rich sources for exploration. The chapter has also suggested a need for continued attention to disinformation studies, as well as for studies in other areas. Calls for media literacy have expanded to address disinformation, but further research is also needed to better understand the role of media competence development in youth civic education (see Chapter 5).

While some scholarship is exploring the relationships between news and youth engagement in politics as more traditionally conceived such as through voting and in the courts, for example, more research is needed that explores how social media and news are mobilized in efforts to lower the US voting age, and how media are leveraged to involve young people in court cases, as exemplified in the Held vs. Montana case (NYRA, 2011).

Much of the research into youth, news, and politics is filled with caution and concern, both for young people themselves and for the larger societies of which they are a part. Of course, it is important to note that there are numerous young people like Sariel Sandoval and Claire Vlases who were introduced at the beginning of this chapter and who are leveraging news and social media to express themselves, to unite with other young people and youth-centric organizations, and to bring about positive change. They and others like them need a continued commitment on the part of scholars, advocates, educators, and caregivers to support them. Adults and young people need to work across generations to establish guidelines and policies governing disinformation, to find ways to bring youth perspectives into educational and political settings, and to bring media platforms into greater accountability. And while it can be difficult to predict what it would mean for young people to take a more active role in bringing about the changes they wish to see, the advocates, caregivers, educators, and scholars who are interested in this subject area tend to be in agreement: they have a right to try.

References

Aashka, D., Boardman, E., & Schwartz-Henderson, L. (2020). *Targeting Greta Thunberg: A case study in online mis/disinformation*. The German Marshall Fund of the United States. https://www.gmfus.org/news/targeting-greta-thunberg-case-study-online-misdisinformation

Allcott, H., & Gentzkow, M. (2017). Social media and fake news in the 2016 election. *Journal of Economic Perspectives, 31*(2), 211–236.

Amnå, E. (2012). How is civic engagement developed over time? Emerging answers from a multidisciplinary field. *Journal of Adolescence, 35*(3), 611–627.

Appleby, K. D. (2013). Controlling information with propaganda: Indoctrinating the youth in nazi Germany. *Dalhousie Journal of Interdisciplinary Management*, 9(1), Article 1. https://ojs.library.dal.ca/djim/article/view/2013vol9Appleby

Baym, G. (2005). The daily show: Discursive integration and the reinvention of political journalism. *Political Communication*, 22(3), 259–276. https://doi.org/10.1080/10584600591006492

Bengtson, V. I., Cutler, N. E., Mangen, D. J., & Marshall, V. W. (1985). Generations, cohorts, and relations between age groups. In R. H. Binstock, & E. Shanas (Eds.), *Handbook of aging and the social sciences* (pp. 304–338). Van Nostrand Reinhold.

Bengtsson, S., & Johansson, S. (2020). A phenomenology of news: Understanding news in digital culture. *Journalism*, 1464884919901194. https://doi.org/10.1177/1464884919901194

Bennett, W. L., & Segerberg, A. (2013). *The logic of connective action: Digital media and the personalization of contentious politics*. Cambridge University Press.

Boczkowski, P., Michelstein, E., & Matassi, M. (2017, January 4). *Incidental news: How young people consume news on social media*. 50th Hawaii International Conference on System Sciences, University of Hawaii at Manoa. https://scholarspace.manoa.hawaii.edu/items/922ba71b-203a-4538-8df8-257c3bab3c44

Boulianne, S., Lalancette, M., & Ilkiw, D. (2020). "School strike 4 climate": Social media and the international youth protest on climate change. *Media and Communication*, 8(2), 208–218. https://doi.org/10.17645/mac.v8i2.2768

Boulianne, S., & Theocharis, Y. (2020). Young people, digital media, and engagement: A meta-analysis of research. *Social Science Computer Review*, 38(2), 111–127.

Bowman, B. (2019). Imagining future worlds alongside young climate activists: A new framework for research. *Fennia - International Journal of Geography*, 197(2), Article 2.

Bowyer, B. T., Kahne, J. E., & Middaugh, E. (2017). Youth comprehension of political messages in YouTube videos. *New Media & Society*, 19(4), 522–541. https://doi.org/10.1177/1461444815611593

Boykoff, J. (2006). Framing dissent: Mass-media coverage of the global justice movement. *New Political Science*, 28(2), 201–228. https://doi.org/10.1080/07393140600679967

Braungart, R. G., & Braungart, M. M. (1986). Life-course and generational politics. *Annual Review of Sociology*, 12(1), 205–231. https://doi.org/10.1146/annurev.so.12.080186.001225

Brosius, A., Ohme, J., & de Vreese, C. H. (2022). Generational gaps in media trust and its antecedents in Europe. *The International Journal of Press/Politics*, 27(3), 648–667. https://doi.org/10.1177/19401612211039440

Brough, M. (2020). *Youth power in precarious times: Reimagining civic participation*. Duke University Press.

Buckingham, D. (2002). *The making of citizens: Young people, news and politics*. Routledge. https://www.taylorfrancis.com/books/mono/10.4324/9780203132272/making-citizens-david-buckingham

Buckingham, D. (2017, January 12). Fake news: Is media literacy the answer? *David Buckingham*. https://davidbuckingham.net/2017/01/12/fake-news-is-media-literacy-the-answer/

Carter, C. (2004). Scary news: Children's responses to news of war. *Mediactive*, 3, 67–84.

Cheruiyot, D., Wahutu, J. S., Mare, A., Ogola, G., & Mabweazara, H. M. (2021). Making news outside legacy media. *African Journalism Studies*, 42(4), 1–14. https://doi.org/10.1080/23743670.2021.2046397

Christensen, C. L. (2013). Engaging, critical, entertaining: Transforming public service television for children in Denmark. *Interactions: Studies in Communication & Culture, 4*(3), 271–287. https://doi.org/10.1386/iscc.4.3.271_1

CIRCLE. (2019). *The gun violence prevention movement fueled youth engagement in 2018*. Tufts University. https://circle.tufts.edu/latest-research/gun-violence-prevention-movement-fueled-youth-engagement-2018-election

CIRCLE. (2020). *Poll: Young people believe they can lead change in unprecedented election cycle*. https://circle.tufts.edu/latest-research/poll-young-people-believe-they-can-lead-change-unprecedented-election-cycle

CIRCLE. (2022). *Young women of color continue to lead civic and political engagement*. https://circle.tufts.edu/latest-research/young-women-color-continue-lead-civic-and-political-engagement

CIRCLE. (2024). *Youth civic engagement: What Is It?* https://circle.tufts.edu/understanding-youth-civic-engagement/what-it

Clark, L. (2023, June 15). *Meet the kids behind the historic Montana climate trial*. E&E News by POLITICO. https://www.eenews.net/articles/meet-the-kids-behind-the-historic-montana-climate-trial/

Clark, L. S., & Marchi, R. (2017). *Young people and the future of news: Social media and the rise of connective journalism*. Cambridge University Press. https://books.google.com/books?hl=en&lr=&id=WD41DwAAQBAJ&oi=fnd&pg=PA24&dq=info:7Z5VPHvKHtEJ:scholar.google.com&ots=R11lB_n-lm&sig=kdSOqQkHYw7Vev_TSINY_FjO4UM

Cohen, C. J., & Kahne, J. (2011). *Participatory politics: New media and youth political action*. Macarthur Foundation. http://ictlogy.net/bibliography/reports/projects.php?idp=2180&lang=es

Costera Meijer, I., & Groot Kormelink, T. (2015). Checking, sharing, clicking and linking. *Digital Journalism, 3*(5), 664–679. https://doi.org/10.1080/21670811.2014.937149

Darcy, O. (2023, April 21). Analysis: The demise of BuzzFeed News marks the end of an era for digital media | CNN Business. *CNN*. https://www.cnn.com/2023/04/21/media/buzzfeed-news-digital-media-demise/index.html

DiResta, R., Shaffer, K., Ruppel, B., Sullivan, D., Matney, R., Fox, R., Albright, J., & Johnson, B. (2018). The tactics & tropes of the Internet Research Agency. *New Knowledge*. https://digitalcommons.unl.edu/senatedocs/2/?ref=reneediresta.com

Edgerly, S. (2017). Seeking out and avoiding the news media: Young adults' proposed strategies for obtaining current events information. *Mass Communication and Society, 20*(3), 358–377. https://doi.org/10.1080/15205436.2016.1262424

Faris, R. M., Roberts, H., Etling, B., Bourassa, N., Zuckerman, E., & Benkler, Y. (2017). Partisanship, propaganda, and disinformation: Online media and the 2016 U.S. presidential election. Berkman Klein Center for Internet & Society. https://papers.ssrn.com/sol3/papers.cfm?abstract_id=3019414

Fillol, J., & Pereira, S. (2020). Crianças, jovens e notícias: Uma revisão sistemática da literatura a partir da communication abstracts. *Comunicação e Sociedade, 37*, 147–168. https://doi.org/10.17231/comsoc.37(2020).2429

Flanagan, C. A., & Sherrod, L. R. (1998). Youth political development: An introduction. *Journal of Social Issues, 54*(3), 447–456. https://doi.org/10.1111/j.1540-4560.1998.tb01229.x

Freelon, D., & Lokot, T. (2020). Russian disinformation campaigns on Twitter target political communities across the spectrum. Collaboration between opposed political groups might be the most effective way to counter it. *Misinformation Review, 1*(1). https://dash.harvard.edu/handle/1/42401973

Freelon, D., & Wells, C. (2020). Disinformation as political communication. *Political Communication*, *37*(2), 145–156. https://doi.org/10.1080/10584609.2020.1723755

Gerber, A., Green, D., & Shachar, R. (2003). Voting may be habit-forming: Evidence from a randomized field experiment. *American Journal of Political Science*, *47*(3), 540–550.

Gil de Zúñiga, H., Weeks, B., & Ardèvol-Abreu, A. (2017). Effects of the news-finds-me perception in communication: Social media use implications for news seeking and learning about politics. *Journal of Computer-Mediated Communication*, *22*(3), 105–123. https://doi.org/10.1111/jcc4.12185

Gordon, H. R., & Taft, J. K. (2011). Rethinking youth political socialization: Teenage activists talk back. *Youth & Society*, *43*(4), 1499–1527. https://doi.org/10.1177/0044118X10386087

Greenberg, B. S., & Brand, J. E. (1993). Television news and advertising in schools: The 'Channel One' controversy. *Journal of Communication*, *43*(1), 143–151. https://doi.org/10.1111/j.1460-2466.1993.tb01252.x

Grinberg, N., Joseph, K., Friedland, L., Swire-Thompson, B., & Lazer, D. (2019). Fake news on Twitter during the 2016 US presidential election. *Science*, *363*(6425), 374–378.

Guess, A., Nagler, J., & Tucker, J. (2019). Less than you think: Prevalence and predictors of fake news dissemination on Facebook. *Science Advances*, *5*(1), eaau4586.

Hanson, A. B., & Brown, M. (2023, August 14). Young environmental activists prevail in first-of-its-kind climate change trial in Montana. *AP News*. https://apnews.com/article/climate-change-youth-montana-trial-c7fdc1d8759f55f60346b31c73397db0

Harvard Youth Poll. (2021). *Harvard Youth Poll, 42nd Edition*. Harvard Kennedy School. https://iop.harvard.edu/youth-poll/42nd-edition-fall-2021

Hendershot, H. (Ed.). (2004). *Nickelodeon nation: The history, politics, and economics of America's only TV channel for kids*. NYU Press.

Hendrickx, J. (2023). The rise of social journalism: An explorative case study of a youth-oriented Instagram news account. *Journalism Practice*, *17*(8), 1810–1825. https://doi.org/10.1080/17512786.2021.2012500

Hermida, A. (2020). Post-publication gatekeeping: The interplay of publics, platforms, paraphernalia, and practices in the circulation of news. *Journalism & Mass Communication Quarterly*, *97*(2), 469–491. https://doi.org/10.1177/1077699020911882

Hoffmann, M., & Jamal, A. (2014). Political attitudes of youth cohorts. In M. Lynch (Ed.), *The Arab uprisings explained: New contentious politics in the Middle East* (pp. 273–295). Columbia University Press. https://doi.org/10.7312/lync15884-014

Hooghe, M. (2004). Political socialization and the future of politics. *Acta Politica*, *39*(4), 331–341. https://doi.org/10.1057/palgrave.ap.5500082

Howard, P. N., Kollanyi, B., & Woolley, S. C. (2016). Bots and automation over Twitter during the US election. *Computational Propaganda Project: Working Paper Series*. https://demtech.oii.ox.ac.uk/wp-content/uploads/sites/12/2016/11/Data-Memo-US-Election.pdf

Howard, P. N., Neudert, L.-M., Prakash, N., & Vosloo, S. (2021). *Digital misinformation/disinformation and children*. https://www.unicef.org/globalinsight/media/2096/file/UNICEF-Global-Insight-Digital-Mis-Disinformation-and-Children-2021.pdf

Jensen, H. S. (2013). TV as children's spokesman: Conflicting notions of children and childhood in Danish children's television around 1968. *The Journal of the History of Childhood and Youth*, *6*(1), 105–128.

Jimenez, C., Clark, L. S., & Ramirez, J. (2023). "We know about things too": Exploring the labors of love involved in cultivating youth voice in online youth civic engagement programs with Youth of Color. *Youth & Society.* https://doi-org.du.idm.oclc.org/10.1177/0044118X231207973

Jones, J. P. (2010). *Entertaining politics: Satiric television and political engagement.* Rowman & Littlefield Publishers.

Kahne, J., & Middaugh, E. (2012). Digital media shapes youth participation in politics. *Phi Delta Kappan, 94*(3), 52–56. https://doi.org/10.1177/003172171209400312

Kalogeropoulos, A., Fletcher, R., & Nielsen, R. K. (2019). News brand attribution in distributed environments: Do people know where they get their news? *New Media & Society, 21*(3), 583–601. https://doi.org/10.1177/1461444818801313

Kligler-Vilenchik, N., & Literat, I. (2018). Distributed creativity as political expression: Youth responses to the 2016 U.S. Presidential election in online affinity networks. *Journal of Communication, 68*(1), 75–97. https://doi.org/10.1093/joc/jqx005

Kligler-Vilenchik, N., Tenenboim-Weinblatt, K., Boczkowski, P. J., Hayashi, K., Mitchelstein, E., & Villi, M. (2022). Youth political talk in the changing media environment: A cross-national typology. *The International Journal of Press/Politics, 27*(3), 589–608. https://doi.org/10.1177/19401612211055686

Kruikemeier, S., & Shehata, A. (2017). News media use and political engagement among adolescents: An analysis of virtuous circles using panel data. *Political Communication, 34*(2), 221–242. https://doi.org/10.1080/10584609.2016.1174760

Langbein, J. H., Lettow, R., & Smith, B. P. (2009). *History of the common law: The development of Anglo-American legal Institutions.* Aspen Publishers.

Lee, N.-J., Shah, D. V., & McLeod, J. M. (2013). Processes of political socialization: A communication mediation approach to youth civic engagement. *Communication Research, 40*(5), 669–697. https://doi.org/10.1177/0093650212436712

Lee-Wright, P., Phillips, A., & Wtischge, T. (2012). *Changing journalism.* Routledge. https://scholar.google.com/scholar_lookup?title=Changing+Journalism&author=P+Lee-Wright&author=A+Phillips&author=T+Witschge&publication_year=2012#d=gs_cit&t=1716665010474&u=%2Fscholar%3Fq%3Dinfo%3A4E9XaqwLUNcJ%3Ascholar.google.com%2F%26output%3Dcite%26scirp%3D0%26hl%3Den

Loader, B. (Ed.). (2007). *Young citizens in the digital age: Political engagement, young people and new media.* Routledge.

Loader, B. D., Vromen, A., & Xenos, M. A. (2014). Introduction. In B.D. Loader, A. Vromen, & M.A. Xenos (Eds.),*The networked young citizen: Social media, political participation and civic engagement.* Routledge.

Madden, M., Lenhart, A., & Fontaine, C. (2017). *How youth navigate the news landscape Pew report* (p. 30). Knight Foundation, Data & Society. https://knightfoundation.org/reports/how-youth-navigate-the-news-landscape

Maheshwari, S., & Isaac, M. (2024, February 22). Instagram's uneasy rise as a news site. *The New York Times.* https://www.nytimes.com/2024/02/22/technology/instagram-news-site.html

Mampaey, J., De Wit, K., & Broucker, B. (2021). The delegitimation of student protest against market-oriented reforms in higher education: The role of mass media discourse. *Studies in Higher Education, 46*(3), 523–533. https://doi.org/10.1080/03075079.2019.1643304

Marchi, R. (2012). With Facebook, blogs, and fake news, teens reject journalistic "objectivity. *Journal of Communication Inquiry, 36*(3), 246–262. https://doi.org/10.1177/0196859912458700

Marwick, A., & Lewis, R. (2017). *Media manipulation and disinformation online* (p. 106). New York: Data & Society Research Institute. https://www.posiel.com/wp-content/uploads/2016/08/Media-Manipulation-and-Disinformation-Online-1.pdf

Matsa, K. E. (2022, October 21). More Americans are getting news on TikTok, bucking the trend on other social media sites. *Pew Research Center.* https://www.pewresearch.org/fact-tank/2022/10/21/more-americans-are-getting-news-on-tiktok-bucking-the-trend-on-other-social-media-sites/

Mayer, J. (2017, December 21). A conservative nonprofit that seeks to transform college campuses faces allegations of racial bias and illegal campaign activity. *New Yorker.*

Mayer, K. U. (2009). New directions in life course research. *Annual Review of Sociology, 35*(1), 413–433. https://doi.org/10.1146/annurev.soc.34.040507.134619

McDevitt, M., & Chaffee, S. (2002). From top-down to trickle-up influence: Revisiting assumptions about the family in political socialization. *Political Communication, 19*(3), 281–301. https://doi.org/10.1080/01957470290055501

Middaugh, E., Clark, L. S., & Ballard, P. J. (2017). Digital media, participatory politics, and positive youth development. *Pediatrics, 140*(Suppl 2), S127–S131. https://doi.org/10.1542/peds.2016-1758Q

Mihailidis, P. (2018). *Civic media literacies.* Routledge.

Milkman, R. (2017). A new political generation: Millennials and the post-2008 wave of protest. *American Sociological Review, 82*(1), 1–31. https://doi.org/10.1177/0003122416681031

Miller-Idriss, C. (2020). *Hate in the homeland: The new global far right.* Princeton University Press.

Myers, S. L., & Grant, N. (2023, February 14). Combating disinformation wanes at social media giants. *The New York Times.* https://www.nytimes.com/2023/02/14/technology/disinformation-moderation-social-media.html

Newman, N., Fletcher, R., Eddy, K., Robertson, C. T., & Nielsen, R. K. (2023). *Digital news report 2023.* https://policycommons.net/artifacts/4164711/digital_news_report_2023/4973510/

NYRA. (2011, June 23). *Voting Age Status Report—NYRA.* https://www.youthrights.org/issues/voting-age/voting-age-status-report/

O'Brien, K., Selboe, E., & Hayward, B. M. (2018). Exploring youth activism on climate change: Dutiful, disruptive, and dangerous dissent. *Ecology and Society, 23*(3). https://www.jstor.org/stable/26799169

Onimisi, T. (2024). Electoral violence, youth participation, and the Nigerian general election: Lessons for the future. *Ife Social Sciences Review, 32*(1), 78–88.

Padilla, Y. A., Hylton, M. E., & Sims, J. L. (2022). Promoting civic knowledge and political efficacy among low-income youth through applied political participation. *Journal of Community Engagement and Scholarship, 12*(2), Article 2. https://doi.org/10.54656/KRYI6242

Painter, J., Kangas, J., Kunelius, R., & Russell, A. (2024). The journalism in climate change websites: Their distinct forms of specialism, content, and role perceptions. *Journalism Practice, 18*(4), 954–973. https://doi.org/10.1080/17512786.2022.2065338

Papacharissi, Z. (2015). *Affective publics: Sentiment, technology, and politics.* Oxford University Press.

Parker, K., Graf, N., & Igielnik, R. (2019). *Generation Z looks a lot like Millennials on key social and political issues.* Pew Research Center. https://www.pewsocialtrends.org/2019/01/17/generation-z-looks-a-lot-like-millennials-on-key-social-and-political-issues/

Penney, J. (2019). 'It's so hard not to be funny in this situation': Memes and humor in U.S. youth online political expression. *Television & New Media, 21*(8), 791–806. https://doi.org/10.1177/1527476419886068

Peters, C., Schrøder, K. C., Lehaff, J., & Vulpius, J. (2022). News as they know it: Young adults' information repertoires in the digital media landscape. *Digital Journalism*, *10*(1), 62–86. https://doi.org/10.1080/21670811.2021.1835986

Poot, F., & Bauwens, J. (2023). 'Like the oceans we rise': News frames on youth for climate. *YOUNG*, *31*(2), 107–123. https://doi.org/10.1177/11033088221115964

Raby, R., Caron, C., Théwissen-LeBlanc, S., Prioletta, J., & Mitchell, C. (2018). Vlogging on YouTube: The online, political engagement of young Canadians advocating for social change. *Journal of Youth Studies*, *21*(4), 495–512. https://doi.org/10.1080/13676261.2017.1394995

Røsok-Dahl, H., & Kristine Olsen, R. (2024). Snapping the news: Dynamic gatekeeping in a public service media newsroom reaching young people with news on snapchat. *Journalism*, 14648849241255701. https://doi.org/10.1177/14648849241255701

Rubin, B. C., Hayes, B., & Benson, K. (2009). 'It's the worst place to live': Urban youth and the challenge of school- based civic learning. *Theory into Practice*, *48*(3), 213–221.

Russell, A. (2016). *Journalism as activism: Recoding media power*. Polity.

Shah, D. V., McLeod, D. M., Rojas, H., Cho, J., Wagner, M. W., & Friedland, L. A. (2017). Revising the communication mediation model for a new political communication ecology. *Human Communication Research*, *43*(4), 491–504. https://doi.org/10.1111/hcre.12115

Sreekumar, T. T., & Vadrevu, S. (2013). Online political memes and youth political engagement in Singapore. *AoIR Selected Papers of Internet Research*. https://spir.aoir.org/ojs/index.php/spir/article/view/8770

Strasser, M. A., Sumner, P. J., & Meyer, D. (2022). COVID-19 news consumption and distress in young people: A systematic review, *Journal of Affective Disorders*, *300*, 481–491. https://doi.org/10.1016/j.jad.2022.01.007

Thorson, K. (2020). Attracting the news: Algorithms, platforms, and reframing incidental exposure. *Journalism*, *21*(8), 1067–1082. https://doi.org/10.1177/1464884920915352

Timberg, C., Romm, T., & Greene, J. (2020, March 2). Tech firms take a hard line against coronavirus myths. But what about other types of misinformation? *Washington Post*. https://www.washingtonpost.com/technology/2020/02/28/facebook-twitter-amazon-misinformation-coronavirus/

Tufekci, Z. (2017). *Twitter and tear gas: The power and fragility of networked protest*. Yale University Press.

Twumasi, N. (2024, January 16). 8 questions for Sariel Sandoval & Claire Vlases. *Time for Kids*. https://www.timeforkids.com/g56/8-questions-for-sariel-sandoval-and-claire-vlases-g5/

UNICEF. (2020). *Pandemic participation: Youth activism online and the COVID-19 crisis*. https://www.unicef.org/globalinsight/stories/pandemic-participationyouth-activism-online-covid-19-crisis

Unigwe, C. (2019, October 5). It's not just Greta Thunberg: Why are we ignoring the developing world's inspiring activists? *The Guardian*. https://www.theguardian.com/commentisfree/2019/oct/05/greta-thunberg-developing-world-activists

Urdal, H. (2006). A clash of generations? Youth bulges and political violence. *International Studies Quarterly*, *50*(3), 607–629. https://doi.org/10.1111/j.1468-2478.2006.00416.x

Vasquez, M. (2017, May 7). Inside a stealth plan for political influence. *The Chronicle of Higher Education*. HTTP://WWW.CHRONICLE.COM/ARTICLE/INSIDE-A-STEALTH-PLANFOR/240008?CID=WB&UTM_SOURCE=WB&UTM_MEDIUM=EN&ELQTRACKID=A07B9E4B33404E09847AA3B1FA45DFF5&

ELQ=4577011384504BCF995CF40B0400F064&ELQAID=13827&ELQAT=1&ELQCAMPAIGNID=5761

Villi, M., Aharoni, T., Tenenboim-Weinblatt, K., Boczkowski, P. J., Hayashi, K., Mitchelstein, E., Tanaka, A., & Kligler-Vilenchik, N. (2022). Taking a break from news: A five-nation study of news avoidance in the digital era. *Digital Journalism*, *10*(1), 148–164. https://doi.org/10.1080/21670811.2021.1904266

Vodafone Foundation Germany. (2020). 'Studie Zu Desinformation in Der Coronakrise: Mehr Junge Menschen Regelmäßig Mit Falschnachrichten Konfrontiert'. www.vodafone-stiftung.de/desinformation-jugend-coronakrise/

von Zabern, L., & Tulloch, C. D. (2021). Rebel with a cause: The framing of climate change and intergenerational justice in the German press treatment of the Fridays for future protests. *Media, Culture & Society*, *43*(1), 23–47. https://doi.org/10.1177/0163443720960923

Vraga, E. K., Thorson, K., Kligler-Vilenchik, N., & Gee, E. (2015). How individual sensitivities to disagreement shape youth political expression on Facebook, *Computers in Human Behavior*, *45*, 281–289. https://doi.org/10.1016/j.chb.2014.12.025

Vromen, A., Loader, B. D., Xenos, M. A., & Bailo, F. (2016). Everyday making through Facebook engagement: Young citizens' political interactions in Australia, the United Kingdom and the United States. *Political Studies*, *64*(3), 513–533. https://doi.org/10.1177/0032321715614012

Watts, R. J., Griffith, D. M., & Abdul-Adil, J. (1999). Sociopolitical development as an antidote for oppression—Theory and action. *American Journal of Community Psychology*, *27*(2), 255–271. https://doi.org/10.1023/A:1022839818873

Watts, R. J., & Hipolito-Delgado, C. P. (2015). Thinking ourselves to liberation?: Advancing sociopolitical action in critical consciousness. *The Urban Review*, *47*(5), 847–867. https://doi.org/10.1007/s11256-015-0341-x

Wood, M. C. (2007). Nature's trust: A legal, political and moral frame for global warming. *Boston College Environmental Affairs Law Review*, *34*(3), 577–603.

Wood, M. C. (2009). Advancing the sovereign trust of government to safeguard the environment for present and future generations (part 1): Ecological realism and the need for a paradigm shift. *Environmental Law*, *39*, 43.

Yani, A. A. (2021). An examination of Indonesia's anti-terrorism policy during the covid 19: The rise of digital-based terrorism propaganda among youths. *Hasanuddin Journal of Social & Political Sciences*, *1*(2), 77–85.

Yosso, T. J., & Solorzano, D. G. (2006). Leaks in the Chicana and Chicano educational pipeline. Latino Policy & Issues Brief. Number 13. In *UCLA Chicano Studies Research Center (NJ1)*. UCLA Chicano Studies Research Center. https://eric.ed.gov/?id=ED493404

Youniss, J., Bales, S., Christmas-Best, V., Diversi, M., McLaughlin, M., & Silbereisen, R. (2002). Youth civic engagement in the twenty-first century. *Journal of Research on Adolescence*, *12*(1), 121–148. https://doi.org/10.1111/1532-7795.00027

Zukin, C., Keeter, S., Andolina, M., Jenkins, K., & Delli Carpini, M. (2006). *A new engagement: Political participation, civic life, and the changing American citizen*. Oxford University Press.

11 Learning

Fashina Aladé

Children growing up today have an endless array of media choices that are labeled as "educational." But what does this mean, exactly, and can media really support children's learning? In short, yes. Decades of research suggest that when content is developmentally appropriate, backed by a curriculum grounded in empirical evidence, and presented in engaging ways, children can indeed learn from media. This chapter critically examines the role of educational media in shaping children's learning experiences, with a focus on both traditional platforms such as educational television and emerging digital technologies like educational apps. This chapter also highlights the gaps in existing research when it comes to understanding the differential impact of educational media on diverse learners.

What Is Educational Media?

To answer this question, we must first look back at the early days of television. In 1961, Newton Minow, the newly appointed chairperson of the Federal Communication Commission, delivered a keynote address to the National Association of Broadcasters (Kamp, 2020). He noted that, at its worst, television could be described as a "vast wasteland" full of violence, frivolous humor, and commercialism. That soundbite went on to fuel decades of critics determined to prove that television was destroying American society. But as Kamp explains, that was not in fact the point of Minow's speech. He went on to describe how television could do better, could be better. And he specifically noted that children's television had the greatest potential to reinvent itself, "to teach, to inform, to uplift, to stretch, to enlarge the capacities of our children" (Minow, 1961, as cited in Kamp, 2020, p. 5).

Over the years, numerous terms have been used to refer to television programs that are intended to educate or benefit children, and these terms often refer to a wide array of programming (Fisch, 2004). The Children's Television Act of 1990 defined "educational/informational" programming as content that would "further the positive development of the child in any respect, including the child's cognitive/intellectual or emotional/social needs" (FCC, 1991, p. 2114). While this act was monumental in that it was the first to provide any sort of legal guidance on children's television production and broadcasting, many scholars argued that this definition was too broad and left too much room for interpretation. For example, Kirkorian and Anderson (2008) argued, "Although many programs may be unintentionally educational, and others may teach messages not normally endorsed by a curriculum (e.g., glorifying violence), these should not be considered 'educational.'" These authors instead offered a much more stringent definition, describing educational media as "curriculum-driven products developed around a deliberate plan to teach" (Kirkorian et al., 2008, p. 188). Likewise, in this chapter, we focus on media content that has deliberate and intentional learning goals.

Despite diverse definitions, it is generally agreed that educational television serves as a form of *informal education*. Unlike formal education, which occurs in the classroom, informal education takes place outside of school, involves experiences that are not part of a school curriculum, and often must compete with other activities to gain children's attention and engagement. Fisch (2004) explains that educational television is intended to supplement formal education by: (1) exposing children to topics that they might not otherwise encounter; (2) providing compelling experiences that encourage children to spend additional time exploring concepts that they are learning about in school; (3) encouraging positive attitudes toward academic subjects, especially among populations that are less likely to pursue those subjects on their own; and (4) motivating children to engage actively in learning both inside and outside of the classroom.

In the late 1990s, Anderson (1998) set out to end the debate once and for all and provide the empirical evidence to make it clear that the term "educational television" is not, in fact, an oxymoron. He reviewed several decades of research on educational television that shows that when developmentally appropriate content is coupled with entertaining program formats, children benefit. This has been shown across a wide range of educational outcomes including school readiness (Anderson et al., 2001), literacy skills (Linebarger et al., 2004), mathematics skills (Fisch & McCann, 1993), science skills (Dingwall & Aldridge, 2006), and prosocial skills (Mares & Woodard, 2005). Table 11.1 provides a non-exhaustive summary of the types of content children have been shown to learn from educational television programs, with accompanying research studies that have demonstrated effectiveness in each area.

Table 11.1 Types of content children learn from educational media.

Type of Content	Example Learning Goals	Example Research Articles with Supporting Evidence
Literacy	Letter recognition, phonics, vocabulary	Linebarger et al. (2004) Penuel et al. (2012) Wright et al. (2001)
Mathematics	Counting, addition/subtraction, shape and pattern recognition	Fisch and McCann (1993) Watson et al. (2021)
Science	Animal habitats, weather patterns, plant life cycles, the scientific method	Aladé and Nathanson (2016) Bonus et al. (2023)
Problem-Solving	Critical thinking, logical reasoning, persistence	Anderson et al. (2000) Fisch et al. (2024)
Social-Emotional Skills	Sharing, empathy, conflict resolution	Friedrich and Stein (1973) Oades-Sese et al. (2021)
Cultural Awareness/Reduction of Stereotypes	Customs, languages, global geography, social justice and equity	Gorn et al. (1976) Johnston and Ettema (1982)
Computing and Engineering	Simple coding, computational thinking, how machines work	Leonard et al. (2016) Pila et al. (2019)

Source: Author

Today's Digital Learning Environment

In the time since Anderson's seminal article, our media landscape has changed dramatically. Children now have access to educational content across a wide range of analog and digital devices. While television/video viewing remains the top digital activity for children age zero to eight, Common Sense Media's 2020 report shows that children's media use in the United States is increasingly splintered across multiple devices (Rideout & Robb, 2020). Similar trends hold true across much of Europe, East Asia, and Australia (see, for example, Dinleyici et al., 2016; Gou & Dezuanni, 2018; Hasanagić et al., 2020; Pedersen et al., 2022). In 2018, Piotrowski took up the mantle of extending Anderson's powerful metaphor and explained that, like its predecessor, "educational media" also is not an oxymoron (Piotrowski, 2018). When age-appropriate, curriculum-backed content is delivered in an engaging way, children benefit, no matter how small or large the screen.

For young children especially, educational media is one of the most popular types of content children engage with. Parents see educational media as a relatively harmless, and perhaps even beneficial, way to occupy their children's attention, often relying on this tool when they need to accomplish other chores or tasks.

Interactive vs. Passive or Receptive Media

A common refrain heard from both families and educators is that having young children play a game on a tablet is better than having them watch television "passively." Is interactive media better for learning than more traditional media like television, which is often labeled as "passive" media? In short: not always.

A research team from Northwestern University (Aladé et al., 2016) conducted an experiment to test this question in the context of early math learning. Preschool-aged children either played an interactive game on a tablet or watched a non-interactive video that displayed the same content. The children who played the game interactively were better able to apply the math skill to a very similar task. But the children who watched the non-interactive video performed better when asked to apply the math skill to a new situation. Researchers concluded that interactivity is helpful for practicing a specific skill (similar to the benefits of rote memorization in elementary school) but that watching content non-interactively allows children to learn the lesson in a more holistic way that can be more easily applied to new contexts.

Other studies have shown similar results (Schroeder & Kirkorian, 2016). In fact, some leading developmental psychologists and educational media experts recommend referring to television and video as "receptive" rather than "passive" media. The term receptive media more accurately reflects the fact that young children's brains are still highly activated when they watch television (Anderson & Davidson, 2019). Cumulatively, this body of research suggests that parents should not feel pressured to buy their children tablets at an early age. While the interactive features of educational apps and games can be helpful in certain learning contexts, high-quality content delivered via traditional platforms like television can be just as effective for learning new skills and concepts.

How Do Children Learn from Educational Media? Theoretical Frameworks

Although research clearly demonstrates that children *can* learn from television, explanations as to *how* children learn from television are limited. Early research on children's learning from media was grounded in theories from the field of psychology, most commonly Bandura's Social Cognitive Theory and Vygotsky's Sociocultural Theory of Cognitive Development.

While those theories are most certainly still important for setting the stage and understanding the developmental context of young media users, they are applicable to understanding any effects of media on children. In this chapter, we turn to the few existing theories that have been specifically developed to explain children's learning from educational media.

The Capacity Model

In response to the dearth of theoretical explanations available that specifically addressed children's learning from educational media, Fisch (2000, 2004) put forth the ***capacity model*** to explain how children extract and comprehend educational content from television programs. The model is based on the idea that viewers' comprehension of television draws on the limited capacity of working memory. If the demands of processing a television program exceed the capacity of working memory, comprehension is impaired. That is, encoding, storage, and retrieval of the information all suffer (Fisch, 2000). The demands of processing are compounded by the nature of the medium itself. Unlike reading, the viewer's experience with television involves processing both auditory and visual information at the same time, and it is not self-paced. Instead, the viewer's processing must be employed in a way that fits the pace of the program (Fisch, 2000).

According to the model, working memory resources are culled from three sources: 1) processing of the narrative, 2) processing of educational content, and 3) distance—the degree to which the educational content is integral or tangential to the narrative. *Narrative content* is defined as the story content of the program whereas *educational content* is defined as the underlying educational concept or message that the program is intended to convey. When the educational content is tangential to the central narrative of the program, the two parallel processes of comprehension compete for limited resources in working memory. The result is that the educational content cannot be processed as deeply as it otherwise might be, and comprehension of the educational content is likely to be impaired. On the other hand, when the distance between narrative and educational content is small, the two parallel processes become complementary rather than competitive, and comprehension is likely to be strengthened. Factors that allow for more efficient processing of either type of content (e.g., familiarity with the content, prior knowledge related to the content) will reduce the demands of processing that type of information. Thus, competition is reduced, resulting in more efficient and more effective processing.

The model introduces the principle of *narrative dominance*, the idea that priority is given to comprehension of narrative over educational content, to help determine the allocation of cognitive resources when viewing (Fisch, 2000). The principle of narrative dominance makes it clear that processing of the narrative can never be abandoned, and so children's comprehension of the educational content is dependent upon their comprehension of the narrative content. In other words, if they struggle to process the basic storyline, it is unlikely they will be able to process the embedded educational lesson.

Several studies have found empirical support for the tenets of the capacity model. Nichols (2011) tested the effects of distance and pace within the framework of the capacity model. She manipulated the pace of the program and the distance between the narrative and educational content in programs for 3- to 5-year-olds and found that slow pace and low distance resulted in greatest comprehension of both narrative and educational content. Piotrowski (2014b) found that story schema development was a positive predictor of comprehension of both narrative and educational content. Children with greater story schema skills were more easily able to comprehend the narrative content, which in turn allowed for greater allocation of resources to processing the educational content. Aladé and Nathanson (2016) tested several predictions about the relationship of viewer characteristics to both narrative comprehension and educational content comprehension. They found that verbal ability, short-term memory, and prior knowledge had an indirect influence on educational content comprehension through narrative comprehension, supporting the principle of narrative dominance.

Transfer and Preparation for Future Learning

While the capacity model speaks to children's ability to comprehend the educational content of a television program, numerous studies have shown that even when comprehension is strong, children are not always able to *transfer* the information they've learned to new contexts. Transfer is a cognitive process that involves learning something in one context, understanding and remembering that new information, and then applying it to a new context. This idea of transfer is really the crux of our education system—to be truly successful post schooling, students must not only learn what is taught to them, but then be able to apply that knowledge to new situations they encounter in their everyday lives and careers.

Research has shown that very young children often have difficulty transferring content they learn from media. Barr (2010) describes this issue as a 2D to 3D transfer problem—to learn from screen-based media, children must be able to see something represented in two-dimensional form (i.e., on a television or tablet screen) and then apply that information to the three-dimensional world. In a seminal study, McCall et al. (1977) found that 18- to 36-month-olds were able to imitate some of the behaviors they viewed on a television set, but they did not imitate the behaviors as well as children who saw those same behaviors modeled in person. This difficulty in learning from televised models became known as the *video deficit effect*. Many studies have replicated the video deficit effect over the years (see Barr, 2010, for a review). Interestingly, 6-month-old infants do not show evidence of video deficit. It peaks around 15 months of age, and then somewhere between 36 months and 5 years (depending on the difficulty of the task), children become able to imitate equally well from screen-based and real-life models (Barr, 2010).

Does the video deficit effect mean that there is no point in children under age 5 watching educational media? Not at all. Studies have shown there are many factors that can help ameliorate the video deficit for young children, such as repetition, prior experience, and social contingency (Barr, 2010). Moreover, educational media is not meant to replace in-person learning. In fact, Bonus (2023) posits that rather than a tool for immediate learning and transfer, educational media may be most effective as *preparation for future learning* (PFL).

The PFL framework was first introduced by Bransford and Schwartz (1999) as an alternative to traditional explanations of transfer. Unlike traditional methods of assessing transfer, which often require students to transfer material to a new context after a single instance of learning, PFL considers that learning experiences are meant to be iterative and compounded. Therefore, under the PFL paradigm, transfer is assessed after at least two complementary learning instances. For example, research has shown that students who are given a homework assignment where they have to use a new set of skills and *then* attend a formal lecture on the same topic perform better on a subsequent transfer task compared to students who only attend the lecture (Schwartz & Bransford, 1998). The researchers explain that this method of multiple learning instances allows participants to "transfer in" their knowledge across interventions (i.e., from the homework assignment to the lecture) before they are required to "transfer out" that knowledge on formal assessments (i.e., from the lecture to the exam). Bransford and Schwartz (1999) explain that proper sequencing is critical under the PFL framework—initial learning interventions should provide foundational knowledge that helps participants organize and process information introduced in later interventions.

Recent studies have specifically used the PFL paradigm to investigate learning in the context of educational media. As discussed earlier, Fisch (2004) describes educational media as informal learning meant to complement or supplement formal learning. Therefore, PFL may be a particularly helpful framework for assessing transfer from educational media when it complements other offline instructional formats. Bonus (Bonus, 2023; Bonus et al., 2023) was the first to apply and test the PFL paradigm specifically with educational media. Bonus et al. (2023) found that children learned more from a hands-on science activity when they watched educational television before (vs. after) completing the activity. This newly burgeoning body of work suggests that educational television might be particularly useful for introducing new topics to children that they will then encounter again later either from their teachers at school or in other informal learning contexts.

Active Playful Learning

Active Playful Learning (APL) is a framework for understanding how children learn new content or skills through intentional play, especially through guided play where adults help children explore and discover their way through a set of clearly defined learning goals (Fletcher et al., 2024). APL is an especially helpful theoretical framework for this chapter because it is grounded in both the science of learning and the importance of culturally sensitive pedagogy. As Fletcher et al. (2024) explain, the principles of APL are guided by a three-part model: (1) cultural and community values; (2) the *how* of learning; (3) the *what* of learning.

Cultural and Community Values. A primary principle of APL is that the best learning environments combine the science of learning with the importance of cultural and community values that are relevant to the learner. There is an emphasis here on co-designing new learning tools with members from the target community. As Fletcher and colleagues write, "pedagogical practices, learning activities, and spaces designed to spark playful learning will be most effective when local representatives (e.g., residents, grassroots organizations, community leaders) have a voice at the table" (Fletcher et al., 2024, p. 311).

The How of Learning. The second component of the APL model is a suite of characteristics that describe effective guided play. According to Zosh et al. (2018) guided play should be active, engaging, meaningful, socially interactive, iterative, and joyful. When these a learning environment meets all of these characteristics *and* includes clear learning goals, active playful learning is achieved (Fletcher et al., 2024).

The What of Learning. In a recent national policy report, Hirsh-Pasek et al. (2020) identified six core competencies that students today need to excel and be prepared for the modern world of work. These competencies, collectively known as *the 6Cs* are:

- Collaboration—The ability to form relationships and work together
- Communication—Competence in expressing oneself and getting ideas across to others clearly
- Content—The substance of what is taught in school, i.e., literacy, math, science, etc.

- Critical thinking—Being able to solve a problem using the information at hand
- Creative innovation—Curiosity that drives exploration and innovation
- Confidence—Having the courage and tenacity to persist in the face of adversity

The APL framework can be applied to many types of learning environments, both analog and digital, but is especially helpful for thinking about the design of effective educational media. As discussed earlier, to truly be called "educational media" digital content should be developed with a clear curriculum or set of learning goals in mind (i.e., the what of learning). In thinking about how educational media is different from formal educational tools, many of the characteristics of guided play (i.e., the how of learning) should come to mind. Virtually all media for children is designed to be engaging and joyful; after all, if children do not find a program entertaining, they simply won't turn it on. Educational apps and games are also typically designed to be both active and iterative, allowing for children to manipulate game features that support practice and repetition of key skills. And many of the best educational programs feature opportunities for meaningful engagement and social interactivity—from classic television shows like *Mister Rogers' Neighborhood*, *Blues Clues*, and *Dora the Explorer*, which utilized direct address to the audience and invited children to respond from their living rooms, to modern online games that invite interaction and collaboration between players. Finally, though this is less ubiquitous in the world of educational media, programs that successfully engage diverse audiences must be designed in a way that reflects cultural and community values. A few recent educational television shows provide excellent examples of how this can be done; *Molly of Denali*, *Rosie's Rules*, and *Alma's Way* were each developed to highlight specific cultures, and importantly, were created with iterative input from individuals from those respective communities.

What Factors Support Children's Learning from Media?

From the theoretical frameworks reviewed above and the decades of research on children's learning from media, there are a few key strategies that we can confidently say are supportive of children's learning.

Repetition

Children learn best from screens when they are familiar with the content and can map new ideas onto familiar ones. Adults may feel annoyed when children want to watch their favorite movie or television episode over and over and over again, but this practice is actually very supportive of their learning. Comprehending new content shown on screen is hard work for young developing brains. It requires a lot of mental capacity to encode and retain all of the information presented in even a relatively short 11-minute episode. *Blue's Clues,* which first aired in 1996, was an innovative preschool television show in that it used repetition as a central part of their curriculum. Extensive research was done on this program, and one of the most notable findings was that children who watched the same episode for five consecutive days did not tend to lose interest and indeed learned much more than their peers who watched the episode only once (Crawley et al., 1999).

Engaging Characters

The characters featured in children's media content can be an important conduit for learning. Children (and adults) often form strong, friendship-like attachments with their favorite media characters, known as ***parasocial relationships*** (Calvert & Richards, 2014; Rubin & McHugh, 1987). Studies have shown that children learn more from these trusted familiar characters than from unfamiliar characters who present the same content (Gola et al., 2013; Lauricella et al., 2011).

Likewise, viewers who feel a strong emotional connection to the characters presenting the educational content in a television show are likely to learn more from viewing than their peers who have not developed those strong relationships after viewing the exact same content (Aladé, 2018; Richards & Calvert, 2017).

Compelling and Comprehensible Narratives

Narrative is a powerful tool for persuasion and other media effects (Moyer-Gusé & Nabi, 2010; Slater, 2002). Because educational media often serves the dual purposes of entertaining and educating, even the most well-designed educational media curriculum is unlikely to be successful if there is no compelling storyline to draw viewers in. At the same time, because we know that children will allocate their working memory first and foremost to the narrative (Fisch, 2000, 2004), it is important that the narrative is easily understood by young viewers. Successful educational media will include a developmentally appropriate narrative that draws viewers in, coupled with educational content that is well-integrated into the story.

Social Contingency

In line with the principles of active playful learning, successful educational media programs often include some aspects of social contingency. Even in television programs, which may be considered more passive than newer digital technologies, strategies like direct address—where a character speaks directly to the viewer and invites them to respond back—have successfully been used to invite children to engage actively in the viewing experience (Piotrowski, 2014a). Newer digital media like games and apps offer even more potential for socially contingent interactions, whether by playing together with friends or by connecting with virtual characters.

Cross-Platform Learning

Studies show that when children engage with the same characters and encounter the same content across multiple platforms, this maximizes learning outcomes. For example, if a young child watches an episode of *Sesame Street* and then plays one of the freely available *Sesame Street* games on the PBS Kids website or app, they are likely to learn more than if they watch the show or play the game alone (Fisch et al., 2016). The effectiveness of cross-platform learning, also sometimes referred to as transmedia learning (Alper, 2013), is likely due, in part, to simple repetition, but may also connect back to the PFL framework and that idea that multiple learning interventions result in greater transfer of knowledge (Bonus, 2023).

Do *All* Children Learn from Educational Media?

While many scholars have argued for the importance of considering race, ethnicity, culture, and other aspects of identity when researching the effectiveness of educational media, we unfortunately have very limited research available to help answer this question. To date, most research on children's learning from media has been conducted using what Jordan and Prendella (2019) call "WEIRD" (Western, Educated, Industrialized, Rich, and Democratic) samples. When studies do include racial-ethnic diversity amongst their participants, race is often ignored or treated as a control variable so that results can be discussed across all participants.

One thing we do know is that *access* is a critical prerequisite for learning. Children who don't have access to an educational media program certainly cannot benefit from it. In the United States, access to newer digital technologies and critical infrastructure like high-speed internet mirrors many other demographic disparities, with urban, White, educated, and higher-socioeconomic status families having greater access, on average, than their rural, non-White, lower-socioeconomic status counterparts. Similar patterns associated with wider reflections of income inequalities occur throughout the world. Content distribution platforms often exacerbate these access disparities. For example, a 2021 analysis of the most downloaded children's educational apps found that free apps had lower markers of educational quality compared to paid apps (Meyer et al., 2021).

In some countries, public broadcasting efforts help to ameliorate access issues. In the United States, for example, many educational television programs and accompanying online games are produced via public media stations and made freely available via public broadcasting channels and free apps like the PBS KIDS app. Analytic reviews and recontact studies (the latter describing a research approach in which young research participants are recontacted later in life and invited to participate in additional research to examine change over time) have consistently shown that these programs, typically funded through the U.S. Department of Education's Ready To Learn initiative, are highly effective for learners across demographics (Hurwitz & Schmitt, 2019; Lowenstein et al., 2019). Countries like Canada and the UK have similar systems for providing free educational content to families. However, public media access is far less universal in the global south.

Beyond access, we also know that media depictions of one's ingroup and outgroups contribute to how children develop their ethnic-racial identities and generally make sense of the world around them (Berry & Asamen, 1993; Rogers et al., 2021). Most research that examines the impact of racial depictions in media on children has done so with a focus on negative effects. For example, studies examining Black children's and adolescents' exposure to stereotypical depictions of Black characters found that increased exposure was related to lower self-esteem, less satisfaction with one's appearance, less confidence in one's abilities, more negative feelings about one's ethnic-racial group, and poorer academic performance (Gordon, 2016; Martins & Harrison, 2012; Rogers et al., 2021; Ward, 2004). Similar findings have been shown with Latine (Rivadeneyra et al., 2007) and Native American (Fryberg et al., 2008) adolescents. A few studies have also found similar effects in the positive direction. Watching favorable depictions of one's ethnic-racial group can have a positive impact on children's self-perceptions and views about their ethnic-racial group (McDermott & Greenberg, 1984). An early exploratory study found that, for girls especially, exposure to Black TV characters whom they liked and viewed very positively, was associated with more positive feelings about themselves (Stroman, 1986). Similarly, Black adolescents who felt strong identification with Black television characters were found to have greater satisfaction with their own appearance (Ward, 2004). And there is certainly a desire for more positive depictions of characters of color. Black parents, especially, say they want their children to be exposed to more positive media representations that reflect the race and culture of their families (McClain & Mares, 2021).

Summarizing this body of work, it is clear that media depictions impact children's ethnic-racial identities and their attitudes toward others. What is not clear is how the development of these ethnic-racial attitudes and identities via media representation impacts children's screen-based learning. A few studies on children's learning from educational media have considered race/ethnicity in more intentional ways, but the evidence has been inconclusive.

Calvert and colleagues (Calvert et al., 2007) conducted an experiment to investigate Latine and White children's participation with and learning from an episode of *Dora the Explorer*. Contrary to their hypotheses, Latine children were not more likely to identify with Dora, a Hispanic/Latine character, than White children. In fact, the White children in the study were more likely to perceive themselves as similar to Dora than the Latine children. These differing levels of identification and perceived similarity ultimately did not matter for children's learning. Across gender and race, children who actively responded to Dora's cues (e.g., by speaking aloud or engaging in pretend play when prompted) were the ones who showed better comprehension and recall of the program content. Lennon (2023) also conducted an experiment to see whether young children would learn more from a science show where the main character matched their race and gender. Black children watched two episodes from two different science programs: *Ada Twist, Scientist*, which features a Black/African American girl, and *Justin Time*, which features a White/Caucasian boy and were tested on their learning of the concepts taught in both shows. Here again, neither race nor gender were predictive of children's learning.

Interestingly, these findings are in direct contrast to much of the literature on ***culturally responsive pedagogy***, which has consistently shown that in other educational settings, having one's culture reflected in educational materials, teachers, and role models leads to positive outcomes for young learners (Howard, 2021). Although our very limited body of literature on the impact of race and culture in children's learning from educational media seems to suggest that race and gender of characters are not particularly strong drivers of children's learning, it is possible that, as a field, we have not yet figured out how to measure these effects. It may be that the influence of characters' race, culture, etc. is occurring at such an implicit level that our current methods are inadequate for capturing these effects. It may also be that the impact is happening via long-term exposure, whereas most studies of children's learning from media use short term, single-exposure methods, often focusing on one program at a time. Future research should consider children's cumulative media exposure, using longitudinal methods and considering the breadth of their media use. For example, perhaps viewing many diverse representations of characters modeling learning and problem solving across the preschool years could lead to better academic achievement later in life. This is a much-needed area for future research. And while traditionally there have not been many examples of diverse representation in children's educational media to study, in recent years, many new programs have been developed that feature diverse, authentic, and culturally specific media characters (see Table 11.2). These programs are ripe fodder for researchers who wish to study the impact of diverse representation in children's educational media.

Table 11.2 Children's educational television programs with an explicit focus on diversity and representation that are currently in production.

Program (First Year of Production)	Target Age	Brief Description
Sesame Street (1969)	2–5	For more than 50 years, Sesame Street has kept diversity and representation as a core feature of its production. Originally designed to reach urban US children in a setting that would feel familiar, over the decades they have gone on to co-produce international productions around the world that attend to the needs of children in their unique geopolitical circumstances.
Molly of Denali (2019)	4–8	Molly of Denali follows the adventures of 10-year-old Molly Mabray, an Alaska Native girl of Gwich'in, Koyukon, and Dena'ina Athabascan descent. The show is notable for its authentic portrayal of Alaska Native culture and traditions, and it emphasizes the importance of community, nature, and family. The curriculum is focused on informational literacy, helping children develop research and critical thinking skills. Molly and her friends use both modern technology and traditional knowledge to solve problems, and they often rely on storytelling and cultural practices passed down by elders in their community.
Alma's Way (2021)	4–6	Alma's Way is an animated series about 6-year-old Alma Rivera, who lives in the Bronx. The show emphasizes the importance of thinking things through, promoting critical thinking and problem-solving skills in young viewers. As she learns to solve problems, Alma celebrates her Puerto Rican heritage and the diverse community that surrounds her, giving the show a rich cultural backdrop.
Rosie's Rules (2022)	3–6	Rosie's Rules is an animated series featuring 5-year-old Rosie Fuentes and her blended, multi-cultural, Mexican-American family. Rosie explores the world around her, learning important lessons about how things work in her family, community, and society. The show is designed to teach preschoolers early social studies concepts, like family dynamics, cultural traditions, and community roles, and Rosie's daily adventures often highlight themes of diversity and inclusion.

(Continued)

Table 11.2 (Continued)

Program (First Year of Production)	Target Age	Brief Description
Work it Out Wombats! (2023)	3–6	Work It Out Wombats! follows the adventures of three sibling wombats who live in a playful and diverse community called the Treeborhood. The wombats tackle various challenges, encouraging young viewers to use creative and logical approaches to "work it out," delivering a core curriculum focused on computational thinking. Though it features a cast of animated animal characters, the series was developed with a strong "culture and inclusion" plan that emphasizes the importance of having a diverse team developing stories that authentically reflect their audience members. The Treeborhood features characters from a variety of species and backgrounds, mirroring the values of inclusivity and respect for differences. Each character has unique traits, abilities, and perspectives, promoting the idea that everyone contributes something valuable to the community.

Source: Author

References

Aladé, F. (2018). *Character portrayals in STEM-focused educational television shows and their impact on children's attitudes towards STEM* (Publication No. 10822173) [Doctoral dissertation, Northwestern University]. ProQuest Dissertations & Theses Global.

Aladé, F., Lauricella, A. R., Beaudoin-Ryan, L., & Wartella, E. (2016). Measuring with Murray: Touchscreen technology and preschoolers' STEM learning. *Computers in Human Behavior, 62*, 433–441. https://doi.org/10.1016/j.chb.2016.03.080

Aladé, F., & Nathanson, A. I. (2016). What preschoolers bring to the show: The relation between viewer characteristics and children's learning from educational television. *Media Psychology, 19*(3), 406–430. https://doi.org/10.1080/15213269.2015.1054945

Alper, M. (2013). Developmentally appropriate new media literacies: Supporting cultural competencies and social skills in early childhood education. *Journal of Early Childhood Literacy, 13*, 175–196. https://doi.org/10.1177/1468798411430101

Anderson, D. R. (1998). Educational television is not an oxymoron. *Annals of the American Academy of Political and Social Science, 557*, 24–38. http://www.jstor.org/stable/1049440

Anderson, D. R., Bryant, J., Wilder, A., Santomero, A., Williams, M., & Crawley, A. M. (2000). Researching Blue's clues: Viewing behavior and impact. *Media Psychology*, 2, 179–194. https://doi.org/10.1207/s1532785xmep0202_4

Anderson, D. R., & Davidson, M. C. (2019). Receptive versus interactive video screens: A role for the brain's default mode network in learning from media. *Computers in Human Behavior*, 99, 168–180. https://doi.org/10.1016/j.chb.2019.05.008

Anderson, D. R., Huston, A. C., Schmitt, K. L., Linebarger, D. L., & Wright, J. C. (2001). Early childhood television viewing and adolescent behavior: The recontact study. *Monographs of the Society for Research in Child Development*, 66(1), 1–143.

Barr, R. (2010). Transfer of learning between 2D and 3D sources during infancy: Informing theory and practice. *Developmental Review*, 30, 128–154.

Berry, G. L., & Asamen, J. K. (1993). *Children and television: Images in a changing socio-cultural world*. Sage Publications.

Bonus, J. A. (2023). Conceptualizing U.S. Educational television as preparation for future learning. *Journal of Children and Media*, 17(1), 97–116. https://doi.org/10.1080/17482798.2022.2134899

Bonus, J. A., Dore, R. A., Wilson, J. M., Freiberger, N., & Lerner, B. (2023). Of scientists and superheroes: Educational television and pretend play as preparation for science learning. *Journal of Applied Developmental Psychology*, 89, 101603. https://doi.org/10.1016/j.appdev.2023.101603

Bransford, J. D., & Schwartz, D. L. (1999). Rethinking transfer: A simple proposal with multiple implications [research-article]. *Review of Research in Education*, 24, 61–100. https://ezproxy.msu.edu/login?url=https://search.ebscohost.com/login.aspx?direct=true&db=edsjsr&AN=edsjsr.1167267&site=eds-live

Calvert, S. L., & Richards, M. N. (2014). Children's parasocial relationships. In A. Jordan, & D. Romer (Eds.), *Media and the well-being of children and adolescents* (pp. 187–200). Oxford University Press.

Calvert, S. L., Strong, B. L., Jacobs, E. L., & Conger, E. E. (2007). Interaction and participation for young Hispanic and Caucasian girls' and boys' learning of media content. *Media Psychology*, 9, 431–445. https://doi.org/10.1080/15213260701291379

Crawley, A. M., Anderson, D. R., Wilder, A., Williams, M., & Santomero, A. (1999). Effects of repeated exposures to a single episode of the television program Blue's clues on the viewing behaviors and comprehension of preschool children. *Journal of Educational Psychology*, 91(4), 630–637. https://doi.org/10.1037/0022-0663.91.4.630

Dingwall, R., & Aldridge, M. (2006). Television wildlife programming as a source of popular scientific information: A case study of evolution. *Public Understanding of Science*, 15, 131–152.

Dinleyici, M., Carman, K. B., Ozturk, E., & Sahin-Dagli, F. (2016). Media use by children, and parents' views on children's media usage. *Interactive Journal of Medical Research*, 5(2), e18. https://doi.org/10.2196/ijmr.5668

FCC. (1991). Report and order: In the matter of policies and rules concerning children's television programming. *Memorandum Opinion and Order*, 2111–2127.

Fisch, S. M. (2000). A capacity model of children's comprehension of educational content on television. *Media Psychology*, 2, 63–91. https://doi.org/10.1207/S1532785XMEP0201_4

Fisch, S. M. (2004). *Children's learning from educational television*. Lawrence Erlbaum.

Fisch, S. M., Damashek, S., & Aladé, F. (2016). Designing media for cross-platform learning: Developing models for production and instructional design. *Journal of Children and Media*, *10*(2), 238–247. https://doi.org/10.1080/17482798.2016.1140485

Fisch, S. M., Fletcher, K., Abdurokhmonova, G., Davis, L., Fisch, N., Fisch, S. R. D., Jurist, M., Kestin, R., Pesch, A., Seguì, I., Shulman, J., Silton, N., Tomforde, J., Volpe, C., Wright, C. A., & Hirsh-Pasek, K. (2024). "I wonder, what if, let's try": Sesame Street's playful learning curriculum impacts children's problem solving. *Journal of Children and Media*, *18*(3), 334–350. https://doi.org/10.1080/17482798.2024.2356958

Fisch, S. M., & McCann, S. K. (1993). Making broadcast television participative: Eliciting mathematical behavior through "Square one TV. *Educational Technology Research and Development*, *41*(3), 103–109. http://www.jstor.org/stable/30218390

Fletcher, K., Wright, C. A., Pesch, A., Abdurokhmonova, G., & Hirsh-Pasek, K. (2024). Active playful learning as a robust, adaptable, culturally relevant pedagogy to foster children's 21st century skills. *Journal of Children and Media*, *18*(3), 309–321. https://doi.org/10.1080/17482798.2024.2356956

Friedrich, L. K., & Stein, A. H. (1973). Aggressive and prosocial television programs and the natural behavior of preschool children. *Monographs of the Society for Research in Child Development*, *38*, 1–64. http://www.jstor.org/stable/1165725

Fryberg, S. A., Markus, H. R., Oyserman, D., & Stone, J. M. (2008). Of warrior chiefs and Indian princesses: The psychological consequences of American Indian mascots. *Basic and Applied Social Psychology*, *30*(3), 208–218. https://doi.org/10.1080/01973530802375003

Gola, A. A. H., Richards, M. N., Lauricella, A. R., & Calvert, S. L. (2013). Building meaningful parasocial relationships between toddlers and media characters to teach early mathematical skills. *Media Psychology*, *16*, 390–411.

Gordon, M. K. (2016). Achievement scripts: Media influences on black students' academic performance, self-perceptions, and career interests. *Journal of Black Psychology*, *42*(3), 195–220. https://doi.org/10.1177/0095798414566510

Gorn, G. J., Goldberg, M. E., & Kanungo, R. N. (1976). The role of educational television in changing the intergroup attitudes of children. *Child Development*, *47*, 277–280. https://doi.org/10.2307/1128313

Gou, H., & Dezuanni, M. (2018). Towards understanding young children's digital lives in China and Australia. *Comunicar: Media Education Research Journal*, *26*(57), 81–89. https://files.eric.ed.gov/fulltext/EJ1192375.pdf

Hasanagić, S., Papović, M., & Kovačević, S. (2020). *Children's media habits and parental attitudes*. UNICEF.

Hirsh-Pasek, K., Hadani, H., Blinkoff, E., & Golinkoff, R. M. (2020). *A new path to education reform: Playful learning promotes 21st-century skills in schools and beyond*. Big Ideas Policy Report, Issue.

Howard, T. C. (2021). Culturally responsive pedagogy. In J. A. Banks (Ed.), *Transforming multicultural education policy and practice: Expanding educational opportunity* (pp. 137–163). Teachers College Press. https://books.google.com/books?id=OEROEAAAQBAJ

Hurwitz, L. B., & Schmitt, K. L. (2019). Raising readers with ready to learn: A six-year follow-up to an early educational computer game intervention. *Computers in Human Behavior*, 106176. https://doi.org/10.1016/j.chb.2019.106176

Johnston, J., & Ettema, J. S. (1982). *Positive images: Breaking stereotypes with children's television*. Sage.

Jordan, A., & Prendella, K. (2019). The invisible children of media research. *Journal of Children and Media*, *13*(2), 235–240. https://doi.org/10.1080/17482798.2019.1591662

Kamp, D. (2020). *Sunny days: The children's television revolution that changed America*. Simon & Schuster.

Kirkorian, H. L., & Anderson, D. R. (2008). Learning from educational media. In S. L. Calvert & B. J. Wilson (Eds.), *The handbook of children, media, and development* (pp. 188–213). Wiley-Blackwell. https://doi.org/10.1002/9781444302752.ch9

Kirkorian, H. L., Wartella, E. A., & Anderson, D. R. (2008). Media and young children's learning. *The Future of Children*, *18*, 39–61. https://www.jstor.org/stable/20053119

Lauricella, A. R., Gola, A. A. H., & Calvert, S. L. (2011). Toddlers' learning from socially meaningful video characters. *Media Psychology*, *14*, 216–232.

Lennon, M. (2023). *Young Black children's learning from and awareness of race and gender representation in preschool STEM television shows* [Doctoral dissertation, Northwestern University]. ProQuest Dissertations & Theses Global.

Leonard, J., Buss, A., Gamboa, R., Mitchell, M., Fashola, O. S., Hubert, T., & Almughyirah, S. (2016). Using robotics and game design to enhance children's self-efficacy, STEM attitudes, and computational thinking skills. *Journal of Science Education and Technology*, *25*(6), 860–876. https://doi.org/10.1007/s10956-016-9628-2

Linebarger, D. L., Kosanic, A. Z., Greenwood, C. R., & Doku, N. S. (2004). Effects of viewing the television program between the lions on the emergent literacy skills of young children. *Journal of Educational Psychology*, *96*, 297–308. https://doi.org/10.1037/0022-0663.96.2.297

Lowenstein, D., Johnson, P., & Fragale, M. (2019). Ready to learn and public media: Improving early learning outcomes for America's children. In S. Pasnik (Ed.), *Getting ready to learn*. Routledge. https://doi.org/10.4324/9780203701973

Mares, M.-L., & Woodard, E. (2005). Positive effects of television on children's social interactions: A meta-analysis [article]. *Media Psychology*, *7*(3), 301–322. https://doi.org/10.1207/s1532785xmep0703_4

Martins, N., & Harrison, K. (2012). Racial and gender differences in the relationship between children's television use and self-esteem: A longitudinal panel study. *Communication Research*, *39*, 338–357. https://doi.org/10.1177/0093650211401376

McCall, R. B., Parke, R. D., Kavanaugh, R. D., Engstrom, R., Russell, J., & Wycoff, E. (1977). Imitation of live and televised models by children one to three years of age. *Monographs of the Society for Research in Child Development*, *42*(5), 1–94. https://doi.org/10.2307/1165913

McClain, A. K., & Mares, M.-L. (2021). Media messages: Intersections of ethnic-racial and media socialization in African American families. *Research in Human Development*, *18*(4), 311–329. https://doi.org/10.1080/15427609.2021.2010491

McDermott, S., & Greenberg, B. (1984). Parents, peers and television as determinants of Black children's esteem. *Communication Yearbook*, *8*, 164–177.

Meyer, M., Zosh, J. M., McLaren, C., Robb, M., McCafferty, H., Golinkoff, R. M., Hirsh-Pasek, K., & Radesky, J. (2021). How educational are "educational" apps for young children? App store content analysis using the four pillars of learning framework. *Journal of Children and Media*, *15*(4), 526–548. https://doi.org/10.1080/17482798.2021.1882516

Minow, N. (1961, May 9, 1961). *Television and the public interest* [Keynote Address]. American Archive of Public Broadcasting. https://americanarchive.org/special_collections/newtonminow

Moyer-Gusé, E., & Nabi, R. L. (2010). Explaining the effects of narrative in an entertainment television program: Overcoming resistance to persuasion. *Human Communication Research*, *36*, 26–52.

Nichols, C. (2011). *How fast can they learn? Testing educational and narrative content acquisition through the capacity model*. International Communication Association.

Oades-Sese, G. V., Cahill, A., Allen, J. W. P., Rubic, W.-L., & Mahmood, N. (2021). Effectiveness of sesame Workshop's little children, big challenges: A digital media SEL intervention for preschool classrooms. *Psychology in the Schools*, *58*(10), 2041–2067. https://doi.org/10.1002/pits.22574

Pedersen, J., Rasmussen, M. G., Olesen, L. G., Klakk, H., Kristensen, P. L., & Grøntved, A. (2022). Recreational screen media use in Danish school-aged children and the role of parental education, family structures, and household screen media rules. *Preventive Medicine*, *155*, 106908. https://doi.org/10.1016/j.ypmed.2021.106908

Penuel, W. R., Bates, L., Gallagher, L. P., Pasnik, S., Llorente, C., Townsend, E., Hupert, N., Dominguez, X., & VanderBorght, M. (2012). Supplementing literacy instruction with a media-rich intervention: Results of a randomized controlled trial. *Early Childhood Research Quarterly*, *27*, 115–127. https://doi.org/http://dx.doi.org/10.1016/j.ecresq.2011.07.002

Pila, S., Aladé, F., Sheehan, K. J., Lauricella, A. R., & Wartella, E. A. (2019). Learning to code via tablet applications: An evaluation of Daisy the Dinosaur and Kodable as learning tools for young children. *Computers & Education*, *128*, 52–62. https://doi.org/10.1016/j.compedu.2018.09.006

Piotrowski, J. T. (2018). Is educational media an oxymoron? In N. A. Jennings & S. R. Mazzarella (Eds.), *20 questions about youth and the media | Revised edition*. Peter Lang.

Piotrowski, J. T. (2014a). Participatory cues and program familiarity predict young children's learning from educational television. *Media Psychology*, *17*, 311–331. https://doi.org/10.1080/15213269.2014.932288

Piotrowski, J. T. (2014b). The relationship between narrative processing demands and young American children's comprehension of educational television. *Journal of Children and Media*, 1–19. https://doi.org/10.1080/17482798.2013.878740

Richards, M. N., & Calvert, S. L. (2017). Media characters, parasocial relationships, and the social aspects of children's learning across media platforms. In R. Barr & D.N. Linebarger (Eds.), *Media exposure during infancy and early childhood* (pp. 141–163). Springer.

Rideout, V., & Robb, M. B. (2020). *The common sense Census: Media use by kids age zero to eight, 2020*. Common Sense Media.

Rivadeneyra, R., Ward, L. M., & Gordon, M. (2007). Distorted reflections: Media exposure and Latino adolescents' conceptions of self. *Media Psychology*, *9*(2), 261–290. https://doi.org/10.1080/15213260701285926

Rogers, O., Mastro, D. E., Robb, M. B., & Peebles, A. (2021). *The inclusion imperative: Why media representation matters for kids' ethnic-racial development*.

Rubin, R., & McHugh, M. (1987). Development of parasocial interaction relationships. *Journal of Broadcasting & Electronic Media*, *31*(3), 279–292.

Schroeder, E. L., & Kirkorian, H. L. (2016). When seeing is better than doing: Preschoolers' transfer of STEM skills using touchscreen games [original research]. *Frontiers in Psychology*, *7*(1377). https://doi.org/10.3389/fpsyg.2016.01377

Schwartz, D. L., & Bransford, J. D. (1998). A time for telling. *Cognition and Instruction*, *16*(4), 475–523. https://doi.org/10.1207/s1532690xci1604_4

Slater, M. D. (2002). Entertainment education and the persuasive impact of narratives. In M. C. Green, J. J. Strange, & T. C. Brock (Eds.), *Narrative impact: Social and cognitive foundations* (pp. 157–181). Lawrence Erlbaum Associates Publishers.

Stroman, C. A. (1986). Television viewing and self-concept among black children. *Journal of Broadcasting & Electronic Media*, *30*(1), 87–93. https://doi.org/10.1080/08838158609386610

Ward, L. M. (2004). Wading through the stereotypes: Positive and negative associations between media use and black adolescents' conceptions of self. *Developmental Psychology*, *40*, 284–294. https://doi.org/10.1037/0012-1649.40.2.284

Watson, J., Hennessy, S., & Vignoles, A. (2021). The relationship between educational television and mathematics capability in Tanzania. *British Journal of Educational Technology*, *52*(2), 638–658. https://doi.org/10.1111/bjet.13047

Wright, J. C., Huston, A. C., Murphy, K. C., St. Peters, M., Piñon, M., Scantlin, R., & Kotler, J. (2001). The relations of early television viewing to school readiness and vocabulary of children from low-income families: The early window project. *Child Development*, *72*, 1347–1366.

Zosh, J. M., Hirsh-Pasek, K., Hopkins, E. J., Jensen, H., Liu, C., Neale, D., Solis, S. L., & Whitebread, D. (2018). Accessing the inaccessible: Redefining play as a spectrum. *Frontiers in Psychology*, *9*. https://doi.org/10.3389/fpsyg.2018.01124

12 Advertising/Commercialization

Regina Jihea Ahn

Barbie, Strawberry Shortcake, Thomas the Train, Sesame Street. If we recall our childhood favorite characters, we did love the whole universe of the characters and extended our love to "purchase" their world. We nagged our parents to buy dolls, t-shirts, or minifigures to enjoy the characters in our imaginary world. We have been exposed to advertising and marketing since we were children. Child-directed marketing and advertising are certainly not brand-new issues. If we look back at the roots of child-targeted marketing, its history began in the mid-1900s. Toy-based programs such as *My Little Pony* and *He-Man* boomed in the 1980s with the lucrative market of licensed media characters (Seiter, 1993; Stern & Schoenhaus, 1990). Market research utilized various types of studies by using interviews, focus groups, and storyboards to fill in underdeveloped insight about children's tastes and preferences. Today, we see more aggressive advertisers' approach to children and even adolescents to make them loyal and become their *Lovemarks*, creating loyalty beyond the reasons (Roberts, 2005). These Lovemarks become not merely commodities but irreplaceable icons that generate high levels of love and respect (Duncan, 2010; Roberts, 2005).

Advertising Everywhere: The Constant Presence in Children's World

Various examples of brands can be found related to child-directed advertising marketing, which has received attention for decades. Disney is a great example of advertising and branding aimed at children and their families. Disney has grown as a symbol of storytelling and creativity for about a century but is also known for creating an entertaining consumer culture (Giroux, 2011). Disney has established its character business, and it has expanded in various directions through merchandise, theme parks, resorts, digital video streaming, and more.

Let's see more recent examples. There have been several children who became social media influencers and brand endorsers. One of the most

DOI: 10.4324/9781003453123-14

popular child influencers in the mid-2010s was Evan Lee, who had about two million followers on his YouTube channel EvanTubeHD in 2018 (Hoy et al., 2018) and has now reached more than 7 million. He opened the gate for many child influencers by sharing his favorite toys and games with young audiences online. His sister, Jillian Lee, also joined EvanTube, and later, she launched her own channel, which also reached about 1.73 million followers. Evan's family worked on various unboxing videos of new toys, which brought excitement and surprises to many child audiences but also raised key questions about the ethics blurring of advertising and entertainment (as will be addressed in this chapter).

Another child influencer, Ryan Kaji, became the highest-paid YouTube star through his channel, Ryan's Toys Review (which was later named Ryan's World), with 17 million followers and 22 million dollars of earnings in 2018 (Robehmed & Berg, 2018). As of 2024 (Rankin, 2024), his net worth is expected to exceed $100 million, with his successful video sharing on YouTube, but also with successful collaboration with toy companies and sponsorships with brands and television broadcast stations (e.g., Nickelodeon). His family's business in toys and accessories featured Ryan and his associated characters from his channel, establishing his own brand for young audiences. These child influencers inspired advertisers to collaborate with these star figures and even created collectible toy brands to be promoted through unboxing videos such as LOL Surprise Dolls (Semuels, 2018).

Children and adolescents are constantly bombarded with many persuasive messages and asked to love certain brands. According to recent statistics (Statista, 2023), the spending on digital advertising aimed at children in 2021 was $2.9 billion worldwide and is estimated to reach $6.41 billion in 2025 (See Figure 12.1). In the United States, social media platforms generated about $11 billion in advertising revenues from child users younger than 18 (Brownstein, 2024). Advertising aimed at children is growing on social media, especially on TikTok. Recent statistics showed that after TikTok was launched, children's advertising exposure on TikTok significantly increased (Lafayette, 2023). While YouTube, YouTube Kids, and broadcast TV were the primary channels where children watched advertising in 2021, this trend has been shifted by TikTok's presence. In 2022, the percentage of advertising exposure through YouTube, YouTube Kids, broadcast TV, video-on-demand, and online streaming videos decreased, while the percentage of TikTok advertising exposure increased from 0% to 16%.

Why do we care about advertising for these young consumers? It is great that children can learn lessons from advertising; however, children are widely considered to be limited processors who are not able to cognitively process persuasive messages with critical lenses (Friestad & Wright, 1994; John, 1999). Therefore, advertisers, policymakers, and

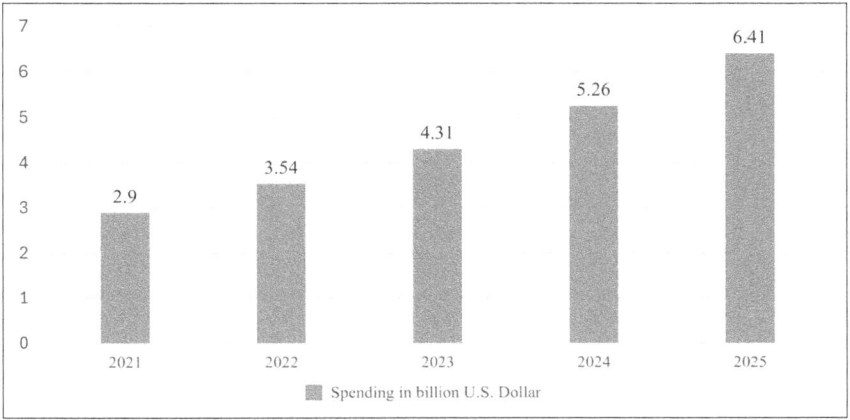

Figure 12.1 Worldwide spending on digital advertising aimed at children.
Note: Chart produced by author using data from Statista, 2023

the government are responsible for protecting this vulnerable consumer group. This chapter will focus on how these young people process advertising messages by age and how advertisers target them. Also, the chapter elaborates on what is missing discussion regarding advertising and DEI (Diversity, Equity, and Inclusivity). The chapter also steps into conversations about artificial intelligence and personalized advertising specifically targeted to young people younger than 18. The chapter aims to provide an understanding of what efforts should be made in the advertising industry for the next generations.

Consumer Socialization

What do children think and know about the ads and other commercial messages that they see? How do they make sense of advertising and marketing? Consumer socialization explains how individuals acquire experiences and knowledge as consumers. Ward (1974) particularly focused on how consumer socialization in childhood can be extended and evolved to their later adult understanding of consumption and the marketplace. The process of consumer socialization not only prepares individuals to be wise and critical consumers but also satisfies social expectations. In other words, consumer socialization is the accumulation of consumer experiences and knowledge that are complicated and mixed with one's roles and norms.

By adopting the definition and conceptualization of consumer socialization by Ward (1974), Moschis and Churchill (1978), and other child development scholars (e.g., Bandura, 1986; Piaget, 1929), John (1999) provided a 25-year review of research on children's consumer socialization and extensively explained how children's consumer skills evolve by age. Friestad and Wright (1994) also adopted the work of previous scholars in consumer socialization and social learning theory and provided a brief overview of how consumer skills develop in childhood. That research has indicated that at the *preoperational age,* when children are between 2 and 7 years old, their cognitive capacity is limited, and they view the surrounding environment with a narrow viewpoint, making it difficult for them to identify advertisers' selling or persuasive intent in advertising. According to Wilcox et al. (2004), children under age 4 to 5 have limited knowledge of how to identify advertising. They may only know it by the differences in length or by recognizing the perceptual features of brands and products. They are not able to process critically what they actually see, which likely makes them accept what they see as "reality." Thus, they are likely to elicit positive attitudes toward advertising, and advertisers try to capture this opportunity to build loyalty with them from when they are young. When children reach the *concrete operational stage* (or analytical stage), generally between 7 to 11 years old, they start perceiving negative aspects of advertising. They recognize advertisers' intent and retrieve consumer experience and information to evaluate advertisers' tactics. Their information processing becomes more abstract and multidimensional than before, and such practice becomes more mature when children enter the *reflective stage*, which is in the range of 11 to 16 years old. In later adolescence, children become more skeptical of various complex advertising messages and social communications.

Over time, children modify their behavior through experience and marketplace knowledge. They learn about how advertising impacts their minds and desires and how to cope with such messages. However, Friestad and Wright (1994) argued that individuals' practices of purchasing, exposure to ads, and reacting to such persuasive attempts facilitate the development of their coping skills toward advertising. Thus, in general, opportunities to practice coping strategies begin during early or middle adulthood. This indirectly explains that recognizing the intent of ads and processing and evaluating them critically is challenging and overwhelming for children and adolescents.

However, today's media landscape and technology make it more challenging for children and adolescents to resist persuasion. First, the boundaries between media are blurred and meaningless. In the past, there was a clear line between toys, games, television programs, and books. Today, children's toys and entertainment can now be played not only through physical objects but also through diverse media technologies. For example, children can enjoy Lego through console gameplay. Warner Bros, TT Games, and The Lego Group launched Lego Dimensions, which is a hybrid version of physical Lego brick and video games (Team, 2015).

Children can play Lego virtually through their smartphones. Recently, Mark Zuckerberg showcased augmented reality Lego, where children can play Legos virtually through Meta Quest 3 (Hollister, 2023). Second, the boundaries between the realms of entertainment, education, and advertising have been blurred as well. Licensed media characters, such as Disney's Mickey Mouse and Minnie Mouse, appear in children's learning apps such as Disney interactive storybooks (e.g., Graser, 2013). Disney utilized the app for children to read and learn 'through' Disney characters from *Frozen, Monsters University*, and *Planes*. The app also attached drawing tools and soundtrack of Disney movies, which enable children to have an immersive experience of the films. Such multi-facets of education and entertainment subtly work as advertising, which could motivate children to consume more Disney movies and merchandise.

Social media influencers' content also makes it easy for advertisers to subtly reach young audiences entertainingly (De Veirman et al., 2019). When social media influencers seamlessly interweave sponsored brands into their user-generated content, the line between entertainment and advertising becomes ambiguous. When Ryan Kaji shares about Carl's Jr.'s StarPals Kids Meal on his channel, or when Charli D'Amelio posts TikTok videos about Dunkin, would children recognize it as advertising? What cues would they use to cope with those messages? Would they care whether they are advertising? The wall between different media forms has collapsed, and this has influenced the form of advertising. Such change has pushed young consumers and their caregivers to be more alert on social media.

Outcomes Associated with Advertising Exposure

Current advertising practices aimed at children and adolescents utilize a feeling of happiness, excitement, and thrill; therefore, the consumer experience is very challenging for young consumers to resist. Since consumers—young or old—are exposed to a tremendous amount of information and advertising every day, we do not always realize how much we need to be alert and cautious with our consumption. This shows how it is potentially quite overwhelming for young children and adolescents. This section reviews outcomes associated with advertising exposure, specifically those that impact young consumers negatively.

Consumerism and Materialism

Critics, parents/caregivers, and consumer advocacy groups have criticized the commercialization of children's everyday lives, in part on the grounds that it can lead to consumerism and materialism (e.g., Hains & Jennings, 2021; Quart, 2004; Seiter, 1993). Accordingly, past studies noted that advertising triggers children's pestering or purchase requests (e.g., Buijzen & Valkenburg, 2003, 2005; De Jans et al., 2019; Moschis & Churchill, 1978). Further, pestering frequently causes parent-child conflicts (De Jans et al., 2019; McDermott et al., 2006). A longitudinal survey of children showed a positive association between advertising exposure and materialism (Opree et al., 2014). Advertising's various appeals and tactics stimulate children's product desires, which lead them to want more of the advertised products. This phenomenon has not only appeared for young children but also for tweens and young teenagers since the late 1990s (Quart, 2004). Marketers found a potential market for young adolescents, even from luxury brands.

Such consumerism and materialism issues are accelerated after a gateway for children to social media is opened. In addition to television advertising, children are constantly exposed to targeted and personalized advertising on social media, particularly on video-streaming sites and influencers' posts (North, 2023). Wherever children and adolescents scroll, they are asked to "buy stuff" millions of times. A few years ago, unboxing videos fueled children's obsession with possessing toys but not playing with toys (Lieber, 2019; Marshall, 2019). Since new toys and gifts are always unboxed in front of child audiences' eyes, their desire to want the product increases, and they start getting obsessed with "owning" the product rather than "using" it.

Children's obsession with product trial and purchase is now extended to cosmetics and skincare. Early this year, a new term called "Sephora Kids" emerged, a phenomenon of tweens and young adolescents purchasing make-up and skincare products excessively at Sephora and Ulta (Kavilanz, 2024; Taylor, 2024). Their purchases of cosmetics and skincare products are even extended to pricey brands such as Drunk Elephant, Glow Recipe, and Laneige. Their temptation is primarily from the exposure of brands through influencers and celebrities on social media. Further, such a phenomenon has been extended to "flex culture," stimulating children and adolescents to experience high-end luxury brands such as Balenciaga, Chanel, Louis Vuitton, and Gucci (Schneier, 2023). Some parents even favorably accept their children's requests to purchase these luxury items. Children's lives are constantly exposed to the realm of comparison, which stimulates them to own and purchase more to fill the gap with people they see on social media.

Another way of accelerating consumerism is transmedia storytelling, branding, and merchandising, which could unlimitedly and unimaginably extend children's universe of consumption. Toy merchandising has a long history, which has been a lucrative market with media characters (e.g., Mickey Mouse, Marvel superheroes). As marketers allow young consumers to enjoy immersive experiences through multiple channels, they allow children to engage in the universe of characters as a whole. See the quote about the power of transmedia storytelling and branding by Jenkins (2006) below.

> A transmedia story unfolds across multiple media platforms, with each new text making a distinctive and valuable contribution to the whole. In the ideal form of transmedia storytelling, each medium does what it does best – so that a story might be introduced in a film, expanded through television, novels, and comics; its world might be explored through gameplay or experienced as an amusement park attraction [...] Reading across the media sustains a depth of experience that motivates more consumption. (pp. 95–96).

Each medium works as a gateway for children to enter the world of media characters, and each of them opens a door for advertisers to market them in a subtle but entertaining way. For instance, there are many ways to engage in the universe of *Harry Potter*. Various media platforms allow audiences to enjoy *Harry Potter* in the forms of books, films, toys (e.g., Legos), games (e.g., Hogwarts Legacy), and theme parks (e.g., Universal Orlando's *Wizarding World of Harry Potter*). Every point of experience becomes an opportunity for children to "consume." Advertisers' approach to such branding makes it difficult for young children to resist. The more they experience such entertainment, the more they are eager to purchase, leading to conflicts with caregivers.

Gender and Sexuality

Children and adolescents are constantly exposed to messages about gender through advertising. While it may be challenging for some to recall specific ads that negatively impact children's perceptions of gender roles and sexuality, this influence has persisted subtly within the advertising industry for decades. One area where this issue is particularly evident is in the marketing of children's toys. Toys are often segregated by gender, and for decades, Barbie has been at the forefront of reinforcing traditional gender roles (Gilblom et al., 2023; Lepore, 2018; Treisman, 2023). As one of the most iconic figures in American history, Barbie has faced numerous protests for promoting stereotypical messages. For example, in 1992, the release of Teen Talk Barbie featured approximately 270 recordings, with Barbie talking primarily about shopping, clothes, and friendships. One of the most controversial recordings stated, "Math class is tough," which received significant public criticism.

In response to these criticisms, Mattel, the company behind Barbie, has taken steps to reflect greater diversity and challenge traditional gender roles through various campaigns. For instance, in celebration of Barbie's 65th anniversary, a new collection featured women athletes, including tennis player Venus Williams (O'Bier, 2024). Additionally, Mattel has partnered with numerous non-profit organizations to support education and research for girls' and women's sports. The company has also introduced different body shapes and careers within the Barbie line, aiming to empower young girls and boost their confidence across a variety of fields (Gilblom et al., 2023).

Nonetheless, young children are still encouraged to conform to specific gender identities, norms, and roles through advertising and toys. In 2015, Target, one of the largest retailers in the United States, removed gender-based signs in the toy aisles (Contrera, 2015). However, it is still common to see dolls, plush toys, and action figures marketed specifically toward boys or girls in today's retail outlets. To address this issue, there is a growing movement toward gender-neutral marketing for children (e.g., California; Segran, 2023). However, we are unsure of the potential impact this may have on the toy industry's landscape and business. Given that gender norms and roles have been ingrained for a long time and gendered toy marketing has a history of about 40 years, transforming gendered advertising and marketing targeted at children poses significant challenges.

Children are also exposed to sexualized messages through advertising and marketing. Around 2009, other toy characters emerged, creating a more diverse and edgier version of the Barbie universe (Gilblom et al., 2023). For example, hyper-sexualized dolls like MGA Entertainment's *Bratz Dolls* suggest that young girls should wear heavy makeup and engage in flirtatious behavior. The concern was not limited to the views of a single individual but has been widely discussed in studies conducted by the American Psychological Association (APA) on the sexualization of girls (American Psychological Association Task Force on the Sexualization of Girls, 2007). These studies highlighted the growing apprehension over how young girls are introduced to toys that are linked to "objectified adult sexuality." More recently, similar concerns have been raised about another toy line by MGA Entertainment, *L.O.L. Surprise! Dolls* (Cavander et al., 2020; Henson, 2020). An issue emerged when it was discovered that the dolls reveal provocative outfits when dripped in cold water, exposing clothing such as suspenders, lingerie, and garters—garments that seem inappropriate for children. Many parents expressed shock and distress by such adult-like attire in toys designed for young children. It is not difficult to observe how sexualized messages can be present in toys marketed toward children today.

While discussions around gender norms, roles, and sexuality are common in children's advertising, there has been limited focus on LGBTQ+ representation. Advertisers have traditionally been cautious about showing the voices of LGBTQ+ gender identity in their advertisements and marketing campaigns since it could lead to backlash from conservative families with children. This is not only happening in advertising aimed at children but also in the overall advertising industry after the backlash of Bud Light's social media campaign, which involved a transgender influencer, Dylan Mulvaney (Guynn, 2024; Holpuch, 2023). Because of this phenomenon, conflicts, and misinformation about LGBTQ+ groups, including youth, are being exacerbated. A recent campaign, which was a collaboration between GLAAD and the Ogilvy Agency, aimed to amplify voices in protecting LGBTQ+ youth from hatred and misinformation (Bloom, 2024). Also, to celebrate various kinds of families, Flamingo Rampant strives to produce publications that focus on various aspects of pride, including positive representations of LGBTQ+ families and communities. This issue should be considered not only as a matter of representation but also as a matter of equality, equity, and citizenship.

Food Choices

According to statistics from 2017 to 2020, approximately 14.7 million children in the United States aged 2 to 19 are affected by obesity (CDC, 2024). This means almost 20% of the country's youth are experiencing this, with 1 out of 5 children meeting a (sometimes critiqued/challenged) clinical definition of obesity. Scholars, critics, and health experts have underscored how media messages, including advertising, contribute to shaping children's unhealthy food habits (Coates et al., 2019; Livingstone & Helsper, 2006; Roberto et al., 2010). Indeed, considering obesity as shameful or as an individual's fault is a social justice issue (see also Chapter 9), and it is important, instead, to critique the role of corporations and other systems that may be putting profits ahead of children's well-being.

Advertisers have promoted unhealthy food and beverages with branded toy marketing since the late 1980s and 1990s. Happy Meal from McDonald's has been viral for many decades because of its iconic red box with food and a shiny plastic toy (Heil, 2019). Many toy and licensed character brands (e.g., Hello Kitty, Power Ranger, Toy Story, etc.) have collaborated with McDonald's, which brought huge success and attraction. Children enjoy positive experiences at McDonald's as a whole, with a moment of bonding with their favorite character toy. Such memories accumulate and contribute to children's positive attitudes and purchase intentions.

Such marketing has intensified as we enter the era of social media and influencers. The boundary between advertisers' and users' content is blurred (van der Bend et al., 2022). Since people love to share what they like, eat, and drink on social media, both advertising and food-related social media content posted by users generate the same advertising effect. A child enjoying a Happy Meal with a toy premium on TikTok plays the same role as a McDonald's television commercial. Mc Carthy et al. (2022), a recent systematic review of unhealthy food marketing, found that interactive food marketing (e.g., social media advertising, advergaming) seemed to have a significant effect on youth's unhealthy food eating habits. This trend was evident in social media influencers' posts of nutritionally poor foods and beverages (Coates et al., 2019; Suciu, 2023). For instance, food marketers have utilized TikTok challenges to generate youth's digital engagement (Brooks et al., 2022). Social media users sharing their own version of the TikTok challenge become 'unofficial brand ambassadors' of those food brands (e.g., Charli D'Amelio's Dunkin endorsement, George, 2020; Williams, 2020). User-generated content from one single TikTok challenge then becomes a collection of massive social media advertising full of joy and excitement. Advergames also subtly imbue persuasive messages about unhealthy food brands and generate positive emotions among children. It is overwhelming for children and teenagers to resist such immersive consumer experiences.

A major concern in food advertising is the disproportionate targeting of Black and Hispanic youth with unhealthy food promotions. This issue is not new; throughout the 1990s and 2000s, neighborhoods with predominantly Black and low-income residents had a significantly higher density of fast-food restaurants and billboards advertising harmful products compared to primarily White neighborhoods (Altman et al., 1991; Block et al., 2004). Unfortunately, this pattern of targeted marketing continues to persist today. In 2019, it was reported that fast food restaurants, including McDonald's and Domino's, invested over $1.5 billion in television advertising targeted at Black and Latine children (Harris et al., 2019). According to Harris et al. (2019), Black youth watched 75% more "junk food" ads compared to White youth. As for Latine youth, preschool-aged children viewed more fast-food ads than older groups on Spanish-language television channels. This unfair targeting has been continued since 2011. In the United States, fast-food restaurants are commonly located near Black and Hispanic neighborhoods. Black and Hispanic youth are positioned as more vulnerable consumers who are aggressively targeted both inside and outside their homes by fast-food brands. This discriminatory exposure of ads toward specific racial and ethnic groups remains an issue that needs to be addressed with the support of consumer advocacy groups and regulations.

Smoking

Another harmful consequence of youth-targeted advertising is triggering youth smoking/vaping behavior. This behavior by itself is very appealing to young consumers because they are not legally allowed to purchase or use (e)cigarettes. However, in reality, a significant number of adolescents are exposed to tobacco advertising and, more recently, e-cigarette advertising (Pettigrew et al., 2023). Interestingly, it turned out that adolescents are particularly susceptible to tobacco advertising, not just merely receptive to general advertising (Hanewinkel et al., 2010). A positive association has been observed between adolescents' e-cigarette use and advertising exposure (Pettigrew et al., 2023).

As the significant impact of tobacco and e-cigarette advertising continued, lawsuits and orders of the federal courts have intervened (Campaign for Tobacco-Free Kids, 2023; Fox, 2017). Big tobacco companies denied the lethal effect of tobacco on people's health for decades, and such false statements were tackled by the U.S. Justice Department in 1999. The companies were also accused of purposely aiming at younger generations, especially adolescents under the age of 18. In 2006, it turned out that those major tobacco companies had violated civil racketeering laws (RICO), and they were ordered to tell the truth about the harmful effects of tobacco to the public. After a long 11-year battle, tobacco companies eventually launched the "truth" campaign in 2017, acknowledging the truth about the health risks regarding tobacco and its marketing to children.

Recently, one of the representative e-cigarette companies, JUUL, was also accused of targeting children (Kaplan, 2021). Some of the strong evidence is that JUUL attempted to target youth through websites, television channels, and magazines, primarily targeting children under 18. While underage vaping has increased, companies' strategies to appeal to young generations remained. JUUL's e-cigarette products have a sleek design that resembles a smartphone and are advertised with young youth models, a fun vibe, and catchy phrases (e.g., make the switch). In addition to JUUL, other e-cigarette brands utilized similar tactics to make the products appealing to younger generations (e.g., Struik et al., 2020).

Drinking

Alcohol advertising potentially has the same effect on youth. According to a recent study about alcohol advertising on social media, children are exposed to about 40,000 alcohol ads on Instagram and Meta (Alcohol and Drug Association, 2023; Hayden et al., 2023). This study revealed that almost 91% of the sampled ads contained a "shop now" call to action, highlighting good feelings, friendship, and joy. Similar to other youth-oriented advertising tactics, user-generated content and influencers are commonly used to make young people engage in alcohol brands and generate positive attitudes toward the category of alcohol. Such a subtle but aggressive approach of marketing aimed at children makes them feel vulnerable toward drinking and even binge drinking. Alcohol advertising was raised as an issue due to the brands' targeting children in the early 2000s (Teinowitz,

2003), but very few cases regarding their presence and regulations were discussed in the late 2020s.

Gambling

A recently discussed harmful outcome generated by advertising is gambling behavior. Long considered only allowed for adults, it is not difficult to observe that the gambling industry is sneaking into children's entertainment content. A recent study by Backholer and Pathirana (2024) reported how children and adolescents are frequently encouraged to click and install gambling apps. This report provides evidence that less regulation exists to protect young children from harmful marketing approaches. GambleAware, the charity and commissioner of educating risks of gambling through intervention programs, also underscores the blurred boundary between entertainment and gambling (Ungoed-Thomas, 2024). It is crucial to redefine gambling for children because of the grey area between gambling and gambling-like entertainment for children. Rigorous policies and regulations are required for gambling brands, especially for advertising appeals aimed at young people, such as using animated or cartoon figures (Ungoed-Thomas, 2024). For instance, social casino games can be considered gambling, but loot boxes and skins that young game users can obtain by chance also contain the element of gambling (Hing et al., 2020). GambleAware's recent research found that 30% of sample participants, aged 12 to 17, have tried gambling, and 40% of them had an experience playing games that feature gambling components. 46% of participants recalled gambling ads through sports and racing events. The problem is that young people who have engaged in such games incorporating gambling elements are more likely to spend money on various forms of gambling (Hing et al., 2020; Ungoed-Thomas, 2024).

Guidelines to Help Young Consumers Cope with Advertising

To help children and adolescents recognize the intent behind persuasive messages and respond critically to advertising, scholars and educators have developed numerous resources aimed at enhancing advertising literacy (see also Chapter 5). Although past literature offers various definitions, it is often described as the skill set required to identify, evaluate, and cope with advertising messages (Livingstone & Helsper, 2006; Nelson, 2016). Advertising literacy is closely related to persuasion knowledge, focusing specifically on advertising (Hudders et al., 2016). Some scholars argue that advertising literacy is a subset of media literacy, which refers to the "specific knowledge and skills that promote critical understanding and use of media" (Jeong et al., 2012, p. 455). Several non-profit organizations aim to educate children, parents, and teachers about the nature of advertising. Notable organizations include Common Sense Media (CSM), the Media Education Lab (MEL), Media Literacy Now (MLN), MediaSmarts, and the National Association for Media Literacy Education (NAMLE).

Identifying Sponsorship Disclosure

The first step to cope with advertising is to identify where the advertising messages are coming from. Advertisers are the source of messages that lead to their sales and profits. Unfortunately, it is often difficult for children to differentiate between organic content (e.g., user-generated content or social games) and advertising, especially when the lines between entertainment and advertising blur, as seen in influencer marketing and advergames. On social media, recognizing sponsorship disclosure on user-generated content could activate adolescents' critical thinking, often leading to a negative response to advertising (van Dam & van Reijmersdal, 2019; van Reijmersdal et al., 2020). van Reijmersdal et al. (2020) demonstrated that such early disclosures enhance young consumers' ability to recognize sponsored material. Hashtags can subtly reveal the advertisers behind content created by influencers or creators.

To ensure children can identify advertising through these disclosures, in the United States, the Federal Trade Commission (FTC), a government body dedicated to consumer protection, and the Children's Advertising Review Unit (CARU), a self-regulatory organization, issue guidelines, recommendations, and even enforce rules related to sponsorship disclosure. CARU's mission is to ensure that the advertising industry operates responsibly when targeting children under 13. They emphasize that disclosures must be presented in a manner that is easy for young audiences to understand. As sponsorship disclosure is one of the clearest methods of signaling the commercial nature of content, CARU, along with several watchdog organizations and consumer advocacy groups, actively monitors advertisers across media platforms where children and adolescents are the primary audience, such as social media or social gaming sites (CARU 2016, 2017; Hsu, 2019; Stanton, 2023).

While there are no specific child-focused regulations at the EU level for sponsorship disclosure in advergames or social media influencer content, general regulations such as the Digital Services Act and guidelines from the European Advertising Standards Alliance help indirectly protect children by ensuring transparency and accountability in advertising, particularly for child-targeted content (EASA, 2023; European Commission, 2024). However, some countries, such as France, have implemented additional child-specific regulations (Le Pechon-Joubert & Imatte, 2023).

Understanding Advertisers' Tactics, Biases, and Representation

It is equally important to evaluate how advertisers target young consumers and to identify which advertising messages contain biases or omit essential information about the brands. Extensive research has focused on improving children's advertising literacy in various advertising environments (e.g., An et al., 2014; Hudders et al., 2016; Hwang et al., 2018; Lou et al., 2020; Nelson, 2016; Nelson et al., 2020; Rozendaal et al., 2011; Stanley & Lawson, 2020). These studies highlight the need to teach children not only to recognize persuasive intent and advertising tactics but also to "pause and reflect" on the hidden biases and underlying sources behind these messages (Hwang et al., 2018; Rozendaal et al., 2011).

To persuade young consumers, advertisers often employ popular figures such as celebrities, peer endorsers, and media characters (De Veirman et al., 2019). Through these influential figures, brands transfer their values and create a strong association between children and the brand. Children are likely to form *parasocial relationships* with these figures, viewing them as trusted sources of information and guidance for making purchasing decisions. Social media influencers, in particular, are relatable to young audiences, fostering a sense of intimacy through ongoing interactions. These repeated interactions can lead to peer modeling and social learning, influencing children's attitudes, beliefs, and behaviors. It is essential to educate children on how influential figures can shape their attitudes and behaviors.

When consuming advertised products, young consumers often adopt the embedded values associated with the brands. Advertising may promote messages about gender roles, perpetuate stereotypes related to race or ethnicity, or create excitement around harmful products for children. Ads typically showcase the positive aspects of brands, and this selective presentation of information can mislead young audiences into accepting these messages without question.

Understanding Advertising Personalization Through AI Algorithms

It is also crucial to understand how advertisers utilize AI algorithms to attract and appeal to children. By understanding such principles in the advertising industry, children could better respond to commercial messages in their lives. The advertising industry has been transformed by the rapid growth of innovation and technology in artificial intelligence (Chuan et al., 2023; Fernández-Gómez & Feijoo, 2024). Accordingly, many experts have raised concerns about using children's consumer data for personalized advertising (Chuan et al., 2023; Fernández-Gómez & Feijoo, 2024). To make ads more relevant to each consumer, advertisers use "user-centric" and "content-centric" machine learning methods. These methods help predict what each consumer might be interested in purchasing or watching. By analyzing consumers' past online behavior, such as browsing history, social media responses, and ad clicks, AI algorithms recommend content for consumers to watch. Social media platforms also use algorithms to show content that matches users' interests and preferences. This consumer data allows advertisers to predict consumer behavior and develop profiling systems (Shumanov & Johnson, 2021). For example, when children search for skincare products, they are more likely to encounter related skincare or beauty advertisements through email, social media, and search engine results. Therefore, understanding how AI algorithms function in personalization is crucial for young consumers to gain a deeper insight into the nature of advertising.

As AI-generated content and virtual personae become more prevalent on social media (Heygate, 2024; Yang, 2024), additional caution is needed to protect children and adolescents. AI-generated social media influencers can now interact with followers in ways that closely mimic human behavior, making it challenging to discern the underlying selling intent, especially for younger audiences. When AI-generated cartoon characters, which are part of a brand, are introduced to children without clear advertising disclosures, it may blur the lines between what is considered content and what is a promotional message. Moreover, the rise of advanced generative AI techniques, such as deepfake ads featuring celebrities, increases the risk of children and adolescents being unable to differentiate between real and fabricated content. Therefore, it is essential to teach children and adolescents AI literacy, in addition to advertising literacy, to help them effectively navigate and mitigate the potentially harmful effects of AI-driven advertising.

Creating Subvertisements

In addition, engaging children in 'creative advertising' activities, where they take on the role of advertisers, can deepen their understanding of the advertiser's perspective and strategies. This approach is particularly useful for confronting brands whose products negatively impact children. For example, Nelson (2016) conducted an advertising literacy intervention for primary school students, where they created healthy food advertisements using their own characters, health claims, and promotional techniques. She further expanded this model to include Jamaican parents and adolescents by introducing the creation of "subvertisements" (Nelson et al., 2020). Subvertisements are counter-advertising messages designed to challenge or disrupt the intentions of marketers (Dery, 1993). By allowing children to become creators rather than passive consumers, this approach empowers them to engage with advertisements more critically and meaningfully.

Conclusion

This chapter explores the pervasive influence of advertising on children and its potential negative impacts on their well-being. It also identifies a critical gap in Diversity, Equity, and Inclusion (DEI) efforts within child-directed advertising, particularly in relation to gender, sexuality, and race/ethnicity. The chapter further outlines strategies to help children identify and understand the persuasive tactics used in advertisements. To better support young consumers navigating the commercialized world, regulators, scholars, and educators must consider children's perspectives and evolving media technologies when developing policies and educational programs.

References

Alcohol and Drug Association (2023, May 16). Alcohol ads on social media target teens and young people. https://adf.org.au/insights/alcohol-social-media-youth/

Altman, D. G., Schooler, C., & Basil, M. D. (1991). Alcohol and cigarette advertising on billboards. *Health Education Research*, 6(4), 487–490. https://doi.org/10.1093/her/6.4.487

American Psychological Association Task Force on the Sexualization of Girls. (2007). *Report of the APA Task Force on the Sexualization of Girls*. https://www.apa.org/pi/women/programs/girls/report

An, S., Jin, H. S., & Park, E. H. (2014). Children's advertising literacy for advergames: Perception of the game as advertising. *Journal of Advertising*, 43(1), 63–72. https://doi.org/10.1080/00913367.2013.795123

Backholer, K., & Pathirana, N. L. (2024). *#DigitalYouth: How children and young people are targeted with harmful product marketing online*. Deakin University. https://iht.deakin.edu.au/wp-content/uploads/sites/153/2024/06/Digital-Youth-brief-Final-2.pdf

Bandura, A. (1986). *Social foundation of thought and action: A social cognitive theory*. Prentice Hall Inc.

Block, J. P., Scribner, R. A., & DeSalvo, K. B. (2004). Fast food, race/ethnicity, and income: A geographic analysis. *American Journal of Preventive Medicine*, 27(3), 211–217. https://doi.org/10.1016/j.amepre.2004.06.007

Bloom, A. (2024, April 12). *GLAAD and Ogilvy launch "Protect This Kid" campaign in support of LGBTQ youth*. GLADD. https://glaad.org/glaad-and-oglivy-launch-protect-this-kid-campaign-in-support-of-lgbtq-youth/

Brooks, R., Christidis, R., Carah, N., Kelly, B., Martino, F., & Backholer, K. (2022). Turning users into 'unofficial brand ambassadors': Marketing of unhealthy food and non-alcoholic beverages on TikTok. *BMJ Global Health*, 7(6), e009112. https://doi.org/10.1136/bmjgh-2022-009112

Brownstein, M. (2024, January 2). *Targeting kids generates billions in ad revenue for social media*. The Harvard Gazette. https://news.harvard.edu/gazette/story/2024/01/social-media-platforms-make-11b-in-ad-revenue-from-u-s-teens/

Buijzen, M., & Valkenburg, P. M. (2003). The unintended effects of television advertising: A parent-child survey. *Communication Research*, 30(5), 483–503. https://doi.org/10.1177/0093650203256361

Buijzen, M., & Valkenburg, P. M. (2005). Parental mediation of undesired advertising effects. *Journal of Broadcasting & Electronic Media*, 49(2), 153–165. https://doi.org/10.1207/s15506878jobem4902_1

Campaign for Tobacco-Free Kids (2023, November 8). *U.S. racketeering verdict big tobacco guilty as charged*. https://www.tobaccofreekids.org/what-we-do/industry-watch/doj

CARU (2016, September 12). *'EvanTube' YouTube channels to disclose sponsored videos as advertising following CARU inquiry*. https://bbbprograms.org/media-center/dd/evantube-youtube-channels-to-disclose-sponsored-videos-as-advertising-following-caru-inquiry

CARU (2017, October 18). *CARU examines YouTube channel 'Ryan Toys Review,' recommends more prominent disclosures of ad content*. https://bbbprograms.org/media-center/dd/caru-examines-youtube-channel-ryan-toys-review-recommends-more-prominent-disclosures-of-ad-content

Cavander, L., Bartholomew, K., & Gaffney, A. (2020, August 19). *LOL Surprise! doll outrage has child commissioner, families calling for removal from shelves*. ABC Australia News. https://www.abc.net.au/news/2020-08-19/outrage-builds-over-sexualised-lol-surprise-kids-dolls/12572752

CDC (2024). *Childhood obesity facts*. https://www.cdc.gov/obesity/childhood-obesity-facts/childhood-obesity-facts.html

Chuan, C. H., Tsai, W. H. S., & Yang, J. (2023). Artificial intelligence, advertising, and society. *Advertising & Society Quarterly*, 24(3). https://dx.doi.org/10.1353/asr.2023.a911198

Coates, A. E., Hardman, C. A., Halford, J. C., Christiansen, P., & Boyland, E. J. (2019). Social media influencer marketing and children's food intake: A randomized trial. *Pediatrics*, 143(4), e20182554. https://doi.org/10.1542/peds.2018-2554

Contrera, J. (2015, August 9). *Target will stop separating toys and bedding into girls' and boys' sections*. The Washington Post. https://www.washingtonpost.com/news/arts-and-entertainment/wp/2015/08/09/target-will-stop-separating-toys-and-bedding-into-girls-and-boys-sections/

De Jans, S., Van de Sompel, D., Hudders, L., & Cauberghe, V. (2019). Advertising targeting young children: An overview of 10 years of research (2006–2016). *International Journal of Advertising*, 38(2), 173–206. https://doi.org/10.1080/02650487.2017.1411056

De Veirman, M., Hudders, L., & Nelson, M. R. (2019). What is influencer marketing and how does it target children? A review and direction for future research. *Frontiers in Psychology*, 10, 498106. https://doi.org/10.3389/fpsyg.2019.02685

Dery, M. (1993). *Culture jamming: Hacking, slashing, and sniping in the empire of signs*. Open Media.

Duncan, K. (2010). *Marketing greatest hits: A masterclass in modern marketing ideas*. A&C Black.

EASA (2023). *EASA best practice recommendation on influencer marketing*. https://www.easa-alliance.org/wp-content/uploads/2018/04/EASA-BPR-ON-INFLUENCER-MARKETING-2023.pdf

European Commission (2024, February 23). *Questions and answers on the Digital Services Act (DSA)*. https://ec.europa.eu/commission/presscorner/detail/en/qanda_20_2348

Fernández-Gómez, E., & Feijoo, B. (2024). Children's advertising literacy in the current digital landscape. In *Advertising literacy for young audiences in the digital age: A critical attitude to embedded formats* (pp. 1–14). Springer Nature Switzerland.

Fox, M. (2017, November 27). *Big Tobacco finally tells the truth in court-ordered ad campaign.* NBC News. https://www.nbcnews.com/health/health-news/big-tobacco-finally-tells-truth-court-ordered-ad-campaign-n823136

Friestad, M., & Wright, P. (1994). The persuasion knowledge model: How people cope with persuasion attempts. *Journal of Consumer Research, 21*(1), 1–31. https://doi.org/10.1086/209380

George, C. (2020, September 5). *How Charli D'Amelio became the face of TikTok.* The New Yorker. https://www.newyorker.com/culture/cultural-comment/how-charli-damelio-became-the-face-of-tiktok#:~:text=Her%20first%20major%20viral%20moment,performances%20seem%20casual%20and%20unlabored

Gilblom, K., Buckley, T., & Townsend, M. (2023). *Mattel goes to the movies.* Bloomberg Businessweek. https://www.bloomberg.com/features/2023-barbie-movie-mattel/?embedded-checkout=true

Giroux, H. A. (2011, August 21). *How Disney magic and the corporate media shape youth identity in the digital age.* Truthout. https://truthout.org/articles/how-disney-magic-and-the-corporate-media-shape-youth-identity-in-the-digital-age/

Graser, M. (2013, November 14). *Disney turns to apps like 'Frozen' storybook to get kids into movie theaters* https://variety.com/2013/digital/news/disney-turns-to-apps-like-frozen-storybook-to-get-kids-into-movie-theaters-1200833254/

Guynn, J. (2024, May 22). *Expect fewer rainbow logos for LGBTQ Pride Month after Target, and Bud Light backlash.* USA Today. https://www.usatoday.com/story/money/2024/05/22/target-bud-light-boycott-pride-month-2024/73737866007/

Hains, R. C., & Jennings, N. A. (Eds.). (2021). *The marketing of children's toys: Critical perspectives on children's consumer culture.* Palgrave Macmillan.

Hanewinkel, R., Isensee, B., Sargent, J. D., & Morgenstern, M. (2010). Cigarette advertising and adolescent smoking. *American Journal of Preventive Medicine, 38*(4), 359–366. https://doi.org/10.1016/j.amepre.2009.12.036

Harris, J. L., Frazier, W., Kumanyika, S., & Ramirez, A. G. (2019). *Increasing disparities in unhealthy food advertising targeted to Hispanic and Black youth.* UConn Rudd Center for Food Policy and Health. https://media.ruddcenter.uconn.edu/PDFs/TargetedMarketingReport2019.pdf

Hayden, L., Brownbill, A., Angus, D., Carah, N., Tan, X. Y., Hawker, K., Dobson, A., & Robards, B. (2023). *Alcohol advertising on social media platforms - A 1-year snapshot.* Foundation for Alcohol Research and Education. https://fare.org.au/alcohol-advertising-on-social-media-platforms/

Heil, E. (2019, November 6). *The Happy Meal, a triumph of marketing blamed for childhood obesity, is turning 40.* The Washington Post. https://www.washingtonpost.com/news/voraciously/wp/2019/11/06/the-happy-meal-a-triumph-of-marketing-blamed-for-childhood-obesity-is-turning-40/

Henson, M. (2020, August 25). *Sexualized toys created for children: A disturbing trend, not a coincidence.* Washington Examiner. https://www.washingtonexaminer.com/opinion/2600038/sexualized-toys-created-for-children-a-disturbing-trend-not-a-coincidence/

Heygate, J. (2024, July 2). *FTC attorney urges brands to assess risks of AI influencers on children.* Campaign US. https://www.campaignlive.com/article/ftc-attorney-urges-brands-assess-risks-ai-influencers-children/1879351

Hing, N., et al. (2020). *NSW Youth Gambling Study 2020.* NSW Responsible Gambling Fund. https://www.gambleaware.nsw.gov.au/supporting-someone/supporting-young-people/gaming-gambling-and-young-people

Hollister, S. (2023, September 27). *The Meta Quest 3 lets you play with virtual Legos in your real living room.* The Verge. https://www.theverge.com/2023/9/27/23892690/meta-quest-3-lego-bricktales-oculus

Holpuch, A. (2023, November 21). *Behind the backlash against Bud Light*. The New York Times. https://www.nytimes.com/article/bud-light-boycott.html

Hoy, M. G., Childers, C. C., & Evans, N. J. (2018). Unboxing parents' understanding of sponsored child influencer videos. In *American Academy of Advertising Conference Proceedings (Online)* (pp. 122–122).

Hsu, T. (2019, September 4). *Popular YouTube toy review channel accused of blurring lines for ads*. The New York Times. https://www.nytimes.com/2019/09/04/business/media/ryan-toysreview-youtube-ad-income.html

Hudders, L., Cauberghe, V., & Panic, K. (2016). How advertising literacy training affect children's responses to television commercials versus advergames. *International Journal of Advertising*, 35(6), 909–931. https://doi.org/10.1080/02650487.2015.1090045

Hwang, Y., Yum, J. Y., & Jeong, S. H. (2018). What components should be included in advertising literacy education? Effect of component types and the moderating role of age. *Journal of Advertising*, 47(4), 347–361. https://doi.org/10.1080/00913367.2018.1546628

Jenkins, H. (2006). *Convergence culture: Where old and new media collide*. NYU Press.

Jeong, S. H., Cho, H., & Hwang, Y. (2012). Media literacy interventions: A meta-analytic review. *Journal of Communication*, 62(3), 454–472. https://doi.org/10.1111/j.1460-2466.2012.01643.x

John, D. R. (1999). Consumer socialization of children: A retrospective look at twenty-five years of research. *Journal of Consumer Research*, 26(3), 183–213. https://doi.org/10.1086/209559

Kaplan, S. (2021, May 25). *Juul bought ads appearing on Cartoon Network and other youth sites, suit claims*. The New York Times. https://www.nytimes.com/2020/02/12/health/juul-vaping-lawsuit.html

Kavilanz, P. (2024, March 12). *The 'Sephora kid' trend shows tweens are psyched about skincare. But their overzealous approach is raising concerns*. CNN Business. https://www.cnn.com/2024/03/12/business/sephora-kid-tweens-skincare-obsession/index.html

Lafayette, J. (2023, January 18). *TikTok gaining on YouTube as key way to reach kids*. Broadcasting + Cable. https://www.nexttv.com/news/tiktok-gaining-on-youtube-as-key-way-to-reach-kids

Le Pechon-Joubert, F., & Imatte, L. (2023, December). *French Law no. 2023-451 of June 9, 2023 sets out a legal framework for influencers, their agents, the advertisers and the platform that distributes their content. The deciphering below offers a quick overview of the main new features of this law*. De Gaulle Fleurance. https://www.degaullefleurance.com/en/the-influencers-law-analysis-by-de-gaulle-fleurance/

Lepore, J. (2018, January 15). *When Barbie went to war with Bratz*. The New Yorker. https://www.newyorker.com/magazine/2018/01/22/when-barbie-went-to-war-with-bratz

Lieber, C. (2019, March 22). *Toy unboxing videos have taken over YouTube. Some experts say they exploit kids*. Vox. https://www.vox.com/the-goods/2019/3/22/18275767/toy-unboxing-videos-youtube-advertising-ethics

Livingstone, S., & Helsper, E. J. (2006). Does advertising literacy mediate the effects of advertising on children? A critical examination of two linked research literatures in relation to obesity and food choice. *Journal of Communication*, 56(3), 560–584. https://doi.org/10.1111/j.1460-2466.2006.00301.x

Lou, C., Ma, W., & Feng, Y. (2020). A sponsorship disclosure is not enough? How advertising literacy intervention affects consumer reactions to sponsored influencer posts. *Journal of Promotion Management*, 27(2), 278–305. https://doi.org/10.1080/10496491.2020.1829771

Marshall, L. (2019, December 3). *Unboxing videos fueling kids' tantrums, breeding consumerism*. CU Boulder Today. https://www.colorado.edu/today/2019/12/03/unboxing-videos-fueling-kids-tantrums-breeding-consumerism

Mc Carthy, C. M., de Vries, R., & Mackenbach, J. D. (2022). The influence of unhealthy food and beverage marketing through social media and advergaming on diet-related outcomes in children—A systematic review. *Obesity Reviews*, 23(6), e13441. https://doi.org/10.1111/obr.13441

McDermott, L., O'Sullivan, T., Stead, M., & Hastings, G. (2006). International food advertising, pester power and its effects. *International Journal of Advertising*, 25(4), 513–539.

Moschis, G. P., & Churchill, G. A. Jr (1978). Consumer socialization: A theoretical and empirical analysis. *Journal of Marketing Research*, 15(4), 599–609. https://doi.org/10.1177/002224377801500409

Nelson, M. R. (2016). Developing persuasion knowledge by teaching advertising literacy in primary school. *Journal of Advertising*, 45(2), 169–182. https://doi.org/10.1080/00913367.2015.1107871

Nelson, M. R., Powell, R., Ferguson, G. M., & Tian, K. (2020). Using subvertising to build families' persuasion knowledge in Jamaica. *Journal of Advertising*, 49(4), 477–494. https://doi.org/10.1080/00913367.2020.1783725

North, A. (2023 November 14). *The world wants your kids to buy stuff. Here's how to help them be less materialistic*. Vox. https://www.vox.com/23944882/kids-money-shopping-allowance-parenting-consumer-culture

O'Bier, T. (2024, May 22). *Barbie collection honors Venus Williams and other women athletes*. KSBY. https://www.ksby.com/life/good-news/barbie-collection-honors-venus-williams-and-other-women-athletes

Opree, S. J., Buijzen, M., van Reijmersdal, E. A., & Valkenburg, P. M. (2014). Children's advertising exposure, advertised product desire, and materialism: A longitudinal study. *Communication Research*, 41(5), 717–735. https://doi.org/10.1177/0093650213479129

Pettigrew, S., Santos, J. A., Pinho-Gomes, A. C., Li, Y., & Jones, A. (2023). Exposure to e-cigarette advertising and young people's use of e-cigarettes: A four-country study. *Tobacco Induced Diseases*, 21. http://www.doi.org/10.18332/tid/172414

Piaget, J. (1929). *The child's concept of the world*. Londres, Routledge & Kegan Paul.

Quart, A. (2004). *Branded: The buying and selling of teenagers*. Basic Books.

Rankin, S. (2024, August 15). *He's got 83 billion views, but can 12-year-old Ryan Kaji open a movie?* The Hollywood Reporter. https://www.hollywoodreporter.com/business/digital/ryans-world-youtube-success-movie-1235973202/

Robehmed, N., & Berg, M. (2018, December 3). *Highest-paid YouTube stars 2018: Markiplier, Jake Paul, PewDiePie and more*. Forbes. https://www.forbes.com/sites/natalierobehmed/2018/12/03/highest-paid-youtube-stars-2018-markiplier-jake-paul-pewdiepie-and-more/

Roberto, C. A., Baik, J., Harris, J. L., & Brownell, K. D. (2010). Influence of licensed characters on children's taste and snack preferences. *Pediatrics*, 126(1), 88–93. https://doi.org/10.1542/peds.2009-3433

Roberts, K. (2005). *Lovemarks: The future beyond brands*. Powerhouse Books.

Rozendaal, E., Lapierre, M. A., Van Reijmersdal, E. A., & Buijzen, M. (2011). Reconsidering advertising literacy as a defense against advertising effects. *Media Psychology*, 14(4), 333–354. https://doi.org/10.1080/15213269.2011.620540

Schneier, M. (2023, February 8). *The toddlers in the $600 high-tops luxury brands target kids, and the parents are buying*. The Cut. https://www.thecut.com/2023/02/childrens-luxury-fashion.html

Segran, E. (2023, December 19). *Can putting Barbies next to G.I. Joes help with kids' gender stereotypes?* Fast Company. https://www.fastcompany.com/90998395/can-putting-barbies-next-to-g-i-joes-help-with-kids-gender-stereotypes

Seiter, E. (1993). *Sold separately: Children and parents in consumer culture*. Rutgers University Press.

Semuels, A. (2018, November 29). The strange phenomenon of L.O.L. Surprise Dolls. The Atlantic. https://www.theatlantic.com/technology/archive/2018/11/lol-surprise-dolls-and-mystery-toys/576970/

Shumanov, M., & Johnson, L. (2021). Making conversations with chatbots more personalized. *Computers in Human Behavior*, 117, 106627. https://doi.org/10.1016/j.chb.2020.106627

Stanley, S. L., & Lawson, C. (2020). The effects of an advertising-based intervention on critical thinking and media literacy in third and fourth graders. *Journal of Media Literacy Education*, 12(1), 1–12.

Stanton, R. (2023, May 16). *Advertising watchdog slams Roblox because of paid-for influencers shilling Robux without disclosure 'children can understand.'* PC Gamer. https://www.pcgamer.com/advertising-watchdog-slams-roblox-because-of-paid-for-influencers-shilling-robux-without-disclosure-children-can-understand/

Statista (2023). *Kids digital ad spend worldwide 2021-2031*. https://www.statista.com/statistics/1326893/children-digital-advertising-spending-worldwide/

Stern, S. L., & Schoenhaus, T. (1990). *Toyland: The high-stakes game of the toy industry*. Contemporary Books.

Struik, L. L., Dow-Fleisner, S., Belliveau, M., Thompson, D., & Janke, R. (2020). Tactics for drawing youth to vaping: Content analysis of electronic cigarette advertisements. *Journal of Medical Internet Research*, 22(8), e18943. http://www.doi.org/10.2196/18943

Suciu, P. (2023, February 17). *YouTube influencers promoting junk food To kids*. Forbes. https://www.forbes.com/sites/petersuciu/2023/02/17/youtube-influencers-promoting-junk-food-to-kids/

Taylor, M. (2024, January 22). 'Sephora kids' and the booming business of beauty products for children. BBC. https://www.bbc.com/worklife/article/20240119-sephora-kids-and-the-booming-business-of-beauty-products-for-children

Team, T. (2015, October 12). *Lego Dimensions & other video games to fuel growth for Time Warner's consumer products business*. Forbes. https://www.forbes.com/sites/greatspeculations/2015/10/12/lego-dimensions-other-video-games-to-fuel-growth-for-time-warners-consumer-products-business/

Teinowitz, I. (2003). *Alcohol industry sued for marketing to children*. Ad Age. https://adage.com/article/news/alcohol-industry-sued-marketing-children/38912

Treisman, R. (2023, July 27). *Is Barbie a feminist icon? It's complicated*. NPR. https://www.npr.org/2023/07/27/1189987314/barbie-movie-feminist-history

Ungoed-Thomas, J. (2024, April 21). *UK children bombarded by gambling ads and images online, charity warns*. The Guardian. https://www.theguardian.com/society/2024/apr/21/uk-children-bombarded-by-gambling-ads-and-images-online-charity-warns

van Dam, S., & van Reijmersdal, E. A. (2019). Insights in adolescents' advertising literacy, perceptions and responses regarding sponsored influencer videos and disclosures. *Cyberpsychology: Journal of Psychosocial Research on Cyberspace*, 13(2), http://dx.doi.org/10.5817/CP2019-2-2

van der Bend, D. L., Jakstas, T., van Kleef, E., Shrewsbury, V. A., & Bucher, T. (2022). Making sense of adolescent-targeted social media food marketing: A qualitative study of expert views on key definitions, priorities, and challenges. *Appetite*, 168, https://doi.org/10.1016/j.appet.2021.105691

van Reijmersdal, E. A., Rozendaal, E., Hudders, L., Vanwesenbeeck, I., Cauberghe, V., & Van Berlo, Z. M. (2020). Effects of disclosing influencer marketing in videos: An eye tracking study among children in early adolescence. *Journal of Interactive Marketing*, 49(1), 94–106. https://doi.org/10.1016/j.intmar.2019.09.001

Ward, S. (1974). Consumer socialization. *Journal of Consumer Research*, 1(2), 1–14. https://doi.org/10.1086/208584

Wilcox, B. L., Wilcox, Kunkel, D., Cantor, J., Dowrick, P., Linn, S., & Palmer, E. (2004). *Report of the APA task force on advertising and children.* https://www.apa.org/pubs/reports/advertising-children

Williams, R. (2020, September 3). *Dunkin' dubs coffee drink 'The Charli' after TikTok's biggest star.* Marketing Dive. https://www.marketingdive.com/news/dunkin-dubs-coffee-drink-the-charli-after-tiktoks-biggest-star/584625/

Yang, A. (2024, January 21). *Parents worry AI-generated influencers are promoting unrealistic beauty standards to kids.* NBC News. https://www.nbcnews.com/tech/internet/parents-worry-ai-influencers-promote-unrealistic-beauty-standards-rcna134814

Index

Note: **Bold** page numbers refer to **tables** and *Italic* page numbers refer to *figures* and page numbers followed by 'n' refer to notes.

academic achievement 123, 221
access/use 16–28, 87–91; current state of affairs 22–24; research trends 17–22; selected cases 24–27
action 87, 93
active mediation 17, 67–71, **72**, 73, *73*, 74–78
active playful learning (APL) 216–218; cultural and community values 216; how of learning 216; what of learning 216–217
adolescence/adolescents 4–8, 12, 13, 16, 17, 19–22, 24, 25, 27, 28, 54, 69, 119, 120, 123, 126, 134, 143, 144, 146–148, 150–153, 162–166, 168, 169, 171, 175–177, 193, 194, 220, 229, 230, 232–235, 238–241, 243; media 40, 164; programming 41, 43, 45, 47, 52–54; use of smartphones to cope with stress 25, **26**
advertising 102, 105, 125, 229–244; advertisers' tactics, biases, and representation 242; constant presence, children's world 229–231; consumerism and materialism 233–235; consumer socialization 231–233; drinking 239–240; exposure 230, 233–240; food choices 237–238; gambling 240; gender and sexuality 235–237; guidelines to help young consumers 240–243; industry 231, 235, 237, 241, 242; literacy 85, 240, 242, 243; messages 231, 240–242; personalization through AI algorithms 242–243; smoking 238–239; sponsorship disclosure, identifying 241; subvertisements, creating 243
African Americans 131, 133, 165, 173–175
agency 9, 12, 17, 18
aggression 4, 11, 14, 68, 71, 111, 121, 162–177
aggressive behavior 166, 168
Aladé, F. 121, 214
algorithmic literacy 85
algorithmized self 22
American Indians 130, 173
American Psychological Association (APA) 40, 236
Anderson, C. A. 167
Anderson, D. R. 210
appearance ideals 144–147, 150
Arab/MENA youth 130
Asian American/Pacific Islander (AAPI) youth 129–130
"asset-based" framing 96

Backholer, K. 240
Barr, R. 214
Barris, Kenya 37
Bechdel-Wallace test 49
BeReal 24
Black adolescents 128, 131, 220
Black children 128, 153, 220, 221
Black youth 128, 129, 131, 173, 238
Bobo doll studies 11

bodies 14, 143–148, 151, 154, 155; dissatisfaction 145, 146, 150, 153, 155; neutrality 154, 155; positivity 154–155
body image 14, 143–156; development and appearance concerns 147–148, **148–149**; disability 146–147; gender and gender identity 145–146; gender minority youth 153–154; media effects on 149–154; objectification theory 151–152; physically disabled youth 154; race and ethnicity 144–145; racial and ethnic minority youth 153; social comparison theory 151; tripartite model 150–151
Bond, B. J. 91, 123
Bonus, J. A. 215
Botha, S. 91
Bradshaw, C. P. 175
Bransford, J. D. 215
Buckingham, D. 190
Burgess, M. C. R. 164

capacity model 213, 214
careers 42, 123, 214, 236
Carter, C. 190, 192
caste-based activism 24
character prominence 39
Chen, L. 68, 71, 73, 75
child-directed marketing 229
childproof 105
Children's Express 190
Children's Internet Protection Act (CIPA) 105
Children's Online Privacy Protection Act (COPPA) 103–105, 108
children's programming 41, 42, 44, 45, 47, 51, 52, 54, 67
children's rights approach 8
Children's Television Act of 1990 209
Cho, S. 174
Christensen, C. L. 190
Churchill, G. A. Jr. 231
Cingel, D. P. 171
cisgender 40, 41, 56, 146, 152; peers 123, 126, 154
civic engagement 89, 92, 95, 186, 195, 200
Clampitt, Bob 190
Clark, C. C. 39

Code of Practice for Online Safety 106
Cohen, R. 155
Collier, K. M. 68, 71
commercialization 229–244; consumerism and materialism 233–235; drinking 239–240; food choices 237–238; gambling 240; gender and sexuality 235–237; smoking 238–239
commodity activism 186
Common Sense Media 4, 89–90, 211, 241
communication 16, 17, 84–86, 101, 103, 119, 216; privacy 101
community values 216, 217
community violence 166
concrete operational stage 232
consumer socialization 231–233
content analysis 39, 46, 51, 54, 91, 154, 164
Convention on the Rights of the Child: Article 12 of 107
Cooke, M. C. 170
co-participatory research 111
COPPA 2.0 105
co-viewing/co-using/co-use 17, 67, 68, 70, 71, **72, 73**, 77
Coyne, S. M. 123, 126, 168
creation 87
critical media literacy 86–88
cross-platform learning 219
Croteau, D. 5
cultivation theory 38, 119
cultural/culture 19, 37, 74–76, 88, 94, 96, 103, 125, 131, 169, 217, 219–221; contexts 13, 74, 75; studies 9, 10; trauma 95, 96
culturally responsive pedagogy 221
cyberbullying 4, 14, 68, 73, 104, 106, 163, 171–177; general effects, adolescent victims 172–175, *174*; perpetrators and bystanders 175–176; victimization 172–174; victims 173, 175–177

The Daily Show 191
Daniels, E. A. 153
data 85
dataveillance 102
Day, K. 77
decisional privacy 101

deficit-based framing 96
desensitization 165
developmental psychology 6, 7, 10
differential susceptibility to media effects model 120
differential susceptibility to media influence (DSMM) framework 11, 12
digital advertising *231*
digital citizenship 20, 95
digital cultures 24, 27, 28
digital divide 23, 92
digital inequalities 18, 56
digital landscape 93, 100, 103, 108, 113
digital learning environment 211–212
digital literacy 85, 86, 109, 134
digital media 9, 13, 16, 27, 67, 68, 86, 100, 187, 194, 195, 199
digital platforms 85, 108
Digital Platforms Inquiry, Australia 108
digital play 9
Digital Services Act (DSA) 105
digital sexual practices **26**
digital technologies 17, 74, 76, 107
discrimination 132, 134
disinformation 14, 186, 187, 194, 196–198, 201
diverse media representations 90, 91
diverse representations 162, 177, 221
diversity 90–92
diversity, equity, and inclusion (DEI) 86–88, 244
Döring, N. 124
Duvernay test 50
dyadic communication process 69

early adolescence 7, 150, 151
educational/education 4, 20, 85, 92, 94–97, 110, 111, 165, 174, 177, 233; content 213, 214; media 209–211, **211**, 212, 213, 215, 217–221; systems 95, 96; technology 23; television 121, 210, 216, 219
empowerment perspective 85
England, D. 121
entertainment media 36, 39, 44, 45, 47, 91
equitable media literacy practice (EMLP) 93, 94

equity 92–94
Espinoza, G. 173
ethnic/racial groups 51–53, 120, 126, *127*, 128–130, 132, 144, 145, 164–166, 174, 176, 177, 238
ethnic/racial identity 13, 40, 51, 54, 126, 128–131, 133, 153, 173, 220; and social media 131–134; and traditional media 126–131
ethnic/racial minorities 91, **126**, 127, 131; adolescent programming 53; adolescents programming 52; children's programming 51–53; quality of 52–54; quantity of 51–52; video games 52, 53–54
Eurocentric appearance standards 145
evaluation, media content 87
exploitative tactics 102
exposure effects: empirical evidence of 122–123
extinction rebellion 200

fearful 165
female characters 41–44, 121, 164, 176
First Edition 190
Fisch, S. M. 213, 214
Fletcher, K. 216
Fredrickson, B. L. 152
"Freedom Writers" 53
Freelon, D. 196
Friestad, M. 232
Fryberg, S. A. 130

gamer-gate 167
gay and lesbian-oriented (GLO) media 46
gender 10, 11, 13, 14, 16, 17. 37, 38, 40–44, 54, 88–91, 119–121, 123, 125, 162, 163, 171–173, 176, 177, 221, 235; identity 18, 40, 42, 44, 50, 119, 120, 124, 126, 133, 145, 187, 236; norms 124, 125, 236; stereotypes 42, 43
gender minorities 38, 41, 42, 154; individuals 40; youths 146. 153, 154
gender portrayals: nature of 120–122
General Data Protection Regulation (GDPR) 104, 108
generational or cohort approaches 194

global crises 76
Global Kids Online project 4
Global North 21, 27, 28, 95
Global South 28, 88
González-Velázquez, C. A. 128
Gordon, H. R. 192
Greitemeyer, T. 168

Haidt, J. 20, 169
harms/harmful content 8, 9, 105–107
Harriger, J. A. 154
Harris, J. L. 238
Harvey, C. 91
Harwood, J. 37
Hendershot, H. 190
Hirsh-Pasek, K. 216
Howard, T. C. 197
human development research 193
"Hunger Games" movie 38

identification concept 11
identity development 131–132
identity-empowering environment 57
identity groups 39, 49, 176
identity work 119; theoretical perspectives linking media consumption and 119–120
inclusion 17, 94–95
industries 5
Infocomm Media Development Authority (IMDA) 106, 107
informal education 210
informational privacy 101, 102
information literacy 85
Instagram 24, 192
internet access 22, 105
interventions 66, 102, 168, 187, 215
intervention strategies 77, 78
investigative mediation 68
Ismail, F. R. 173

Jenkins, H. 235
Jensen, H. S. 190
Jimenez, C. 199
Jipguep, M.-C. 166
John, D. R. 231
Jordan, A. 216
Joseph, C. 169

Kamp, D. 209
Kelly, Jack 191

kidfluencers 20
Kids Online Safety Act (KOSA) 105
Kirwil, L. 75
Klein, H. 51
Koch, T. 76
Kowalski, R. M. 171
Krcmar, M. 170, 171

Laible, D. 66
laissez-faire mediation 73
Last Week Tonight with John Oliver 191
Latina culture 145
Latine children 221, 238
Latino adolescents 173, 175
Latinx adolescents 56, 129
Latinx youth 129
learning 209–223; active playful learning (APL) 216–217; capacity model 213–214; compelling and comprehensible narratives 218; cross-platform learning 219; digital learning environment 211–212; educational media 209–210, **211**, 212–217, 219–221, **222–223**; engaging characters 218; interactive *vs.* passive or receptive media 212; preparation for future learning (PFL) 214–216; repetition 217–218; social contingency 218–219; transfer for future learning 214–216
Legault, L. 155
"The Legend of Tarzan" 53
Lennon, M. 221
Lewis, R. 196
LGBTQIA+/LGBTIQ+/LGBTQ+/LGBTQ/LGBT/LGB representation 47, 48, 50, 57n2, 91, 104, 186, 236–237
life course scholars 194
Limber, S. P. 171
lineage or socialization approaches 193
literacies 18, 84–85, 87, 216, 243
Livingstone, S. 4, 9, 101
Loader, B. D. 195
Lowenberg 194
Lwin, M. O. 69, 73, 75

mainstreaming, media 38
male characters 41–43, 167, 176

Manago, A. 125
Mares, M.-L. 129
marginalized identities 144–147
marginalized social groups 152–154
marketing strategies 4
Marwick, A. 196
Masterman, L. 87
Mazières, A. 41
McCall, R. B. 214
Mc Carthy, C. M. 238
media consumption 67, 119, 134, 152
media effects 5, 10; theories 37
media entertainment 49
media literacy 19, 71, 78, 84–86, 86, 87–90, 93–95, 198, 201, 240, 241
media literacy education 84–97; access and 88–90; definitions and conceptualization 84–86; diversity, equity, and inclusion (DEI) 86–88; diversity and 90–92; equity and 92–94; inclusion and 94–95; trauma-informed equity-minded asset-based model (TEAM) for 95–97
media platforms 76, 95, 201, 235, 241
media practice model 120
media psychology 10
media representations 13, 36–37, 39–41, 49, 55, 87, 91, 124, 144; emergent themes 55–57; gender, sexual orientation, and race/ethnicity 40–44, 54–55; gender identity representation 40–41; inclusive media (representation) research practices 56; incorporate young voices 56–57; media effect theories 38–39; media selection theories 37–38; minoritized gender representation 42–44; quantity and quality typologies 39–40; sexual identity representation 44–50; sexual minority portrayals 47–50; sexual minority representation 44–47; social media and newer communication technologies 55–56; theoretical approaches 37–39
media selection theories 37–38
Media/Society (Croteau) 5
media stereotypes 6
media technologies 74, 79, 244
mediated contact theories 38, 39

mediation: gendered aspect 21
media use 8, 16, 17, 20, 21, 24, 25, 67, 68, 70, 78, 123, 129, 152, 221
media users 5, 11
media violence 162, 163, 166, 168, 169, 171, 176, 177; effects of 162, 166, 169, 176
meta-analysis research 79n1
middle childhood 147, 148
Miller-Idriss, C. 196
minoritization experiences 41
minoritized gender representation 42–44; adolescent programming 41; children's programming 41, 42–43; quality of 42–44; quantity of 41–42; video games 41–44
minoritized groups 37, 39, 40, 48, 51, 52, 152, 166
minoritized youth 14, 38, 54, 55, 84, 91
Minow, Newton 209
Mitchell, K. J. 133
mobile media 24
modeling 66, 67
The Model of Intuitive Media Exemplars (MIME) 170, 171
monitoring 68
moral foundations theory (MFT) 169–171
morality 169
moral panics 17
moral reasoning 14, 162, 168–171, 175
Moschis, G. P. 231
Mügge, D. O. 168
multimedia literacies 85
multi-risk individuals 168
MySpace 24

Narratio Fellowship 91
narrative content 213, 214
narrative dominance 213
Nathanson, A. I. 214
National Association for Media Literacy Education (NAMLE) 84, 86, 88, 90, 94, 241
Native American/Indigenous youth 130
negative roles, media 12
negative roles, technology 12
new media literacies 85

"news-finds-me" attitude 189
News for Children 190
news literacy 85
news/politics 185–201; disinformation, dark side of youth participation 196–198; researching young people, frameworks 192–194; responding to disinformation 198; signs of hope 200–201; social change, organizations role 198–200; and young people 188–192; youth, vote, and courts 198–200; youth and social movements 195–196
Newsround 190
Nichols, C. 214
Nick News with Linda Ellerbee 190
Nikken, P. 76
"Normative Whiteness" 53

Oberle, C. D. 155
objectification theory 150, 151
"objective" digital data 102
O'Dell, C. 163
Olweus, D. 171
'one-size-fits-all' approach 78
online aggression 14, 171
online behavior 132, 171, 243
online harassment 104, 173
online platforms 103, 106
online privacy 101–103
online racial discrimination 132–134
online racism 134
Online Safety (Miscellaneous Amendments) Act 106
Online Safety Code 107
online spaces 131, 132
Opree, S. J. 76

Padilla-Walker, L. M. 71
parasocial relationships 218, 242
parental consent 104, 105
parental mediation 17, 24, 25, 27, 66–69, 71, 73–79; effects 73–77; meta-analysis 71, 74; origin and types 66–68; working of 68–73
parental socialization **25**
parents/caregivers 6, 13, 19, 21, 65–79, 106; primary socialization agents 65–66
participation gap 87
"passive" media 212

Pathirana, N. L. 240
Payne Fund studies 162
Penney, J. 196
Personal Data Protection Act (PDPA) 104
personal information 69, 101–104
Peter, J. 11
physical aggression 163–164, 168
physical privacy 101
Piotrowski, J. T. 214
play 8, 9, *65*, 71, 78, 111
policies 100–113; participation of children 107–112, *112*; privacy concept 101–104; protection from harm 104–107
political expression 7, 14, 187, 192, 196, 198, 201
positive roles, media 12
positive roles, technology 12
power: imbalance of 172, 173
Prendella, K. 216
preoperational age 232
preparation for future learning (PFL) 214–216
priming theory 167
Privacy Act 104
privacy concept 101–104
proactivity 73–74
produsers 20
Project Look Sharp (PLS) 89
promotive mediation 73
protectionist perspectives 85
psychological reactance 69
public-private alliance 108

Qi, J. 4
qualitative research 12
quantitative criticism 10
quantitative research 12

race/ethnicity 36, 37, 40–44, 49, 51, 54, 91, 143, 144, 148, 152, 176, 244
racial dignity 134
racial discrimination 132, 133
racial identity 120, 133, 134
Radio Times article 190
Ramasubramanian, S. 91
receptive media 212
reflective stage 232
reinforcement 66, 67

relational aggression 163, 164
religious identity 119, 134
representations 5, 13, 14, 36–57, 90–92, 162, 164–167, 237, 242; of people of color 50; quantity 39, 46, 51, 52; tests and ratings 49; of violence in media 163–165
research traditions: studying young people and media 9–12
research trends, access/use 17–22; affordances, risks, and literacies 18–19; digital citizenship 20–21; gendered aspect 21; overcoming barriers 18; overloaded by new 19–20; young voices, foregrounding 21–22
restrictive mediation 67–71, **72**, 73, **73**, 74, 75, 78
restrictive parental mediation 17–19, 24
revenge porn 173
reverse socialization 79
rights of children 8, 9, 100, 108, 200
rights respecting 9
right to privacy 9
risk factors 166, 168, 173
Rivadeneyra, R. 129
Roberts, T.-A. 152
role models 36, 38, 55, 67, 70, 221
Rollins, D. 55
Romero, A. J. 173
rural-urban divide 22

Safer Internet Programme 105
Sago, A. 155
Sanders-Phillips, K. 166
Scharrer, E. 91, 125
Schooler, D. 153
Schwartz, D. L. 215
screen media 76, 77, 166
screen violence 165, 166
selective mediation 73
self-determination theory 69
self-objectification 43, 150, 152, 155
self-regulation 19
"Sephora Kids" 234
sex education **26**
sexual and gender minority youth (SGMY) 125, 126

sexual identities 4, 13, 25, 28, 44, 55, 90, 91, 119, 134; representation 44–50
sexuality 10, 25, 88, 89, 235, 236, 244
sexual minority groups 44–46, 48, 49
sexual minority portrayals 47–50; children and adolescent programming 47–48; quality of 47–48; video games 48
sexual minority representation 44–47; adolescent programming 45–46; children's programming 44–45; quantity of 44–47; video games 46–47
sexual objectification 151, 152
sexual orientation 37, 40–46, 48, 50, 54, 94, 105
sharenting phenomenon 18
Shaw, A. 46
Shi, J. 68, 71, 75
Shiffman, K. S. 51
Shin, W. 69, 75
Smart Nation initiative, Singapore 108
smartphone coping styles, teens **26**
smartphones 24
Snapchat 24
social classes 90, 91, 120
social cognitive theory 38, 120, 163–164
social comparison theory 150–151; downward comparisons 151; upwards comparisons 151
social construction 8
social contingency 215, 218
social groups 14, 39, 75, 87, 96, 148
social identities 13, 119–134; gratifications 37, 54; theory 37
social inequality 23
social interactions 12, 66–67, 78, 84
socialization 18, 65, 66, 193, 198
social justice 10, 88, 92, 94, 143, 144, 146, 155, 156
social media 4–6, 12, 18–21, 55, 56, 124–126, 131, 132, 134, 148, 150, 154, 176, 177, 186–188, 190–192, 199–201, 233, 234, 237–239, 241, 243; and body positivity 154–155; and ethnic/racial identity 131–134; and gender identity and beliefs 124–126; identity development 131–132; influencers 151, 229, 233, 238, 242;

online racial discrimination 132–134; platforms 5, 100, 102, 105–107, 131, 155, 172, 188, 189, 200, 230, 243
social movements 14, 186, 187, 194, 195, 199–201
social networking sites 176
sociocultural approach 7
socioeconomic status (SES) 76
sociopolitical development 187
Spehar, Vitus 191
Sreekumar, T. T. 196
Strasburger, V. C. 6
stronger endorsement, masculine norms 125
structural disempowerment 19
subvertisements 243
Sun, X. 76
Sunlight Alliance for Action (AfA) 108
symbolic annihilation 146
"synthetic" self 22

Taft, J. K. 192
Taggart 164
Tajfel, H. 37
Tamari, T. 154
tech companies 5
technical mediation 68, 78
technological advancements 109, 134
technology landscape 3
technopanics 17–19, 27
teens: digital expression of sexuality 25, 26; use of media to socialize parents 25
Thompson, R. A. 66
Thorson, K. 190
TikTok 24, 188, *188*, 192; cultures, young people 27
Tompkins, T. L. 123
toy-based programs 229
traditional gender norms 42, 124, 125
traditional gender role attitudes 122
traditional media 126, 129, 130, 151, 212; and ethnic/racial identity 126–131; exposure to 129, 130; and gender identity and beliefs 120–124
traditional screen media 119, 165, 171
transgender 40, 50, 123, 146
transgender and gender diverse (TGD) media experiences 123–124
transgender and gender diverse (TGD) youth 123–126
transmedia storytelling 234, 235
transparency 105–107, 198, 199
trauma-informed equity-minded asset-based model (TEAM) 95–97
Travers, Hugo 191
tripartite model 150–151
Turiel, O. 125
Turner, J. C. 37
Turning Point USA 199
Twitter 24
Tynes, B. M. 133

underrepresentation 52, 91, 130, 162
underrepresented or misrepresented identities 36
UNICEF 8
United Nation's Convention on the Rights of the Child 8, 9, 65
user-generated content 192, 233, 238, 239, 241

Vadrevu, S. 196
Valkenburg, P. M. 11
van Reijmersdal, E. A. 241
video games 8, 14, 39, 41, 43, 46–48, 52–54, 162, 164–167, 171, 176; violence 166–168
violence 4, 14, 162–165, 167, 169–171, 176, 177, 197, 200, 209; representations, in media 163–165; TV and film, aggressive outcomes 165–166; video game 166–168
violent media 14, 166, 170, 177
violent video games 6, 167, 168
Vito Russo test 50
vulnerability 12

Waasdorp, T. E. 175
Waddell, T. F. 46
Wang, B. 71, 174
Wang, M. 74
Ward, S. 231
Warren, S. 125
Watts, R. J. 187
weaker sexist attitudes 125
weak-tie racism 132
Weber, R. 169
Wells, C. 196

Westenberg, J. M. 155
WhatsApp 24
White youth 130–131, 173, 238
Wilcox, B. L. 232
Wise Up! 190
women of color 52, 53, 90, 91, 121
Wright, P. 232

Yang, G. S. 167
young audiences 43, 190, 230, 233, 241, 242
young media users 4, 5, 11, 13, 213
young people: platformized digital cultures 27; TikTok cultures **27**
young/younger children 23, 24, 66, 69, 74, 148, 165, 170, 197, 211, 212, 214, 215, 221, 233–236, 240

youth activism 187
youth development 36, 131
youth involvement 185, 187, 194, 195, 199, 200
youth media: gender identity representation 40–41; racial/ethnic identity representation in 51–54; sexual identity representation 44–50
youth of color 129, 131, 132, 153
youth voice 199, 200
YouTube 24, 192

Zhou, X. 125
Zosh, J. M. 216
ZUMIX 92